Oxford Handbook of Operative Surgery

edited by

G. R. McLATCHIE
Professor of Surgical Sciences
University of Sunderland

Consultant Surgeon
Hartlepool and East Durham Health
Services Trust
The General Hospital
Hartlepool

and

D. J. LEAPER
Professor of Surgery
University of Newcastle
North Tees Hospital
Stockton on Tees

Oxford   New York   Tokyo
OXFORD UNIVERSITY PRESS
1996

Oxford University Press, Walton Street, Oxford OX2 6DP

Oxford   New York
Athens   Auckland   Bangkok   Bombay
Calcutta   Cape Town   Dar es Salaam   Delhi
Florence   Hong Kong   Istanbul   Karachi
Kuala Lumpur   Madras   Madrid   Melbourne
Mexico City   Nairobi   Paris   Singapore
Taipei   Tokyo   Toronto
and associated companies in
Berlin   Ibadan

Oxford is a trade mark of Oxford University Press

Published in the United States
by Oxford University Press Inc., New York

A catalogue record for this book is available from the British Library

Library of Congress Cataloging in Publication Data
(Data available)

ISBN 0 19 262097 5

Typeset by Footnote Graphics, Warminster, Wilts
Printed in Great Britain by
The Bath Press

Preface

This book is a practical guide for the surgeon or surgical trainee about to perform or assist at an operation. The procedures described are those commonly carried out in general, urological and orthopaedic surgical practice with an introduction on perioperative management and anaesthetics. These should also prove of interest to operating department nurses, assistants, and students of medicine. Indications for and complications of procedures are given but more extensive descriptions of these can be found in surgical textbooks to which the reader shold refer.

We emphasize that the book is not for the first-time operator nor does it embrace the philosophy of 'see one, do one, teach one'. Anyone aspiring to be a surgeon must acquire the basic skills of safe knot-tying and familiarity with surgical instruments. Only by witnessing, assisting at, and then performing many procedures within the structure of a formal surgical training course can the trainee develop the skill, judgement, and the ability to select patients correctly—the recipe for safe surgery.

Hartlepool
Stockton on Tees
1996

G. R. M.
D. J. L.

Dedications

For Ross, Cameron, Ailidh, Claire, Calum, Charles, and Alice

Acknowledgements

We are grateful to all who have helped us to produce this book, in particular the staff of Oxford University Press and those readers and reviewers who suggested that we produce a sister volume for the *Oxford Handbook of Clinical Surgery*. For the vascular surgical illustrations we thank Professor Peter Bell of Leicester, Portex for illustrations relating to emergency tracheostomy and Ethicon for illustrations and legends relating to surgical knot-tying. Peter Cox, who drew the illustrations and Paul Rogers who took the photographs deserve special mention as does Kate McLatchie who prepared the manuscript.

Abbreviations

ACE	angiotensin-converting enzyme
AO	Arbeitsgemeinschaft für Osteosynthesefragen
AP	anteroposterior
ARDS	adult respiratory disease syndrome
CBD	common bile duct
CMC	carpometacarpal
COPD	chronic obstructive pulmonary disease
CPAP	continuous positive airways pressure
CVP	central venous pressure
DCS	dynamic compression
DCP	dynamic compression plate
DIP	distal interphalangeal joint
DVT	deep vein thrombosis
ECG	electrocardiogram
ECMO	extracorporeal membrane oxygenation
ERCP	endoscopic retrograde cholangiopancreatography
ESWL	extracorporeal shock-wave lithotripsy
ETT	endotracheal tube
FDP	fibrinogen degradation products
GI	gastrointestinal
HFPPV	high-frequency positive pressure ventilation
HIV	human immunodeficiency virus
ICU	intensive care unit
IM	intramuscular
IMI	intramuscular infusion
IMV	intermittent mandatory ventilation
IPPV	intermittent positive pressure ventilation
IV	intravenous
IVI	intravenous infusion
IVU	intravenous urography
JVP	jugular venous pressure
MCP	metacarpophalangeal
MTP	metatarsophalangeal
NSAID	non-steroidal anti-inflammatory drug
OPSI	overwhelming post-splenectomy infection
PCAS	patient-controlled analgesic system
PCN	percutaneous nephroscopy
PDS	polydioxanone sutre
PEEP	positive end-expiratory pressure
PIP	proximal interphalangeal joint
PR	per rectum
PTE	pulmonary thromboembolism
PVC	polyvinylchloride
SIMV	synchronized intermittent mandatory ventilation
TPN	total parenteral nutrition

Degree of difficulty of procedures

Minor	Usually taking up to 30 minutes
Intermediate	30–45 minutes
Major	45–90 minutes
Extra major	2–4 hours
Complex	Extensive surgery taking more than 4 hours to complete

Contributors

G. Bannister MD FRCS (Orth.)
Consultant Orthopaedic Surgeon, Southmead Hospital, Bristol, Avon

M. Berry MB ChB FFARCS MD
Consultant Anaesthetist (retired), Hartlepool and Peterlee Hospitals NHS Trust, Hartlepool, Cleveland

C. Johnston MA MD FRCA
Consultant Anaesthetist, Southmead Hospital, Bristol, Avon

C. M. E. Lennox MB ChB FRCS (Orth.)
Consultant Orthopaedic Surgeon, Hartlepool and Peterlee Hospitals NHS Trust, Hartlepool, Cleveland

K. Martin RGN BSc (Hons)
Theatre Sister, South Tees Acute Hospitals NHS Trust, Middlesbrough, Cleveland

G. Packer MB ChB FRCS (Orth.)
Consultant Orthopaedic Surgeon, Southend District General Hospital, Westcliffe-on-Sea

J. R. Rhind MB ChB FRCS
Consultant Urologist, North Durham Acute Hospitals NHS Trust

1 Perioperative management and anaesthetics

C. JOHNSTON and
M. BERRY

Introduction 2
Relationship between surgeons and
  anaesthetists 4
Planning an admission to hospital 6
Preoperative assessment of the patient 8
Preoperative assessment of the emergency
  patient 14
Classifications 16
Preparation of the patient for surgery 18
The nature of anaesthesia 20
Drugs in anaesthetic practice 24
Sedative techniques 30
Conduct of a general anaesthetic 32
Morbidity and mortality 40
Postoperative care 42
Postoperative complications 44
Postoperative pain relief 48
Late postoperative complications 52
Intensive care 54
Practical procedures 58

2 INTRODUCTION

The object of this chapter is to give surgeons an understanding of the problems which their patients may cause to the anaesthetist and thus enable them to utilize the anaesthetic, recovery, and intensive care departments of the hospital efficiently during the pre-, peri-, and postoperative care of patients. It is not designed to be a comprehensive textbook of anaesthesia. Practical procedures are described, but these descriptions should be used to jog the memory rather than act as a substitute for practical teaching in the operating theatre. The term 'anaesthetist' will be used to describe medically qualified specialist anaesthetists, known in some countries as anesthesiologists.

4 RELATIONSHIP BETWEEN SURGEONS AND ANAESTHETISTS

The origins of surgery are lost in antiquity. In contrast, anaesthesia is a youthful speciality. The first successful anaesthetic was administered in 1846, the first professor of anaesthesia was appointed in 1933, and the inception of the Royal College of Anaesthetists took place in 1992. Most contemporary anaesthetic drugs and techniques have been introduced within the past 30 years. Anaesthesia is now the largest hospital speciality in the UK with over 2500 consultants. In addition to perioperative care, anaesthetists are involved in the management of patients in obstetric and intensive care units and in the treatment of acute and chronic pain. The comment that surgeons like their anaesthetists to possess three As—ability, availability, and affability, with the emphasis on availability—has become legend, but it should be emphasized that anaesthetists also have their likes and dislikes. A well-organized surgeon who efficiently assesses patients in the out-patient clinic, publishes theatre lists well in advance, and informs the anaesthatist of anticipated problems is the ideal. Surgery is a team process, and good organization, efficient communications, and high morale are as important in the operating theatre as in any other sphere of life where people interact.

PLANNING AN ADMISSION TO HOSPITAL

Nowadays there is considerable pressure on surgeons to reduce the hospital stay of patients. When an operation is booked, surgeons should note how they plan to admit and discharge their patient.

Routes for admission
- Referral to a preoperative clerking or anaesthetic assessment clinic
- Admission to the ward several days before surgery for investigation and assessment
- Admission to the ward on the day before surgery or the morning of the operation
- Admission to a specialized day surgery unit

Preoperative assessment clinics
These have the following *advantages*:
(1) they reduce cancellations on the day of surgery;
(2) the time spent in hospital is reduced;
(3) surgical and anaesthetic techniques can be discussed with patients;
(4) investigations can be organized efficiently;
(5) house officers' time can be utilized efficiently;
(6) when necessary, interpreters, stoma therapists, and acute pain nurses can attend the clinic to discuss problems with the patients.

Their *disadvantages* are as follows:
(1) the assessment may be performed by a different team from the one who ultimately sees the patient in hospital and gives the anaesthetic;
(2) the patient's health may alter between the clinic and admission;
(3) the patient is required to make an additional journey to hospital.

Preoperative advice
The time at which an operation is booked provides an opportunity to advise patients to lose excess weight, give up smoking, and obtain dental treatment. For day cases, important details about when food and drugs can be taken should be emphasized. Fact sheets are useful. Clear communication is vital at this stage.

Planning an operating list

Advance booking of cases allows lists to be organized more efficiently than if the list is made up during the afternoon ward round on the day before surgery. This requires protection of beds for elective surgery.

Communication

The anaesthetic department should be warned at least 24 hours before elective surgery is planned on the very young, the very frail, patients with a family or personal history of anaesthetic complications, patients with potentially difficult airway problems, or staff. The theatre manager should be informed at least 24 hours in advance if surgery involves the use of specialist equipment such as X-ray machines, lasers, or endoscopes if their supply is limited. The director of the intensive care unit (ICU) must be warned at least 48 hours in advance if an operation is planned which is likely to require an elective admission to the ICU. The X-ray department and the physiotherapy department should also be warned if their assistance is likely to be needed.

Order of the list

Priority for early operations should be given to infants and diabetics who do not tolerate prolonged starvation. Major cases of unpredictable length should also be operated upon as early as possible. The patient's details and the side of the operation should be accurate. Badly organized and inaccurate theatre lists cause delays and put patients at unnecessary risk.

PREOPERATIVE ASSESSMENT OF THE PATIENT

'We have now made surgery safe for the patient. Let us make sure the patient is safe for surgery!' Fitness for anaesthesia is a nearly meaningless concept nowadays as virtually anyone can be given an anaesthetic. The question is whether the benefits of surgery outweigh the risks of the anaesthetic. For elective surgery the patient should be as fit as possible. In emergency surgery the patient should be resuscitated as far as possible before the anaesthetic commences.

General characteristics

The physiological age of the patient is far more important than the chronological age. Patients over 80 usually have good cardiovascular systems and are often easier to anaesthetize than patients 20 years younger who have not taken care of themselves.

Obesity
This causes cardiovascular stress and reduces pulmonary reserves. There is an increased risk of regurgitation. In patients weighing over 100 kg venepuncture may be difficult, regional blocks are difficult to perform, and intramuscular injections may prove ineffective if deposited in the surrounding adipose layers.

Racial origin
Genetically inherited conditions are more common in certain races. Examples include sickle cell anaemia in African and Caribbean blacks, porphyria in Scandinavians and white South Africans, and thalassaemia amongst people of Mediterranean origin.

Familial
Sickle cell anaemia, porphyria, pseudocholinesterase deficiency, and malignant hyperpyrexia run in families.

Facial bone physiognomy
Prominent incisor teeth and an underslung chin make endotracheal intubation difficult, particularly when present in a patient with a short neck or limited neck extension.

Dentition
An increasing number of patients have expensive fixed plates or crowns and they do not wish them to be damaged.

Tremors
These may indicate thyrotoxicosis or Parkinson's disease and affect drug selection.

Mentation

Elderly and confused patients usually become worse in the postoperative period as a result of drugs, discomfort, or disorientation. The beliefs of the patient must be considered, particularly if he is a Jehovah's Witness whose views may alter the treatment he receives.

Cardiovascular

Exercise tolerance

Patients who can climb a flight of stairs without stopping rarely cause problems to the anaesthetist. Angina may progress to infarction in the perioperative period as a result of anxiety, hypotension, or variations in medication. A patient with coronary artery disease will tolerate carefully supervised minor surgery, but consideration should be given to improving myocardial perfusion before the patient undergoes major surgery.

Heart murmurs

When associated with signs of heart failure, murmurs must be investigated before an anaesthetic is administered. Antibiotic cover may be required. Signs of heart failure are always important. Most anaesthetics will adversely affect cardiac function and mild failure may be exacerbated. Effective preoperative treatment should be instituted whenever possible.

Arrhythmias

A heart rate above 100 in an adult is almost always pathological and its cause must be sought. Rapid irregular rhythms should be controlled before anaesthesia commences, if possible. Heart rates below 50 suggest conduction abnormalities unless the patient is an athlete. Irregularities superimposed upon a basically regular rhythm may be caused by benign ventricular ectopics. ECGs are a useful investigation in patients over the age of 50 undergoing anaesthesia.

Hypertension

The diastolic pressure should be below 100 before elective surgery. Hypertensive patients may be given anaesthetics, but there is an increased risk of perioperative complications.

Anaemia and polycythaemia

The haemoglobin concentration should usually exceed 8 g/dl; the only exception to this is patients with chronic renal failure, who adapt to lower haemoglobin concentrations and only require transfusion before major surgery. If their anaemia is symptomatic, patients with haemoglobin levels in the 8–10 g/dl range should be transfused preoperatively. Severe polycythaemia increases the operative risk, and perioperative venesection is sometimes recommended.

Bleeding disorders and anticoagulant therapy

These may affect the ease with which the operation is performed and may contraindicate the use of regional anaesthesia and intramuscular medication. Patients with a history of bleeding problems should be investigated before surgery. Patients taking long-term oral anticoagulants are usually changed to heparin for their operation.

Respiratory

Asthma

Asthma can be made worse by anaesthesia. Bronchodilators can be given preoperatively, but histamine-releasing anaesthetic drugs such as tubocurare should be avoided. Many anaesthetic drugs have bronchodilator properties, but sudden bronchoconstriction can occur during induction of anaesthesia or recovery from it. Humidification of the inspired gases prevents drying and crusting of bronchial secretions.

Chronic obstructive pulmonary disease

Patients with emphysema who retain CO_2 control of respiration (pink puffers) are rarely a problem perioperatively. A regional technique of pain relief such as a thoracic or upper lumbar epidural will allow the patient to breath more easily during the postoperative period if abdominal surgery has been performed. Patients whose respiration depends upon their hypoxic drive (blue bloaters) are difficult to anaesthetize. Premedication should be mild or omitted altogether, and postoperative ventilation may be required. Regional or local techniques are desirable when possible, but these patients often find it difficult to lie flat for any length of time. Patients with severe respiratory disease need to be admitted for physiotherapy and assessment several days before surgery.

Upper-airway obstruction

Patients whose upper airways are narrowed by trauma, infection, or neoplasm are at great risk. They should be watched closely preoperatively and only anaesthetized by an experienced clinician.

Difficult intubations

Specialist equipment and personnel may need to be available to assist at these.

Infections

Upper respiratory tract infections are not affected by anaesthesia, and it is safe to anaesthetize a patient with a simple head cold. However, if a patient is febrile or has a productive cough as the result of a chest infection, elective surgery should be delayed as anaesthesia can disseminate infection and lead to serious pneumonia.

Genito-urinary tract/renal failure

Renal failure will affect the selection of drugs used during anaesthesia. High potassium levels can cause cardiac problems and massive protein loss in the nephrotic syndrome may affect the binding of anaesthetic drugs and their efficacy. The dose of certain antibiotics, notably the aminoglycosides, needs to be modified in renal failure. Anaemia is common.

Prostatic hypertrophy

Postoperative pain, bed rest and anaesthetic drugs all contribute to urinary retention in men with prostatic hypertrophy. An indwelling catheter may be necessary for the first postoperative days in patients who are symptomatic preoperatively.

Metabolic

Diabetes

Diabetics controlled by diet alone are not an anaesthetic problem. Non-insulin-dependent diabetics can usually be managed by adjusting the timing and dose of tablets they receive, although they may require insulin after major surgery. Insulin-dependent diabetics will require special perioperative care, which should be discussed with the anaesthetist preoperatively.

Hiatus hernia

This increases the risk of regurgitation and inhalation pneumonitis.

Jaundice

Hepatic failure affects metabolism of anaesthetic drugs, but serious problems only arise in the advanced stage. Patients with ascites will have a serious fluid balance problem in the perioperative period. Liver damage can produce clotting abnormalities.

Steroid therapy

Patients on long-term steroid therapy will have suppressed endogenous steroid production and will not cope with prolonged stress. Steroids are usually prescribed perioperatively and then tailed off. These patients heal poorly and are prone to infection.

Any metabolic disease

Such diseases should be controlled before elective surgery is undertaken. Uncontrolled diabetes, Addison's disease, thyrotoxicosis, or myxoedema can lead to serious complications in the postoperative period. Phaeochromocytoma and apudomas may present during anaesthesia and can be life-threatening.

Drugs

Psychotropic drugs

Several psychotropic drugs interact adversely with anaesthetic agents. This risk must be balanced against the psychiatric effects of stopping them. Lithium prolongs the action of suxamethonium. The tricyclic antidepressants increase the likelihood of cardiac arrhythmias while monoamine oxidase inhibitors interact with inotropic agents and some analgesics to produce severe hypertension.

History of atopy

Allergic reactions to anaesthetic drugs may occur in one in 5000 cases and may be life-threatening. Anaphylactic responses as a result of prior exposure to a drug are particularly severe. A few patients claim that they are 'allergic to anaesthetics'; previous anaesthetic records must be obtained in these cases whenever feasible.

Alcoholism

High alcohol consumption will induce liver enzymes and lead to abnormally high anaesthetic requirements. The postoperative phase may be complicated by delirium.

Drug abuse

This will lead to increased anaesthetic requirements and can cause difficulty with obtaining venous access. Clinical staff must protect themselves particularly carefully against contamination with blood or body fluids. Drug addicts should be tested to see if they are hepatitis B carriers and should be counselled about HIV testing.

Investigations

A full blood count should be obtained if there is a history of unusual diet, chronic bleeding, or previous unexplained anaemia. Abnormal potassium levels can lead to cardiac arrhythmias, and electrolytes should be measured if diuretics are prescribed. An ECG is a useful investigation in most patients over 50 and younger people whose exercise tolerance is poor. Chest X-rays should only be ordered if there is a good indication. All patients should be weighed on admission.

Day case patients

Each day unit has its own admission criteria. Usually patients booked for day surgery should:

- be ASA1 or 2
- not be hypertensive, grossly obese, or at the extremes of age
- have a companion at home and a telephone

Any necessary investigations should be performed before the date of admission.

Cardiovascular resuscitation is essential and can only be omitted in cases where the rate of blood loss exceeds the possibility of replacing it, for example when there is rapid internal bleeding. A full blood count should be obtained as soon as possible and blood should be cross-matched if necessary. Usually, any blood lost should be replaced by blood but otherwise either crystalloid or colloid can be used for resuscitation provided that sufficient volume is administered. Central venous monitoring will assist the assessment of fluid balance. A systolic blood pressure above 100 mmHg and a pulse rate below 100 are desirable before anaesthesia. Serum urea and electrolytes should be measured in all patients with a history of gastro-intestinal upset. Electrolyte disturbances must be corrected, particularly the serum potassium which should lie between 3.3 and 5.0 mmol/l. Potassium levels outside these limits may lead to serious cardiac problems and will affect muscle power. Continuous vomiting may lead to metabolic alkalosis and infection may cause diabetics to develop metabolic acidosis, and this should be treated if possible. Pain should be controlled by intravenous, intramuscular, or local analgesia.

Food

Ideally the patient should be fasted for a minimum of four hours before bringing them to theatre. If the patient has normal intestinal activity, gastric emptying can be speeded up by giving metoclopramide 10 mg IV. H_2-receptor antagonists may be prescribed to reduce gastric acidity with a non-particulate antacid, such as sodium citrate 30 ml, being given at the time of induction.

Postoperative care

When patients are seriously ill, the surgical and anaesthetic teams should liaise as soon as possible to decide whether the patient should be sent to the ICU, sent to the high dependency unit, or returned to the ward postoperatively

Classification of surgical cases

1. **Emergency—immediate operation** Resuscitation is carried out simultaneously with surgical treatment, for example ruptured aneurysm or head, chest, and abdominal injuries. Operation required within 1 hour.
2. **Urgent—delayed operation** Carried out as soon as possible after resuscitation, for example intestinal obstruction, embolism, perforation, major fractures. Operation required within 24 hours.
3. **Scheduled** Early operation necessary, but not immediately required to save life, for example cancer or cardiovascular surgery. Operation required within 3 weeks.
4. **Elective** Procedure at a time to suit both patient and surgeon, for example cholecystectomy, hernia, joint replacement. Patients undergoing elective surgery should only be operated upon when they are fully fit. In contrast, emergency patients are by definition unfit. The aim should be to optimize their condition in the time available.

American Society of Anesthesiologists (ASA) classification of physical fitness

This system is widely employed as a system of indicating the difficulty and risk of anaesthesia.
- *ASA Class 1* A normal healthy person.
- *ASA Class 2* A patient with mild systemic disease. A patient with mild diabetes, controlled hypertension, or obesity would fall into this class. Otherwise fit patients at the extremes of age may be classified ASA2.
- *ASA Class 3* A patient with severe systemic disease that limits activity but is not incapacitating. Examples include severe diabetes with vascular complications, angina pectoris, or healed myocardial infarction.
- *ASA Class 4* A patient with severe systemic disease that limits activity but is not incapacitating. Examples include cardiac failure, peristent angina, severe chronic obstructive pulmonary disease (COPD) or renal failure.
- *ASA Class 5* A moribund patient who is not expected to survive 24 hours without surgery. Examples include ruptured aortic aneurysm or major trauma.
- *Emergency (E)* A patient in one of the preceding classes who is undergoing surgery as an emergency. The risk of surgery is equivalent to a patient in the next-highest category. The letter E is written next to the numerical classification.

PREPARATION OF THE PATIENT FOR SURGERY

The majority of patients are frightened by the prospect of anaesthesia and surgery. Attempts should be made to minimize these fears, and all members of the hospital team can help.

Premedication

Studies suggest that patients obtain more reassurance from a well-conducted preoperative visit than they do from premedicant drugs prescribed without a visit. Patients differ in their desire for preoperative sedation and it should be tailored to the individual patient. Premedication can be prescribed to treat pain, relieve anxiety, produce sedation, reduce salivation, and to treat coexisting medical conditions.

Benzodiazepine drugs are used to reduce anxiety. Diazepam has largely been replaced by temazepam and lorazepam. Temazepam 10–30 mg orally sedates between 30 minutes and 2 hours after a single dose while lorazepam 1–3 mg lasts for up to 8 hours.

Opiates should be employed to treat pain. Those typically used are morphine 0.15 mg/kg, papaveretum 0.3 mg/kg, or pethidine 1.5 mg/kg IVI or IMI.

Antisialogues were necessary when either ether or cyclopropane were administered. Contemporary indications include intra-oral and laryngological procedures, small children, and when ketamine is to be used. These agents also protect against bradycardias. Atropine 0.02 mg/kg, hyoscine 0.008 mg/kg, or glycopyrrollate 0.004 mg/kg are used.

Antihistamines have both sedative and antiemetic properties and therefore make suitable premedicant drugs. Promethazine (Phenergan) 25 mg is used in adults, while trimeprazine (Vallergan) 0.5 mg/kg is popular to sedate children over 2 years old. A few children react against trimeprazine and become pale and hypotensive. Antihistamines are good premedicants for atopic individuals.

Neuroleptic agents include the major tranquillizers and are only occasionally used for premedication. Droperidol has antiemetic and dissociative properties, and is occasionally used as a premedicant.

Acid therapies

Regurgitation and inhalation of stomach contents cause serious morbidity and may lead to death. Pregnant women and patients with hiatus hernias are at particular risk, and an adequate period of preoperative starvation is essential. If the intestine is working normally, stomach emptying may be enhanced by the use of metoclopramide 10 mg IV. An intravenous or oral H_2-receptor antagonist such as ranitidine 50 mg or cimetidine 200 mg can be given to reduce acid secretion and raise the gastric acid pH. A non-particulate antacid such as sodium citrate can be given just prior to anaesthetic induction to raise the pH of the acid left in the stomach.

Bronchodilators

Patients with reversible airways disease may benefit from a bronchodilator such as salbutamol just before induction of anaesthesia.

Antihypertensive agents

Patients on antihypertensive medication should continue to receive their medication throughout the operative period.

Steroids

Patients on steroid treatments need to continue these drugs over the operation period and additional doses may be necessary.

The biochemical mechanisms of anaesthesia remain a mystery. Some drugs act at specific receptor sites on the cell membranes while the actions of anaesthetic vapours appear to depend more upon their physical than their pharmacological properties. The requirements for satisfactory anaesthesia are as follows:

- **Analgesia**
- **Amnesia**
- **Muscular relaxation**

These make up the 'triad of anaesthesia'. The methods available to an anaesthetist for achieving the triad are summarized below.

Regional local anaesthesia

Local anaesthetic neural blockade causes analgesia and muscular relaxation. Amnesia is not essential, but light sedation can be given to an anxious patient. Techniques include epidural, spinal, and brachial plexus blocks. These techniques are regularly employed in orthopaedic and urological surgery, and permit a mother to be awake to enjoy the birth of her child by Caesarean section.

Total intravenous anaesthesia

Combinations of intravenous agents such as opiates and propofol can produce effective anaesthesia with the advantage that atmospheric pollution by anaesthetic gases is avoided and the postoperative respiratory complications of anaesthesia are reduced. Such combinations are often used for day case procedures and can be used for longer anaesthetics. The only single agent to provide the three elements of the triad is ketamine, an anaesthetic with unique properties and mode of action.

Use of volatile agents

A simple type of general anaesthetic follows the sequence

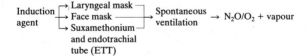

The induction agent provides a smooth transition from alertness to sleep. The main component of the anaesthetic is the anaesthetic vapour which provides amnesia and muscular relaxation. Opiate drugs or local anaesthetic blocks are used to provide pain relief. The relaxation obtained by this method is generally insufficient for intra-abdominal surgery. Muscle

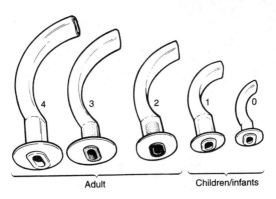

Guedel airway, infant and adult; sizes 0–4.

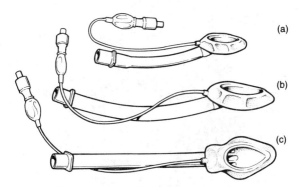

Laryngeal masks: (a) child; (b) female; (c) male.

and adipose tissue absorb the volatile anaesthetic agent and recovery times may be prolonged. However, this technique is relatively safe as patients breathe on their own and will move if the level of anaesthesia is inappropriate for the surgical stimulus. It is essential that the airway remains patent, and a Guedel airway or laryngeal mask can be used during these anaesthetics.

Balanced anaesthesia

This is the most common type of anaesthetic. Separate agents are used to provide the triad effect and the use of muscle relaxants means that the patient must be ventilated. The sequence is

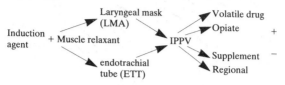

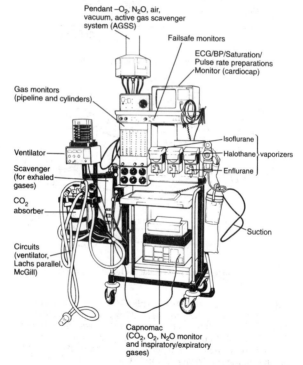

Boyle's anaesthetic machine.

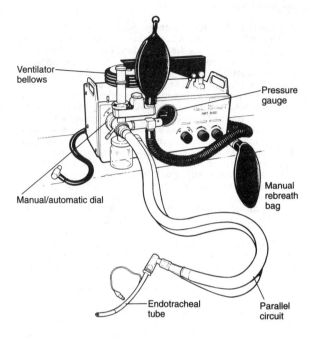

Ventilator bellows

Pressure gauge

Manual/automatic dial

Manual rebreath bag

Endotracheal tube

Parallel circuit

Manley Pulmovent ventilator.

DRUGS IN ANAESTHETIC PRACTICE

Induction agents

Thiopentone (Pentothal, Intraval Sodium) is a barbiturate which is diluted to form a 2.5 per cent solution. It is administered intravenously in a dose of 2–7 mg/kg and acts swiftly to produce unconsciousness which lasts 5–15 minutes. Termination of anaesthetic action occurs when redistribution of this fat-soluble material occurs from brain to adipose tissue and muscle. It must be used cautiously in elderly and severely ill patients where it can cause marked drops in blood pressure. Induction is smooth and well tolerated by most patients. About one in 20 000 patients are allergic to the drug and anaphylactoid reactions to thiopentone are life-threatening. Accidental subcutaneous or intra-arterial injection of thiopentone can produce tissue necrosis. As with other barbiturates, it should not be administered to patients with porphyria.

Propofol (Diprivan) is a phenol derivative bound to a lipid emulsion similar to intralipid. An induction dose of 1–2.5 mg/kg provides unconsciousness for 5–10 minutes. It causes a reduction in peripheral vascular resistance and a resultant drop in blood pressure, which is exaggerated in the elderly and hypovolaemic. Pain on injection may be attenuated by the concomitant injection of a small amount of lignocaine. Patients feel clear-headed when they wake from this drug and often have a sense of well-being. It is used for continuous intravenous anaesthesia and for sedation of patients in critical care units.

Etomidate (Hypnomidate) is an imidazole derivative. It is administered intravenously in a dose of 0.3 mg/kg for induction of intravenous anaesthesia and works in one arm to brain circulation with a duration of action of 6–8 minutes. It is the most cardiostable induction agent and is suitable for use in elderly and sick patients. Pain on injection can be reduced by concomitant administration of lignocaine. Involuntary movements and muscle clonus commonly follow the administration of this drug.

Methohexitone (Brietal) is a short-acting induction agent used in a dose of 1 mg/kg. It produces unconsciousness for 2–3 minutes. It frequently causes pain on injection and this can be treated by dissolving lignocaine in the methohexitone. The addition causes a transient clouding of the solution, but does not affect the activity of the drug. Excitatory phenomena and hiccoughs are common side-effects of this drug.

Ketamine (Ketalar) is a phencyclidine derivative produced in three concentrations of 10, 50, and 100 mg/ml. It can be used to induce anaesthesia in a dose of 1–2 mg/kg IV or 5–10 mg/kg IM. Its actions are different from other anaesthetic drugs as it has a predominant action on the cerebral cortex, producing a dissociative anaesthesia while maintaining respiratory reflexes. It maintains cardiac output and is a suitable induction agent for critically ill patients. It possesses analgesic properties and is suitable as a single agent for producing analgesia and anaesthesia in field locations such as accidents or war. Ketamine causes salivation, and an antisialogue drug should be administered with the premedication or concomitantly. Its main drawback is its tendency to produce hallucinations during the emergence period. These hallucinations can be unpleasant and are only partly eliminated by the use of benzodiazepine sedatives.

Analgesics: opiates

Alfentanil is a potent opiate which is active for only 10–15 minutes and produces cardiovascular stability for intubation.

Fentanyl has a duration of action of about 20–30 minutes. It is commonly chosen for perioperative analgesia and provides cardiovascular stability. The dose varies from 10 µg/kg which is typically used for day cases, to 1000 times this dose, which has been used by cardiac anaesthetists. It is soluble in lipids and can be used for epidural administration.

The common opiates such as **morphine, papaveretum**, and **pethidine** can be used perioperatively and are cheaper and perfectly satisfactory for the majority of general surgery.

Mixed agonist–antagonist opiates such as **pentazocine, buprenorphine, nalbuphine**, and **meptazinol** have been manufactured in an attempt to provide analgesia without producing the common side-effects of nausea, dysphoria, or respiratory depression, but none has proved to be outstandingly effective.

Analgesics: non-opiates

Opiate and non-opiate analgesics can have synergistic effects.

Tramadol is a non-opiate drug which acts at opiate receptors. It is a powerful analgesic which does not cause respiratory depression, but can still cause nausea and vomiting.

The **non-steroidal anti-inflammatory drugs** (NSAIDs) are very effective at treating some types of pain and reduce the requirement for more powerful analgesics. Examples used during anaesthesia include diclofenac, ibuprofen, tenoxicam, and piroxicam. This group of drugs should be avoided if the patient:
- Has a history of peptic ulceration
- Is severely asthmatic
- Is allergic to aspirin
- Has renal problems
- Is taking an ACE inhibitor

Anaesthetic vapours and gases

Ether and **chloroform** were the main anaesthetic drugs for the first century of anaesthesia. They have now been replaced by halothane, enflurane, isoflurane, sevoflurane, and desflurane. These have pungent smells, are very potent, and should only be administered to patients using accurately calibrated vaporizers.

Halothane causes mild cardiac depression and hypotension. Cardiac arrhythmias, notably nodal rhythm and ventricular ectopics, are a known complication of use. Very rarely halothane causes massive hepatic necrosis. Halothane should not be used when repeated anaesthetics are necessary at short intervals, nor should it be used if there has been an unexplained pyrexia after a previous halothane anaesthetic.

Enflurane is a fluorinated ether. It is a cardiac depressant if administered in high concentrations. At lower concentrations, it has little clinical effect on the heart and is probably the agent of choice in seriously ill patients. Recovery from enflurane anaesthesia is rapid.

Isoflurane is an isomer of enflurane. It is an irritant and causes breath-holding if administered in concentrations greater than 2 per cent. It has little effect on the myocardium, but causes peripheral arteriolar dilatation. This drop in systemic blood pressure, while cardiac output and thus oxygen delivery to the tissues are maintained, makes it an ideal agent for inducing hypotension during surgery. Only a small proportion of the drug is metabolized and patients wake rapidly.

Desflurane and **sevoflurane** are newer vapours not in widespread use at the time of writing. Desflurane is very potent and acts rapidly, offering the possibility to day case patients of a gas induction without the need for intravenous drugs and swift recovery.

Anaesthetic vapours are administered to the patient in a 'carrier' gas which may be air, oxygen, or most commonly mixtures of nitrous oxide and oxygen. **Nitrous oxide** is a weak anaesthetic and this limits its role as a single agent. A mixture of 50 per cent nitrous oxide in oxygen (**Entonox**) is widely used as an analgesic in obstetric analgesia and by paramedics. A 70 per cent concentration in oxygen is employed for general anaesthesia and this will render about 99 per cent of patients unconscious. It is a soluble gas and will easily pass into gas-filled body cavities and increase their pressure. Therefore it should be avoided if there is a suspicion of pneumothorax, lung cyst, severe intestinal distension, or intracranial gas. Chronic abusers of the agent may develop pernicious anaemia and peripheral neuropathy. Anaesthetic machines are now equipped with waste gas systems to minimize exposure of medical staff to anaesthetic gases and vapours.

Muscle relaxants

Muscle relaxants enable tracheal intubation and controlled ventilation. Elimination of muscle tone improves operating conditions, particularly during intra-abdominal and thoracic procedures. Muscle relaxant drugs can be classified as either depolarizing or non-depolarizing agents.

Suxamethonium is the only commonly used depolarizing agent in British anaesthetic practice. The drug acts rapidly to stimulate muscle motor end-plates and causes them to depolarize simultaneously. This effect can be detected by the uncoordinated twitching of muscles (fasciculations). A dose of 1mg/kg usually lasts for about 3–5 minutes. This rapid onset, unrivalled by any of the non-depolarizing agents, makes it an invaluable drug for use in an emergency situation when rapid endotracheal intubation is essential. Suxamethonium is metabolized by plasma pseudocholinesterase. The enzyme has genetically determined variants, and delayed breakdown of suxamethonium with prolongation of its action occurs in about one in 15 000 individuals.

The non-depolarizing muscle relaxants have a slower onset and more prolonged period of action. They work by blocking the motor end-plates of muscles, thus preventing access by acetylcholine.

- **Tubocurare** 0.5 mg/kg lasts for about 40 minutes and tends to cause hypotension.
- **Pancuronium** 0.1 mg/kg lasts for about 40 minutes and tends to cause tachycardia.
- **Vecuronium** 0.1 mg/kg lasts for about 15 minutes and has minimal side-effects.
- **Atracurium** 0.5 mg/kg lasts for about 15–20 minutes and has a very consistent duration of action.
- **Mivacurium** 0.15 mg/kg lasts for about 10–15 minutes and is broken down by pseudocholinesterase.

The last three drugs have the fewest side-effects and can be administered as single boluses or by infusion.

Reversal of muscle relaxation

Partial metabolism of the muscle relaxant must have occurred to reduce its levels from peak concentrations. The anticholinesterase drug **neostigmine** 0.05 mg/kg is given to produce a rise in acetylcholine at the neuromuscular junction. A vagolytic drug such as **atropine** 0.02 mg/kg or **glycopyrrollate** 0.008 mg/kg must be concomitantly administered to prevent bradycardias.

Complications of muscle relaxants

Allergic reactions The incidence of serious adverse reactions to the muscle relaxants is quoted at between one in 5000 and one in 20 000. Suxamethonium is the drug most commonly implicated.

Muscle pains These are common following suxamethonium, but are also seen after non-depolarizing agents.

Pseudocholinesterase deficiencies Both suxamethonium and mivacurium are metabolized by pseudocholinesterase, and their action will be prolonged if the enzyme concentration is low as a result of a familial tendency or disease state.

Failure to reverse One cause of difficulty in re-establishing muscle tone may be a relative excess of muscle relaxant.

Awareness This occurs when a patient receives a muscle relaxant but is not rendered unconscious. This may be due to a technical error on the part of the anaesthetist or his equipment, or occasionally because the patient is abnormally resistant to the effect of the hypnotic components of the anaesthetic.

Malignant hyperpyrexia This may be triggered by muscle relaxants, anaesthetic vapours, and neuroleptic drugs (see p. 40).

Sedation differs from general anaesthesia in that the sedated patient will continue to respond to verbal command and laryngeal reflexes are maintained. It can be used in conjunction with local or regional analgesia, or to allow a potentially distressing but non-painful procedure such as gastroscopy to be tolerated. Prolonged sedation is used to keep patients comfortable in ICUs.

Benzodiazepines

Midazolam provides sedation for about 30 minutes but amnesia for rather longer. A typical dose of midazolam is 0.1 mg/kg but the drug should be titrated in 1.0–2.5 mg increments until the desired effect is produced.

Diazepam is presented in either propylene glycol or lipid emulsion. The typical dose of diazepam is 0.2 mg/kg. It is a less potent amnesic agent than midazolam, but produces a similar degree of sedation. The metabolites are active drugs and can lead to prolonged sedation in certain cases.

Lorazepam 1–4 mg is a potent amnesic and sedative agent. Its duration of action of 6–12 hours makes it unsuitable for use during day case surgery or diagnostic procedures.

The action of benzodiazepines can be reversed by **flumazenil** which is a highly specific competitive inhibitor of benzodiazepines at their receptor sites. The dose is titrated against response. It has a short duration of action and patients may apparently recover fully, only to return to their sedated state some 30 minutes later.

Opiates

Opiates and benzodiazepines have synergistic effects. Combinations of fentanyl and midazolam may be useful during mildly uncomfortable procedures, such as invasive radiological investigations or lithotripsy, but must be used with great caution as the side-effects of airway obstruction and respiratory depression occur at low drug doses. In ICUs long-term sedation may be provided by morphine or papaveretum infusions combined with midazolam.

Intravenous anaesthetic agents

Propofol has been used in subanaesthetic doses to provide sedation and sleep to patients undergoing surgery under regional blockade.

Inhalational agents

Entonox (50 per cent nitrous oxide in oxygen) has proved to be a very safe analgesic and sedative drug. The term 'relative analgesia' is employed to describe the administration of 50 per cent nitrous oxide during dental procedures.

Monitoring of sedation techniques

Patients should be carefully supervised during sedation as the borderline between sedation and general anaesthesia is narrow. There should always be someone present whose sole responsibility is to monitor the patient, as airway obstruction or respiratory arrest can easily develop. It is desirable that the patient's pulse and saturation are measured using a pulse oximeter. Full resuscitation facilities must be instantly available and those present must have been trained in airway management.

CONDUCT OF A GENERAL ANAESTHETIC

A general anaesthetic consists of three phases:
- induction
- maintenance
- reversal

Induction

Induction is the most critical phase of the anaesthetic. Hypoxia, regurgitation, hypertension, and hypotension must be avoided. All equipment should be checked and all personnel should be present before the patient arrives in the anaesthetic room. The patient's identity and operation should be confirmed. Intravenous access should be established, except perhaps in infants, where this may be extremely difficult, and small children with airway problems such as croup which may be exacerbated by distress. Monitoring should commence. The options are as follows.

Awake intubation

Local anaesthesia of the upper airways enables direct or fibre-optic laryngoscopy and intubation of patients who are known to have abnormalities of the upper airway or to be difficult to intubate. In rare life-threatening conditions it may be necessary to perform tracheostomy under local anaesthesia before beginning the anaesthetic.

Gas induction

This is also a very safe technique of inducing anaesthesia. Any vapour can be used, but halothane and sevoflurane are the least irritant. Gas inductions are used to induce patients with lower airways problems, e.g. inhaled peanuts, in which case a vapour–oxygen mixture is employed. This is a safe combination with nitrous oxide to induce patients with a needle phobia and children in whom intravenous access is difficult.

Intravenous induction

The dose of induction agent is titrated against the patient's response. Muscle relaxants can then be administered to allow endotracheal intubation, or the patient can continue to breath on a face-mask or laryngeal mask.

Rapid sequence induction

If the patient is at risk of regurgitation of stomach contents, a rapid sequence or 'crash' induction is used. The patient is pre-oxygenated with a well-fitting face-mask for 2–3 minutes and a precalculated dose of induction agent is then injected. As the patient loses consciousness, the anaesthetic assistant applies pressure on the anterior aspect of the cricoid which will occlude the oesophagus between the posterior aspect of the cricoid and the posterior pharyngeal wall. This prevents passive reflux of potentially harmful stomach contents. Suxamethonium is injected intravenously and the airway secured as soon as the fasciculations have ceased. Only after the cuff of the endotracheal tube is inflated is the cricoid pressure released.

Airway management

When prolonged ventilation is required or there is a risk of regurgitation, it is normal to intubate the patient by either the orotracheal or nasotracheal routes. The Brain laryngeal mask is a very effective technique of maintaining a clear airway in patients who are spontaneously breathing, and patients may be ventilated through these masks if they have good lung compliance. Simple short anaesthetics can be effectively conducted using a face-mask.

Ventilation of the lungs using a face-mask is a fundamental medical skill which all doctors should possess. It can be particularly difficult if the patient:

- Has a florid beard
- Has a stocky build and a short neck
- Is very obese or is pregnant
- Is very thin and edentulous
- Has anatomical or pathological deformities of the head or neck

Equipment for airway management

Face-mask

The airway is first cleared by extending the neck and, if necessary, inserting a Guedel airway. The mask is placed on the face from above downwards, fitting the nose into the upper groove of the mask and moulding the cheeks to form a seal. The position of the hand is critical. The little finger should be positioned behind the angle of the jaw to lift the chin upwards. The thumb should be directly opposed to the little finger and press the mask onto the face. The index finger supports the mask and controls its pressure on the face in the horizontal plane. The middle and ring fingers are placed flat on the bone under the chin and should not dig into the soft tissues. Mask-holding is made easier by keeping the elbow straight and locking the wrist, and using the torso muscles to elevate the chin rather than attempting to do this with the arm and forearm muscles.

Laryngeal mask

This airway is inserted into the pharynx and its large volume cuff inflated. A partial seal is produced and patients with good lung compliance can be hand or mechanically ventilated by connecting the breathing circuit to the airway. However, it

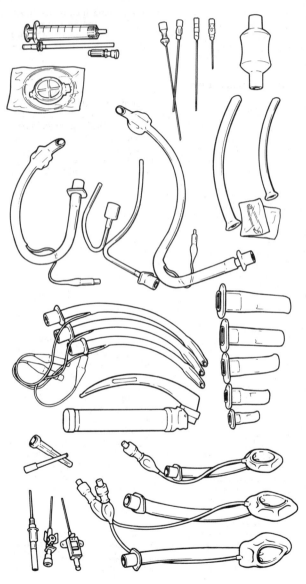

Equipment for airway management.

does not protect against regurgitation of stomach contents and should not be used if the patient may have a full stomach. The mask comes in six sizes; size 4 is usually chosen for adults. The patient must be adequately anaesthetized before the mask is inserted. The laryngeal mask is prepared by deflating and lubricating its cuff. The patient's head is gently extended until the lower jaw falls open. The airway is then steadily inserted into the mouth, pushing up against the hard palate. The mask will slide backwards and downwards into the pharynx. Successful insertion is indicated by a resistance against further insertion. The cuff should be inflated with 10–20 ml of air and the chest should expand when the reservoir bag of the breathing circuit is gently squeezed.

Endotracheal intubation
This is performed so that:
- Ventilation can be assisted
- Neuromuscular blocking agents can be administered
- The respiratory passages can be protected against soiling from regurgitated stomach contents.

Failure to recognize that the tip of the tracheal tube has been inserted into the oesophagus can have fatal consequences.

Adult males are usually intubated using a 9 mm internal diameter oral endotracheal tube (ETT) with the 22 cm mark at the lips; females are intubated with an 8 mm ETT positioned at 20 cm. For younger patients the formula is

length of tube = age in years/2 + 12 cm
internal diameter of tube = age in years/4 + 4.5 cm.

Tracheal intubation should be practised on a model and then performed under supervision. Care needs to be taken to avoid dental damage and undue trauma to the lips and larynx. About one in 80 patients offers problems at intubation, even to skilled anaesthetists. An aid to intubation is the gum rubber bougie which enables an endotracheal tube to be 'railroaded' into a larynx that is hard to visualize.

Complications of intubation include the following.
- Failed intubation: this is not a crisis if adequate oxygenation is maintained by face-mask.
- Oesophageal intubation: this must be recognized immediately as otherwise it may prove fatal.
- Endobronchial intubation: this is recognized by unequal chest movement, lack of breath sounds on the left side of the chest, and low blood oxygen saturations. It is easily remedied by withdrawing the endotracheal tube a short distance.
- Laryngeal damage: rough handling of the endotracheal tube can lead to damage which includes dislocation of the vocal cords. Prolonged intubation may lead to a vocal cord granuloma.
- Sore throat: this is very common.

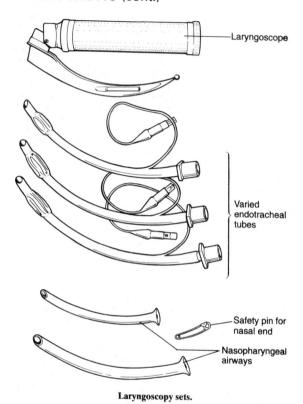

Laryngoscopy sets.

The crisis

The nightmare situation in which one can neither intubate nor ventilate a patient should almost never arise. The following temporizing measures can be used to maintain oxygenation while preparations are made to provide a definitive airway:

- needle cricothyrotomy (see p. 65)
- cricothyrotomy (see p. 66)

Maintenance

During surgery the anaesthetist

- maintains ventilation and oxygenation
- ensures cardiovascular stability

- replaces fluid losses
- ensures that the patient remains unaware
- monitors the patient
- records results

Monitoring

The greatest safety factor in anaesthesia is the continuous presence of an appropriately trained and skilled anaesthetist. Monitors can assist this work, but the principles on which they work must be understood as they may otherwise mislead.

Electrocardiogram (ECG)

The ECG is a sensitive indicator of cardiac rhythm and ventricular ischaemia. Nodal rhythm, sinus bradycardia, and ventricular ectopics are common during surgery and may require treatment.

Pulse oximeter

The pulse oximeter measures the proportion of oxygenated haemoglobin in the circulation. False readings may obtained under the following conditions.

- A pigment on the patient's skin (nail varnish, paint) interferes with light transmission.
- An abnormal haemoglobin is circulating (carboxyhaemoglobin, methaemoglobin).
- Peripheral perfusion is poor.

A pulse oximeter can indicate that a patient is adequately oxygenated, but provides no information about ventilation. A sedated patient being administered oxygen may remain saturated for many minutes despite being apnoeic.

Blood pressure

The blood pressure is influenced by myocardial contractility, intravascular volume, and peripheral vascular resistance. Automatic oscillotonometers are now common and give an impression of accuracy. However, they function poorly if:

- The patient is moving
- A member of the scrub team is leaning on the cuff
- The patient is not in sinus rhythm
- The blood pressure is changing rapidly

They measure trends accurately but single readings cannot be relied upon. Direct intravascular measurement of blood pressure is preferable in patients whose blood pressure may fluctuate. False readings from arterial systems may result from:

- Air bubbles in the monitoring line
- Failure to zero and calibrate the transducer
- Incorrect positioning of the transducer

Central venous monitoring

Central venous lines indicate the volume of the circulation, and are useful during the resuscitation of patients and prolonged surgical procedures (see p. 59).

Pulmonary artery and wedge pressure monitoring

A Swan–Ganz catheter is inserted into the central venous circulation and a small (< 1 ml) balloon at its tip, which floats the tip of the catheter through the right side of the heart and into the pulmonary artery, is inflated. Once the balloon is wedged in the distal segments of the lung, the pressure trace seen indicates the filling pressure of the left side of the heart. Swan–Ganz catheters are useful in managing patients with poor cardiac function (see p. 62).

Capnography

Measurements of carbon dioxide indicate the effectiveness of ventilation and can detect abnormal metabolism, i.e. malignant hyperpyrexia, gas embolism, and ventilator disconnection.

Ventilator disconnect alarm

Unnoticed disconnection of the breathing system in a paralysed ventilated patient causes death. An apnoea alarm may be part of the capnograph or a device such as a pneumotachograph or respirometer which is built into many anaesthetic ventilators.

Oxygen monitor

An oxygen-measuring device, usually a fuel cell, is included in the anaesthetic system to ensure that the oxygen output of the machine is not faulty as a result of incorrect gas supply or mechanical failure.

Neuromuscular monitoring

Nerve stimulation leads to characteristic responses by muscles during the period when the effect of muscle relaxants is wearing off. These responses can be measured by a simple nerve stimulator device or by sophisticated machines such as the 'relaxograph'.

Vapour-monitoring devices

New anaesthetic machines incorporate devices which analyse the inspired and expired concentrations of volatile anaesthetic agents.

Reversal

Once surgery is completed, the patient must regain his airway reflexes as swiftly as possible and then be restored to full consciousness in a pain-free state. Problems associated with this phase of the anaesthetic include the following.

- **Persistent neuromuscular blockade** is caused by suxamethonium apnoea or attempts to reverse non-depolarizing relaxants before they have started to wear off.
- **Partial reversal of neuromuscular block** causes characteristically twitchy movements and the patient has a sensation of suffocation. Additional reversal agent may help.
- **Failure to establish respiration**, despite normal muscle activity, may be due to excess opiates. The respiratory stimulant doxapram or the opiate antagonist naloxone may help to stimulate respiration.
- **Restlessness** (see p. 44).

If the patient does not breathe adequately, he should be resedated, ventilated, and transferred to the ICU until the anaesthetic drugs wear off. Full clinical assessment of such patients is essential to ensure that a serious treatable clinical condition has not gone undiagnosed (e.g. hypoglycaemia, brain haemorrhage).

Minor sequelae of anaesthesia are very common, but only one death per 200 000 surgical procedures can be directly attributed to anaesthesia.

Mortality

The major causes of anaesthetic mortality are:
- Misplacement of an endotracheal tube in the oesophagus
- Disconnection of the breathing system in a paralysed patient
- Failure of an anaesthetist to pay sufficient heed to the patient under his care

Life-threatening conditions associated with anaesthesia

Anaphylactoid drug reactions
About one in 6000 patients may have an adverse drug reaction causing life-threatening cardiovascular collapse, hypoxia, and bronchospasm. Reactions to thiopentone are particularly severe. Treatment involves giving oxygen, adrenaline, fluids, and steroids. The surgical procedure may have to be abandoned. If the patient recovers, attempts should be made to identify the cause of the reaction and skin or radio-allergosorbent (RAS) tests should be performed. The patient must be counselled about the risks of future anaesthetics.

Malignant hyperpyrexia
Diagnosis is made when a patient develops signs of a massive metabolic reaction with a rise in core temperature of 1°C per 30 minutes. Surgery must be completed rapidly, inhalation anaesthetics agents discontinued, and the patient hyperventilated with 100 per cent oxygen and actively cooled. Dantrolene 1 mg/kg is administered and repeated up to a total of 10 mg/kg. Treatment for acidosis and hyperkalaemia must be commenced.

Pneumothorax
Spontaneous, traumatic, or iatrogenic pneumothorax may follow central-line insertion. Positive pressure ventilation and the use of nitrous oxide are both likely to increase the size of a pneumothorax and may produce a build-up of intrathoracic pressure and cardiac tamponade. The presence of a chest drain does not mean that it is working! Tension pneumothorax can be difficult to diagnose in the intubated ventilated patient.

Gas embolism
This is most commonly seen during head and neck surgery with steep head-up tilt, but can occur in any operation where large veins are exposed above the level of the heart. It may also occur during laparoscopic procedures if insufflation gases

are inadvertently injected intravenously. Gas-cooled lasers have also been reported to cause embolism. Nitrous oxide should be discontinued and 100 per cent oxygen administered. Attempts should be made to aspirate air from the right atrium via a CVP line or, *in extremis*, by aspiration from the heart through the chest wall. The left lateral head-down position is recommended.

Attempts should be made to remove all air from venous lines, and this is particularly important when treating infants and neonates. Air in arterial monitoring lines is always dangerous: 1/ml of air flushed through an arterial line has been reported to cause fatal cerebral air embolism.

Upper-airway problems
These may be caused by obstruction, haemorrhage, or inhaled vomit. Adequate personnel, equipment, and training are required to overcome these emergencies.

Less serious morbidity

- Awareness
- Nausea and vomiting
- Dental damage
- Trauma to oropharyngeal soft tissues
- Peripheral nerve lesions
- Discomfort of neck, jaw, groin, and lower back
- Urinary retention
- Muscle pains—commonly associated with use of suxamethonium
- Discomfort from intramuscular injections for premedication or analgesia

Four levels of care are now recognized:
- the recovery room
- the high dependency unit
- the intensive care unit
- the general ward

Recovery room

This unit has a high staff-to-patient ratio with a rapid turnover of patients. The object of the unit is to ensure the following.
- The patients airway is maintained until the anaesthetic wears off and consciousness returns.
- Breathing is adequate.
- The patient remains cardiovascularly stable.
- No harm arises if the patient is restless during the transition from anaesthesia to full consciousness.
- The patient is comfortable and is given additional analgesia if required.
- Irrigation systems and drains are functioning correctly.
- Surgical and anaesthetic staff are informed if a complication develops.

High dependency unit

These units have an intermediate staffing ratio, usually one nurse per three or four patients, and may be located in the recovery unit or the ICU, be a self-contained ward, or be a zone within a general ward. The staff are trained to monitor arterial pressure and CVP, to administer drug infusions and to manage pain-relief techniques such as epidural infusions. Units of this type are particularly suitable for the care of patients following vascular and neurosurgical procedures and major abdominal surgery, and those patients whose preoperative condition gave cause for concern.

Intensive care units

ICUs have high staff-to-patient nursing ratios, constant medical cover, and full monitoring and ventilation facilities. They give cardiovascular and respiratory support to their patients and may additionally provide treatment for renal or hepatic failure.

Day case patients

Day case patients will be discharged from the recovery unit or ward shortly after surgery. Before discharge the patient should:
- Be comfortable
- Should be able to stand erect with his eyes closed
- Be able to dress himself
- Have eaten and drunk without feeling nauseated

The patient may then be discharged home accompanied by a companion. Clear verbal and written postoperative instructions should be given to the patient and he should know how to obtain advice and help in case of postoperative complications. A patient who has received anaesthetic or sedative drugs should not make important business decisions, drink alcohol, work with machinery, or drive a vehicle for at least 24 hours.

Restlessness

Transient disorientation and restlessness is common during emergence from anaesthesia. Serious confusion may be caused by:
- Extreme anxiety before the start of surgery
- Recovery from anaesthesia in aggressive heavy drinkers
- Airway obstruction
- Persistent neuromuscular blockade
- Urinary retention
- Sedative drugs given to patients in pain
- The central effects of atropine, especially in elderly patients
- PAIN

Restlessness should only be attributed to pain after other potential causes have been excluded, as the administration of opiates may mask other conditions.

Respiratory complications

Respiratory depression may be caused by excessive perioperative administration of anaesthetic drugs. Treatment involves assisting respiration with reintubation and ventilation if necessary. If an excess of opiate drugs is thought to be the cause, naloxone 0.1–0.4 mg may be titrated intravenously to see if respiration improves.

Upper airway obstruction causes the patient to struggle to breath. Tracheal tug is visible, the accessory respiratory muscles contract, and 'see-saw' respiration may occur. This may give the impression of good ventilation, even though no breathing is taking place. The airway should be cleared, the oropharynx cleared of secretions, and a Guedel airway inserted to elevate the tongue. Laryngospasm can occur during emergence from anaesthesia and urgent re-intubation may be indicated, using suxamethonium or propofol to relax the vocal cord spasm.

Occasionally, the upper airway is abnormally compressible because of laryngomalacia or an unusually large and floppy epiglottis; such patients may develop an inspiratory stridor and can be helped by providing continuous positive airways pressure (CPAP). Tracheal and laryngeal polyps are a rare cause of postoperative respiratory obstruction.

Pulmonary pathology may become apparent only after positive pressure ventilation has ceased. Left-ventricular failure, fat embolism, and pneumothorax can become symptomatic during the recovery period. Basal atelectasis occurs during general anaesthesia and may progress to lobar pneumonia if the patient is unable to take deep breaths during the postoperative period.

Assessment of respiratory function
- Clinical judgement remains the most useful. The rate, depth, and regularity of breathing can be assessed, and use

of accessory muscles indicates difficulty in breathing.

- Cyanosis is hard to judge clinically under artificial lighting. The pulse oximeter is more reliable. A patient who has an oxygen saturation of less than 90 per cent on room air needs oxygen therapy, and the cause of the poor oxygenation should be sought.
- Blood gases can be measured. Normal end-tidal CO_2 pressure is 5.3 kPa, but it often rises to 7.5 kPa when patients are given opiates. End-tidal CO_2 values above 10 kPa occur in patients developing respiratory failure.
- Peak flow and tidal volume measurements can be useful in the postoperative period, but expiratory efforts may be impeded by opiates and discomfort.
- Chest X-ray films are useful to assess changes associated with pulmonary oedema, infection, inhalation pneumonitis, and pneumothorax. Adult respiratory distress syndrome (ARDS) may develop in patients who have been severely hypovolaemic or septicaemic. X-ray changes reach their maximum 24 hours after clinical changes become apparent and resolve slowly.

Treatment of respiratory problems

Diuretics   If there is evidence of raised JVP or CVP, cardiomegaly, or pulmonary oedema, frusemide 20 mg is suitable as an initial treatment. The patient needs to be mobile to void urine after a rapid diuresis. Alternatively, a catheter should be inserted.

Bronchodilators   Asthmatics and chronic bronchitics commonly wheeze in the postoperative period. Nebulized salbutamol 2.5 mg may make these patients breathe more easily.

Respiratory stimulants   A dose of doxapram (*Dopram*, not to be confused with *dopamine*) administered at the end of the operation has been recommended as a method of encouraging deep respiration and reducing basal atelectasis.

Reversal agents   Respiratory difficulties will be seen if there is residual muscle weakness due to persistent neuromuscular blocking effects.

Physiotherapy   Chest physiotherapy is a traditional medical intervention and certainly encourages the patient to expectorate and take deep breaths.

Ventilation   If symptomatic treatment does not produce improvement, the patient will require reintubation, ventilation, and transfer to an ICU.

POSTOPERATIVE COMPLICATIONS
(*cont.*)

Pain

Patients complaining of pain should be treated by appropriate analgesic drugs. Titration of intravenous opiates gives rapid pain relief.

Nausea and vomiting

These are distressing for the patient and may cause sweating, bradycardia, hypotension, and peripheral vasoconstriction. The usual culprit is opiate analgesia. Parenteral antiemetic drugs include metoclopramide, prochlorperazine, ondansetron, and cyclizine. Hyoscine skin patches have been used. Combinations of antiemetics may help patients who are very nauseated.

Recurarization

The effects of non-depolarizing muscle relaxants may persist beyond the time that the anticholinesterases used to reverse their action are effective. Similar effects are seen if an operation is abruptly terminated and an attempt is made to reverse neuromuscular paralysis when the patient still has high levels of neuromuscular blocking agent. The use of an electrical nerve stimulator should ensure that no patient is left partially paralysed without ventilatory support.

Treatment

It is reasonable to give one additional dose of reversal agent, typically glycopyrrollate 0.5 mg, or atropine 1.2 mg, plus neostigmine 2.5 mg. If this is ineffective, the patient may need to be re-sedated and ventilated until full neuromuscular strength returns. Persistent blockade should lead one to consider whether the patient has a myasthenic syndrome.

Hypotension

Relative hypotension with a normal heart rate and full pulse is normal in a young, sleeping, and comfortable patient. Hypotension and tachycardia indicate hypovolaemia or septicaemia and must be managed aggressively. Hypotension with bradycardia is seen in the nauseated patient, but may also occur with intra-abdominal bleeding. Such patients will look pale and will have a weak pulse. They should be treated by rapid transfusion and returned to theatre to control haemorrhage. Loss of fluid into bowel or soft tissues will require rapid rehydration and monitoring of urine output and CVP. Septicaemia will require rehydration, inotropic and ventilatory support, and the administration of appropriate antibiotics.

Hypertension

This may lead to ventricular failure, myocardial infarction, bleeding at the operating site, damage to vascular anastomoses, and cerebral haemorrhage. It is commonly seen following vascular surgery, or in patients whose routine antihypertensive agent has been inadvertently withdrawn. Rapid emergence from anaesthesia and pain can lead to raised blood pressures. These will usually need to be treated by an appropriate antihypertensive agent.

Shivering

Violent shaking is seen quite commonly following inhalational agents. Its cause is unknown. The patient should be administered high flow oxygen as hypoxia may occur owing to high oxygen consumption during this period.

Sweating

Profuse sweating in the postoperative period may be associated with nausea, incipient cardiac failure due to fluid overload or myocardial infarction, septicaemia, or carbon dioxide retention. Sweaty patients must be observed closely and treated appropriately.

Good-quality pain relief reduces postoperative complications and allows patients to be discharged earlier. The main classes of drugs used in pain relief are opiates, NSAIDs, simple analgesics, and local anaesthetic agents. Antidepressant agents may help to treat chronic pain of central origin. Other drugs, such as alpha-2 adrenergic agents and calcium-channel blockers, are being investigated for their ability to synergize with the analgesic drugs.

Opiates

These may act as agonists, antagonists, or inactive blocking agents at the opiate receptors on the cell membranes. Pure agonists remain the most effective, with morphine, papaveretum, pethidine, and diamorphine being administered postoperatively to the majority of patients. The dose-related side-effects include nausea, vomiting, and dysphonia. Opiates also enhance postoperative respiratory depression and may cause sleep disturbance. Addiction is uncommon when opiates are used to treat acute pain.

Naloxone is a pure antagonist drug which is able to reverse the effects of opiate agonists. Adult (0.4 mg/ml) and neonatal (0.02 mg/ml) preparations are available. Naloxone can be used to reverse respiratory depression associated with opiate overdose, but will also reverse analgesia and may precipitate opiate withdrawal syndromes. The half-life of naloxone is relatively short and the effects of a single intravenous dose wear off after 20 minutes, leading to re-sedation of the patient. Intramuscular administration or a continuous infusion may be necessary to counteract this effect.

Other drugs used to treat pain

NSAIDs reduce pain and inflammation by inhibiting the formation of prostaglandin and thromboxane. A significant number of patients should not be prescribed them (see p. 25). Aspirin and paracetamol remain simple, cheap, and effective.

Benzodiazepines have no intrinsic analgesic properties but may make very frightened patients calmer and more comfortable. Opiate–benzodiazepine combinations may cause significant respiratory depression.

Clonidine is an alpha-2 adrenergic agonist which decreases noradrenaline release from sympathetic nerve terminals. It is used in the treatment of hypertension, migraine, and chronic pain. This group of drugs may reduce opiate requirements in acute pain.

Combinations of analgesic drugs provide a more effective and better quality of pain relief than individual agents.

Methods of administering analgesic drugs

Oral medication is appropriate for many patients, and many classes of drugs come in tablet form.

Drugs can be given **rectally** to patients who are feeling nauseated. Diclofenac and paracetamol suppositories are available

Percutaneous patches of hyoscine are marketed and some opiate patches are under trial.

Intramuscular on demand

The patient is given an injection of opiate if he requests it or the nurse feels that he requires pain relief. The patient must be in pain before analgesia is administered, and this is an inherently unsatisfactory system.

Regular analgesic administration

This may be by regular intramuscular injection or by continuous intravenous infusion. These techniques can allow a patient to remain pain free throughout the postoperative period, but variation in analgesic requirements means that a proportion of patients can become oversedated. Careful patient assessment is essential, and this should include a pain and sedation score, a respiratory rate, and, where possible, oximetry.

Patient-controlled analgesic systems (PCAS)

Pumps have been designed which permit self-administration of drugs by patients. The patient is given a handset which controls delivery of a bolus of opiate and/or local anaesthetic whenever the button is depressed. To prevent overdosage, the pump then 'locks out' for a period before a further dose can be administered. PCAS are usually used to administer intravenous opiates, but they can also be used to deliver drugs subcutaneously, intramuscularly, or epidurally. The patient's vital signs, pain score, and sedation score must be observed regularly. Nausea, vomiting, and dysphoria remain a problem in some patients.

Typical regimens include the following:
- Morphine sulphate 1 mg/ml, bolus 1 mg, lock-out time 5 minutes
- Papaveretum 1 mg/ml, bolus 2 mg, lock-out time 5 minutes
- Pethidine 10 mg/ml, bolus 10 mg, lock-out time 3 minutes

An antiemetic is sometimes mixed with the opiate. This method of pain relief is safe and cost-effective.

Epidural administration

The administration of local anaesthetics and/or opiates by the epidural route has reduced the morbidity following major surgery and greatly improved patient comfort. The patient

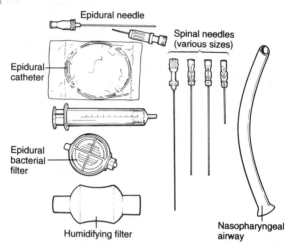

Epidural set and anaesthetic applicator.

can co-operate with physiotherapy and mobilize quickly. Complications include respiratory depression, pruritis, and urinary retention.

Intrathecal opiates

These are often given simultaneously with a perioperative local anaesthetic block and produce prolonged postoperative analgesia. The side-effects are similar to those when the opiate is given by the epidural route.

Local anaesthetic blocks

A local anaesthetic can be continuously administered by an indwelling catheter placed alongside the nerve or by a single-shot technique, in which case bupivacaine is usually chosen as it has a duration of action longer than those of the other local anaesthetics. Wound infiltration ('bupivacaine squirting') is a simple, quick, and effective method of providing postoperative pain relief. Regional blocks used for treatment of postoperative pain include the following.

    Brachial plexus block provides analgesia to the upper limb. It can be approached by the interscalene, supraclavicular, and axillary routes.

    Intercostal blocks provide analgesia in the lower thoracic and upper abdominal region following chest trauma or upper abdominal incision. They are technically simple to perform, but pneumothorax can be caused and absorption of local anaesthetic can rapidly lead to high plasma concentrations.

Inguinal block is effective in the treatment of pain following herniorraphy and orchidopexy.

Penile block can be employed to treat the pain of circumcision.

Caudal block treats perineal pain including haemorrhoidectomy.

Lateral cutaneous nerve block of thigh can reduce the pain of hip surgery.

Femoral nerve block used to relieve quadriceps spasm and the pain of femoral and knee surgery.

Ankle block is useful in foot surgery.

Other techniques of pain relief

Cryotherapy
Direct application of a cryoprobe to a nerve results in the area supplied remaining pain free until the nerve regenerates in weeks or months. A proportion of patients develop dysaesthesiae afterwards.

Transcutaneous electrical nerve stimulation (TENS)
This procedure has been used during childbirth and in the treatment of chronic pain, but is less effective in postoperative pain.

Acupuncture
This is widely used in some oriental societies but is not effective in all patients.

Hypnosis
Again, this is only effective when patient and practitioner are well-matched.

LATE POSTOPERATIVE COMPLICATIONS

Perfusion problems
- Myocardial infarction
- Tissued drips
- Compartment syndromes
- Venous thrombosis

Respiratory complications
- Fat embolism
- Pulmonary embolism
- Basal atelectasis leading to lobar pneumonia
- Hypoxia: analgesia, atelectasis

Anastomotic breakdown

Urinary retention

Renal failure

Infection

Confusion

Complications due to drug imbalances
These are particularly associated with digoxin, antihypertensives, anticonvulsants, and antidepressants.

Drug sensitivity

Indications for elective admission of surgical patients to intensive care include the following.

- Major vascular surgery in patients with poor myocardial function
- Major abdominal surgery especially in obese patients and those with chronic respiratory disease
- Complications of major trauma: fat embolism, ARDS
- Head and neck surgery which may lead to postoperative airway difficulties
- Cardiac and thoracic surgery
- Major neurosurgery
- Fragile elderly patients who have required major surgery
- Sepsis

Ethics of intensive care

Intensive care can now sustain life beyond its natural limits, but at a great psychological and financial cost to the patient, the family, and the community. A holistic approach to the care of a patient with multisystem failure is essential, and the likely outcome of treatment should be regularly reappraised. Patients who survive in a persistent vegetative state represent the worst outcome of intensive care.

Cardiovascular support

The aim of treatment is to optimize oxygen delivery to the tissues by manipulating cardiac output, haemoglobin concentration, and oxygen saturation. Haemoglobin concentration should be maintained above 10 g/dl. Oxygen saturation should be maintained above 90 per cent, and this often requires ventilatory support. Having achieved the first two aims, cardiac output can be improved by having an adequate 'preload'. Right-ventricular preload is equivalent to the CVP. The effect of preloading can be judged by performing a **fluid challenge**. Boluses of fluid are administered in rapid succession to the patient while the CVP is monitored. Initially the fluid will help to expand an underfilled circulation, but optimal filling is achieved when the CVP rises and then remains at an elevated level when a fluid bolus is given. In a normal person the right-sided filling pressure (CVP/JVP) is an indication of the filling pressure of the left side of the heart. However left- and right-ventricular function may differ in patients with compromised left-ventricular function and in severe arteriopaths, and management of these patients may be assisted by measuring left atrial pressures using a Swan–Ganz catheter.

Once filling pressure has been improved, the myocardium can be supported using **inotropic drugs**. Dobutamine 1–40 μg/kg/minute is the most popular inotropic drug as it causes relatively few cardiac arrhythmias. Dopamine 10–50 μg/kg/minute is often administered simultaneously because it can improve renal function. Dopamine is also inotropic in higher doses but causes renal and splanchnic circulatory shutdown to a greater degree than dobutamine. Adrenaline is a powerful inotropic drug but can cause myocardial ischaemia.

Cardiac output is governed by both the power of the myocardium and the peripheral resistance or afterload. High peripheral vascular resistance can be reduced by short-acting drugs such as sodium nitroprusside and glyceryl trinitrate and by longer-duration antihypertensive agents such as hydrallazine and alpha-adrenergic blockers. Septic shock causes peripheral shunting with poor tissue perfusion despite low vascular resistance, but these patients may improve if noradrenaline is administered to raise peripheral resistance. Phosphodiesterase inhibitors such as enoximone combine inotropic properties with reduced peripheral resistance and may be useful.

Cardiac output and peripheral resistance can be measured using a Swan–Ganz thermodilution catheter. Doppler flow or thoracic impedance techniques can measure cardiac output non-invasively. Measurements of mixed venous oxygen saturation correlate well with survival and patients whose Svo_2 can be elevated by about 40 per cent have a better prognosis.

Respiratory support

Many patients who have undergone major surgery become hypoxic in the postoperative period. Opiates and sleep disturbance lead to irregular breathing patterns which peak on the second or third postoperative night. Patients with poor respiratory function will benefit from oxygen therapy for several days postoperatively. Spontaneously breathing patients usually cough and expectorate, but if they cannot clear secretions by themselves, physiotherapy or suction through a minitracheostomy can help. An exhausted patient needs to be ventilated.

The aim of respiratory therapy is to maintain oxygenation on the upper shelf of the oxyhaemoglobin sigmoid dissociation curve and to clear carbon dioxide. Accumulation of carbon dioxide above the normal level of 5.3 kPa is treated by increasing the minute ventilation. If lung function deteriorates, a succession of measures is taken to maintain oxygenation. High inspired oxygen concentrations are toxic to the alveolar cells, while high mean pulmonary inflation pressures result in tamponade of the heart and reduced cardiac filling. Therefore cardiovascular and respiratory therapy must be balanced.

Intensive care ventilators offer many modes of supporting respiration, described by jargon initials. These include the following.

Intermittent positive pressure ventilation (IPPV), also

known as controlled mechanical ventilation: both rate and depth of breathing are controlled by the machine. Multiplying the respiratory rate by the tidal volume gives the patient's minute ventilation.

Intermittent mandatory ventilation (IMV): the patient can breathe on his own for much of the time, but if minute ventilation falls below a certain level the ventilator will take over.

Synchronized IMV (SIMV): if the ventilator does take over from the patient, the inspirations are triggered by efforts made by the patient and are then servo-assisted.

Pressure support: all the patients breathing efforts are servo-assisted so that a greater depth of respiration is achieved than the patient can manage by himself.

Positive end-expiratory pressure (PEEP): a technique to increase mean intrapulmonary pressure and recruit additional alveoli into the respiratory exchange process.

Continuous positive airways pressure (CPAP): analogous to PEEP except that the patient is breathing spontaneously.

High frequency ventilation (HFPPV): large volumes of gas are blown over the lung surface to improve respiratory gas exchange. The technique allows gas exchange to occur at reduced mean airway pressure and this may improve healing of bronchopleural fistulae.

Extracorporeal membrane oxygenation (ECMO): an experimental technique to allow extracorporeal blood oxygenation akin to that occurring during cardiopulmonary bypass. In selected patients it may allow the lungs to be rested while healing occurs.

Renal support

Fluid and electrolyte balance must be monitored and appropriate fluid replacement given. Renal failure can be treated as follows.

Peritoneal dialysis: technically simple but cannot be used immediately following abdominal or thoracic surgery.

Haemodialysis: effective and controllable though technically complex.

Haemofiltration: requires less equipment than haemodialysis but results in large volumes of fluid being haemofiltered which need to be replaced intravenously.

Haemoperfusion: increasingly popular as a technique for postoperative renal support.

All clinicians should develop a pride in undertaking simple practical procedures swiftly, cleanly, and with the minimum discomfort to their patients. The techniques described in this section are only one method of undertaking tasks that may be accomplished in many ways.

Peripheral venous cannulation

An appropriate cannula should be selected: a 22G or 24G is satisfactory for small children and an 18G or 19G cannula is adequate to administer drugs to adults, but a 17G cannula or larger should be inserted if the patient is to receive a post-operative infusion. Patients requiring resuscitation and those undergoing major surgery must have one or more 14G or 12G cannulae inserted. The best drip site is the mid-forearm on the patient's non-dominant side; drips placed near to joints are uncomfortable and more prone to phlebitis. Anaesthetists often cannulate veins on the back of the hand because this is usually straightforward and convenient to them; however, patients find this site uncomfortable and inconvenient.

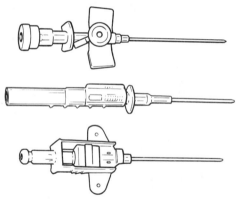

Arterial and intravenous cannulae.

Equipment required
- Disposable towel or drape
- Disposable razor
- Local anaesthetic and syringe
- Intravenous cannula
- Tape or dressing to fasten cannula
- Gloves
- Cleaning agent

Protect the bedclothes with a disposable drape and apply a venous tourniquet to the patient's upper arm, taking care not to pinch the skin. Select a drip site by gently stretching the skin and palpating the veins until one is found that can be ballotted easily; the easiest entry site is at a vein junction. Shaving the area around the cannula will decrease the risk of a hair being inserted along with the cannula and reduce discomfort when the attachment tape is removed. The skin should be cleansed and time allowed for the antiseptic to evaporate. The operator should wear gloves to protect himself against contamination by blood. Local anaesthesia should be used for all children and whenever a cannula larger than 18G is inserted into a conscious adult patient. This can be provided either by prior administration of EMLA cream (a eutectic mixture of lignocaine and prilocaine) or by raising a small intradermal bleb of local anaesthetic (e.g. 1 per cent lignocaine) using a 27G or 28G needle. If the bevel of this needle is reversed, the injection will be nearly painless. The site of skin entry should be away from the vein so that the vein walls are not compressed together. The cannula should be inserted through the skin at an angle of about 20° and then levelled so that entry into the vein is almost horizontal. The bevel of the trocar should be at right angles to the vein. Entry is indicated by appearance of blood in the 'flash chamber', but at least 8 mm of cannula is inserted into the vein before the trocar is withdrawn. The cannula is then gently advanced up the vein, the tourniquet is released, and the drip is secured.

If both walls of the vein are accidentally penetrated, the situation can be salvaged by withdrawing the trocar from the cannula and then slowly withdrawing the cannula until blood is seen entering it, when it should be advanced again in a smooth motion. The trocar should never be reinserted into the patient while the tip of the cannula is in the patient; fragments of plastic can be sheared off. Safety cannulae which prevent needlestick injuries by ensheathing the trocar as it is removed from the cannula are now available.

The cannula should be inspected daily to ensure that the entry site and vein are not tender. Thrombophlebitis is more likely if the cannula is poorly fixed, irritant drugs are injected, or if it remains for more than 72 hours. Glycerol trinitrate (GTN) skin patches have been shown to prolong the useful life of a drip site, but are expensive.

Central venous cannulation

There are numerous central venous cannulation techniques. Peripheral, subclavian, and internal jugular veins are those chosen most frequently. In the hands of an expert, central venous cannulation using subclavian or internal jugular routes carries an acceptable morbidity of 1–2 per cent. However, the poorly instructed practitioner can create havoc. Complications include death, severe haemorrhage, arteriovenous fistula, haematoma, neurological complications, and pneumothorax. The procedure should be taught, not shown. Two routes commonly used in surgical patients will be described.

Peripheral access to central veins

'Long lines' are the safest form of central venous access and can be inserted by anyone competent at venous cannulation. They can be used in patients whose clotting status is uncertain, for instance obstetric patients with pre-eclampsia, and are useful for postoperative fluid monitoring of patients after major surgery. Their disadvantages are that the infusion lines are small bore and long, thus offering considerable resistance to flow, and the tip of the line may not enter the central venous system.

Requirements

As for venous cannulation plus
- Suitable long line, e.g. Drumcath
- Swabs, sterile dressing, and pressure dressing
- Water manometer set or pressure transducer
- An assistant for palpation of the pulse
- A chest X-ray after line insertion

A large vein on the medial aspect of the antecubital fossa is selected. Laterally placed veins usually traverse the clavipectoral fascia and it may prove impossible to feed the line through this barrier. The vein is cannulated in the normal manner and the venous tourniquet is removed. Sterile swabs are placed around the introducer cannula to mop up any leaking blood, the trocar is removed, and the drum cannula is attached to the introducer cannula. The arm is elevated to straighten out the veins and the long line is advanced steadily. Pressure is applied to the ipsilateral jugular veins to prevent the line tip from entering the jugular veins. When a suitable length of cannula has been inserted, the fine-wire guide is withdrawn and the cannula aspirated. During this process the open end of the cannula should be well below mid-thoracic level to prevent air embolism occurring. If blood can be aspirated easily, the cannula can be attached to the measuring system; withdrawing the line a few centimetres usually solves the problem if aspiration is initially impossible. The insertion cannula should then be withdrawn from the vein, leaving only the long line in the patient. A sterile dressing should be applied, followed by a pressure bandage. During this procedure the assistant should palpate the patient's pulse as passage of the central line into the heart may cause arrhythmias; ill patients should be monitored during the procedure. A chest X-ray should be obtained to check the position of the line; this is particularly important if irritant drugs are to be injected as, despite precautions, the line can occasionally pass up into the neck.

Subclavian access to central veins

Mobile patients find the subclavian route the most convenient central venous access. The description that follows is of a Seldinger technique which enables haemofiltration, Swan–Ganz, multilumen CVP, or feeding lines to be inserted. This route is contraindicated if there is a bleeding disorder.

Requirements
- Gown pack and gloves
- Sterile dressing pack
- Sterile towels
- Local anaesthetic, syringe, and needle
- Sutures
- Central venous cannulation set
- Antiseptic
- Sterile saline

The patient should lie flat on a firm bed or couch with his arm by his side. An aide should be available to reassure the patient and monitor his pulse; arrhythmias can occur during the insertion procedure if the guide wire or cannula excites the heart. The foot of the couch should be elevated to ensure that the patient's upper veins are full. The operator should put on gown and gloves, clean the patient's upper torso from neck to shoulder joint and down to the nipple line, and then drape it. The junction of the lateral third of the clavicle with its medial two-thirds is identified and a local anaesthetic skin wheal is raised just inferior to it. Local anaesthetic is then infiltrated in a line from the skin entry point towards the contralateral mid-clavicular point. The introducer needle, attached to a half-full syringe of saline, is inserted in the same direction, passing underneath the clavicle and keeping the point of the needle as horizontal as possible. Dorsal insertion of the tip of the needle can lead to laceration of the subclavian artery or pneumothorax. A free flow of dark-coloured blood indicates successful cannulation.

The syringe is then removed from the introducer needle and replaced by the Seldinger guide wire. Such wires may end in a firm tip, a straight soft tip, or a J soft loop. Either type of soft end can be used, and the wire should pass without resistance. The skin incision is enlarged by nicking the skin with a blade pointed away from where the introducer needle emerges from the skin; the incision should be large enough to accommodate the cannula easily, otherwise insertion will be difficult. The introducer needle is then removed, leaving the guide wire behind. If necessary, a dilator can be passed over the guide wire into the vein and removed again, and the cannula itself is then advanced over the wire. It is essential that the guide wire is gripped at all times and not allowed to slide with the cannula into the circulation. The final stage is to remove the guide wire, connect the ports of the cannula, and measure the CVP.

If the initial insertion attempt fails, a chest X-ray should be obtained to exclude pneumothorax before cannulation of the other side is attempted. After insertion of the line, a check X-ray should be obtained to check the position of the cannula and exclude haemothorax or pneumothorax.

Measurement of the CVP

The CVP is a measure of the filling pressure on the right side of the heart. It can be made using either a water manometer system or a pressure transducer. The water manometer is cheap and simple, but care needs to be taken to measure the CVP from a consistent point. In the supine patient the mid-axillary line is usually used as a zero mark, and a spirit level is employed to ensure that the zero on the patient matches that on the manometer. If the CVP is correctly placed, the fluid level of the manometer should fall rapidly and smoothly to a stable level and then swing with respiration. If a transducer with a display is used, it will be seen that there are four phases to the CVP trace, the *a* and *v* waves and the *x* and *y* descents. A dependent loop should always remain between a manometer or transducer and the central venous line to eliminate the risk of air embolism.

Swan–Ganz catheters

Balloon-tipped flow-directed pulmonary artery catheters, more popularly called Swan–Ganz catheters, may be used in the ICU and the coronary care unit to supplement the information obtained by a central venous line. They may be used to obtain information on left-ventricular filling pressures, cardiac output, peripheral resistance, and mixed venous oxygen saturation. Valuable though this information may occasionally be, the use of these catheters remains controversial and there is no convincing evidence that they improve outcome except in selected groups of seriously ill patients. They are not without their complications, which include pulmonary infarction, pulmonary arterial rupture, and infection.

A catheter sheath is inserted using a technique such as that described above. The ports of the Swan–Ganz are then filled with saline and the catheter is passed through the introducer. At the 10 cm mark, the balloon is inflated with about 0.75 ml of air. A calibrated pressure transducer is attached to the distal port. Advancing the catheter slowly will reveal in turn the waveforms of the atrium, the right ventricle, the pulmonary artery, and the wedged pulmonary capillary trace. The balloon should then be deflated leaving a pulmonary artery trace, which only returns to the wedged position when the balloon is reinflated. A Swan–Ganz catheter must never be left in the wedged position, nor should the balloon be inflated when the tip of the catheter is already wedged.

Arterial sampling and cannulation

The introduction of the non-invasive pulse oximeter has made it easier to obtain useful sequential information about oxygenation in seriously ill patients. However, there remains a place for blood gas measurements to determine carbon dioxide levels, to assess oxygenation in seriously ill patients, and to detect metabolic abnormalities. Such measurements are particularly important in ventilated patients.

Technique

Arterial samples are usually obtained from the radial artery at the wrist, although the femoral artery may be used in critically ill patients. A blood gas sampling syringe should be employed or, if one is not available, a small volume of heparin (1000 units/ml solution) can be aspirated into a 2 ml syringe, the plunger run up and down the barrel two or three times, and then all the heparin ejected except that which is retained in the syringe hub. An assistant should support the patient's hand in dorsiflexion. The artery is identified, the skin cleaned, and a small volume of local anaesthetic injected into the dermis and around the artery. The vessel can then be entered using a 25G needle and the sample gently withdrawn. The syringe is capped, and either analysed immediately or packed into ice. The assistant should maintain firm pressure over the puncture site for at least 5 minutes to ensure that no swelling or bruising occurs.

Repeated blood gas sampling is painful and potentially hazardous to arteries. If it is felt that repeated sampling is likely to be necessary, it is kinder to insert an arterial cannula. Once again the radial artery is usually chosen, but cannulation of the brachial, ulnar, femoral, and dorsalis pedis arteries is possible. A continuous infusion system is required to maintain the cannula patent. It is essential to ensure that the system is flushed and all air excluded. The bedclothes below the site of entry should be protected by a clean drape and the operator ought to wear gloves. A 20G or smaller parallel-sided cannula should be chosen; it is better to avoid those types which have an injection port as someone might be tempted to use this port as access for drug administration. Once again the artery is palpated, the skin is cleaned, and the local anaesthetic is injected. As the cannula is fine bore, the sensation of entering the vessel will be improved if a small skin nick is made before the cannula is inserted. A shallow entry angle should be employed. Direct entry into the artery is desirable, but if it proves impossible to achieve this, the artery can be transfixed, the trocar removed, and the cannula slowly withdrawn until

Welker emergency cricothyrotomy catheter sets

Used for emergency airway access when endotracheal intubation cannot be performed. Airway access is achieved utilizing percutaneous entry (Seldinger) technique via the cricothyroid membrane. Subsequent dilation of the tract and tracheal entrance site permits passage of the emergency airway. NOTE: The 6 mm ID emergency airway (C-TCCS-600) allows use of standard positive pressure ventilation techniques and will also permit spontaneous patient breathing. Supplied sterile in peel-open packages. Intended for one-time use.

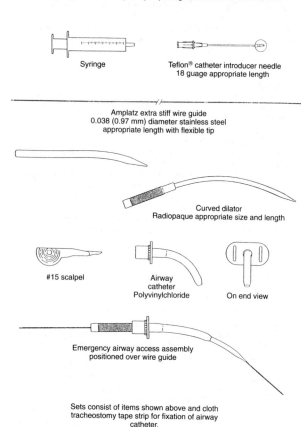

Syringe

Teflon® catheter introducer needle
18 guage appropriate length

Amplatz extra stiff wire guide
0.038 (0.97 mm) diameter stainless steel
appropriate length with flexible tip

Curved dilator
Radiopaque appropriate size and length

#15 scalpel

Airway
catheter
Polyvinylchloride

On end view

Emergency airway access assembly
positioned over wire guide

Sets consist of items shown above and cloth tracheostomy tape strip for fixation of airway catheter.

Emergency cricothyrotomy catheter sets.

free flow of blood occurs. The cannula can then be inserted up the vessel, a process that may be aided by rotating the cannula as it is inserted. The flushing set is then attached to the cannula, ensuring that no small air bubbles are trapped in the taps or line; these could embolize peripherally or even be flushed centrally into the carotid circulation if the rapid flushing system is activated. The flushing system and cannula must be firmly bandaged together; separation of the two parts of the system can lead to serious haemorrhage through the open arterial cannula.

Needle cricothyrotomy

The cricothyroid membrane is identified as the recessed area between the thyroid cartilage and the lower solid bar of cartilage, the cricoid cartilage. This membrane is punctured vertically with a large bore (12G or 14G) cannula. Air aspiration usually indicates correct placement. The cannula is then angulated to 40°, advanced down the trachea, and connected to an oxygen source at 15 litres/minute via either a Y-connector or a side-hole cut in the delivery tubing. Oxygen is then delivered to the patient by intermittently covering the hole for 1 in 5 seconds. An alternative method is to use jet ventilation. Once the ventilation commences the chest should be observed for movement and auscultated for breath sounds. The cannula should then be secured to prevent it from being dislodged. The usefulness of this technique is limited to about 45 minutes. Complications include bleeding, oesophageal perforation, and kinking of the cannula. If the cannula is inadvertently positioned in the soft tissues, ventilation can result in development of subcutaneous and mediastinal emphysema. This method of ventilation may disimpact a foreign body from the larynx.

Minitracheotomy

Again, this is an emergency measure and not a definitive airway. The thyroid cartilage is stabilized using the thumb, index finger and, middle finger while the cricothyroid membrane is identified and an incision made through it. The opening is then dilated to accept a 4 mm tracheal tube. Ideally, a purpose-designed kit such as a Mini-trach should be used, but in an emergency a strong sharp instrument such as a pair of scissors can suffice. Minitracheostomies can be used for both ventilation and suction. Several types of percutaneous tracheostomy sets are now available which allow larger cuffed tracheostomy tubes to be placed for long-term ventilation.

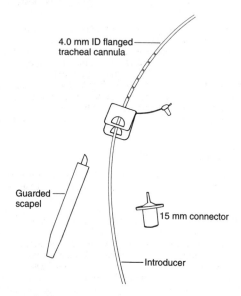

4.0 mm ID flanged tracheal cannula

Guarded scapel

15 mm connector

Introducer

Portex Mini-Trach.

Intra-osseous infusions

The veins of a small child with circulatory collapse are very difficult to cannulate. Intra-osseous infusion should be considered as the method of choice where rapid access to the circulation is required as it requires less time and skill than a venous cutdown. A strong 18 gauge needle at least 40 mm long is inserted at right angles or 60° inferior to the perpendicular either into the anterior surface of the inferior third of the femur 3 cm above the lateral condyle or into the anterior surface of the tibia 2–3 cm below the tibial tuberosity. A very obvious give is felt as the needle penetrates the cortex and enters the bone marrow. It should be possible to aspirate bone marrow through a correctly positioned needle. Choose a limb in which there is no evidence of a fracture proximal to the chosen infusion line. If the needle is correctly sited, crystalloids will run into the bone marrow and rapidly enter the circulation. Blood and colloid solutions may need to be infused under pressure.

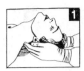

The patient is positioned supine with head, neck and chin fully extended. The operator stands above the head facing the patient's feet.

The skin is cleansed and the position of the cricothyroid membrane located by palpation and marked in ink.

A midline vertical 1cm stab incision is made into the airway through the cricothyroid membrane using the guarded scalpel, cutting edge towards the feet.

The introducer is passed into the trachea.

The cannula is passed over the introducer into the trachea.

The cannula is held in place and the introducer withdrawn.

The cannula is fixed in place with neck tapes.

The suction catheter is passed immediately to clear any existing blood and secretions.

Standard insertion technique.

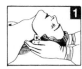

The patient is positioned supine with the head, neck and chin fully extended. The operator stands above the head facing the patient's feet.

The skin is cleansed and the position of the cricothyroid membrane located by palpation and marked in ink.

A midline vertical 1cm skin incision is made with the scalpel.

The 16G Tuohy Needle is fitted to the syringe. With the trachea immobilised the Tuohy Needle is inserted through the cricothyroid membrane. Correct placement is confirmed by aspiration of air.

The syringe is removed and the flexible tip of the guidewire is inserted through the Tuohy Needle into the trachea.

The Tuohy Needle is removed whilst holding the guidewire at skin level once the needle is clear of the skin.

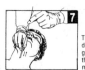

The shoter, large diameter dilator is fed onto the guidewire and passed through the cricothyroid membrane.

The MINI-TRACH cannula is fed, premounted on the curved introducer, onto the guidewire and the cannula introduced into the trachea with firm pressure.

The introducer and guidewire are removed holding the flange in place against the skin.

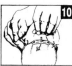

The cannula is fixed in place with neck tapes.

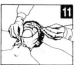

The suction catheter is passed immediately to remove any existing blood and secretions.

Seldinger insertion technique.

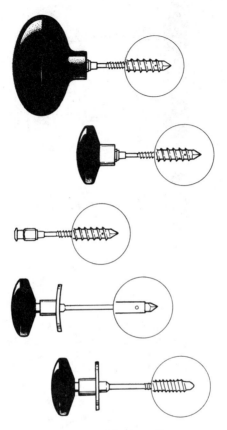

Intra-osseous infusion needles.

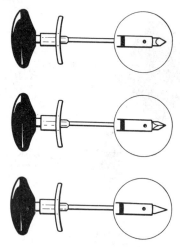

Disposable intra-osseous needles.

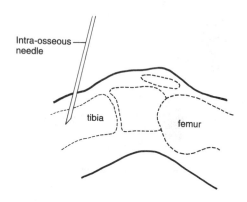

Intra-osseous needle

tibia

femur

Technique for intra-osseous infusion.

Complications

Occasionally cellulitis and even more rarely osteomyelitis may develop at the site of cannulation. Sometimes the needle will fracture, but it is held fast by the cortical bone and the broken fragment does not enter the circulation. Fluids may leak into surrounding tissues, causing a compartment syndrome, if multiple attempts have been made to cannulate a bone.

2 Postoperative complications

Gastrointestinal problems   74
Haemorrhage   76

GASTROINTESTINAL PROBLEMS

Paralytic ileus

After abdominal surgery normal bowel sounds disappear for about 48 hours and usually return on the third or fourth day. This postoperative ileus is due to paralysis of the myenteric plexus and is of two types: intestinal ileus (the commonest) and acute gastric dilatation. Ileus will also occur following peritonitis, abdominal trauma, and immobilization. It may be prolonged in hypoproteinaemic and hypokalaemic patients.

Symptoms
Abdominal distension and vomiting. Absent or 'tinkling' bowel sounds.

Prognosis
Intestinal ileus usually settles with appropriate treatment (see below). Acute gastric dilatation is an emergency. A naso-gastric tube must be passed immediately to prevent inhalation of gastric juices, hypovolaemia, or gastric rupture.

Treatment
Pass a nasogastric tube to empty the stomach of fluid and gas. Maintain continuous aspiration. Ensure adequate hydration by IVI ('drip and suck') and maintain the electrolyte balance. When ileus persists for more than 5–7 days institute TPN.

Nausea and vomiting

These are common symptoms in surgical patients. They may be the result of anaesthetic agents, analgesics, cytotoxic drugs, intestinal ileus, or mechanical obstruction.

Treatment
Ensure nil orally for 4–6 hours before surgery. Exclude mechanical causes and ileus. Give central antiemetics, e.g. metoclopramide (Maxolon) 10 mg orally 8 hourly, 10 mg slow IV, or prochlorperazine maleate (Stemetil) 12.5 mg IV, 25 mg orally. When persistent, pass a nasogastric tube and correct hydration and electrolytes

Diarrhoea

This may occur following an ileus or in association with con-tinuing sepsis (e.g. pelvic abscess). It may also follow specific procedures such as ileo-anal anastomosis, ileal pouch, truncal vagotomy, and right hemicolectomy. The possibility of infec-tion should be remembered; pseudomembranous colitis is commonly forgotten.

Treatment

Identify the cause:
- rectal and ultrasound examination to exclude pelvic abscess
- stool samples for bacteria, protozoa
- microbiology of stools for *Clostridium difficile*.
- Erect/supine abdominal films (obstructive ileus)
  Treat the patient as follows:
- Drainage of a pelvic abscess
- Specific antibacterial or antiprotozoal chemotherapy
- Vancomycin 125 mg orally every 6 hours for 7–10 days
- Drip and suck for ileus
  General measures:
- Replace lost fluids and give codeine phosphate 10–60 mg orally 4 hourly or diphenoxylate hydrochloride (Lomotil) 10 mg orally initially then 5 mg 6 hourly until controlled.

Constipation

This is commonly encountered after elective surgery, particularly in the elderly.

Treatment

Ensure adequate hydration. Limit the use of constipating analgesics after the first 2 days. Ensure adequate dietary fibre. Suppositories or enemas may be indicated depending on the surgery performed. Manual evacuation is rarely necessary. Nevertheless, a *per rectum* examination should not be forgotten.

HAEMORRHAGE

Bleeding after surgery may be arterial or venous. Arterial blood is bright red and spurts in time with the pulse. Venous blood is darker in colour and flows steadily. There can be substantial blood loss (1 litre in 5 minutes) if bleeding is from the large veins.

Types

- **Primary haemorrhage** occurs during surgery and continues.
- **Reactionary haemorrhage** occurs in the first 24 hours (usually after 4–6 hours). It may follow primary haemorrhage or result from the slipping of a ligature or the removal of primary clot as a result of coughing or increasing postoperative blood pressure.
- **Secondary haemorrhage** is due to infection. It occurs about 7–14 days after operation.

Clinical features

There may be visible blood loss into a drainage bottle, onto the bedclothes, etc. The patient is restless, cold, and clammy with an increasing pulse rate. There is pallor and, in continuing bleeding, air hunger (sighing, gasping respirations), thirst, and even blindness.

Blood pressure measurements

Pulse and blood pressure should be recorded every 15–30 minutes. In haemorrhagic shock a fall in blood pressure occurs late, and fit young people can maintain near normal levels for some time despite blood loss. The trend of pulse and blood pressure is the key to blood loss. A rising pulse rate or a 'thready' low volume pulse is an indication of possible blood loss.

Treatment

1. Elevate the foot of the bed; establish an IVI or CVP line.
2. Apply pressure to obvious external bleeding points.
3. Replace lost blood volume with Haemacel or Dextran 70 until whole blood is available. Coagulation problems are minimized if the blood used is as fresh as possible.
4. Arrange for the patient to return to theatre if necessary:
   - to deal with sepsis
   - to ligate the bleeding source
5. Carry out a coagulation screen and treat specific defects in liaison with the haematologist. Clotting factors may be replaced with fresh frozen plasma. Screening is advocated for those patients who have been transfused around 5 units (rule of thumb).
6. Measure urine volume (catheterize the patient).

3 Theatre Procedures

Antibiotic prophylaxis   80
Hypothermia   84
Evaluation of X-rays in surgery   86
Theatre disciplines   88

ANTIBIOTIC PROPHYLAXIS

The principles of antibiotic prophylaxis were laid down in the experiments of John Burke in the early 1960s. He showed that if an appropriate antibiotic was given to an experimental animal before the inoculation of *Staphylococcus aureus,* abscess formation could be prevented. He described a decisive period lasting about 4 hours from the time an incision is made when antibiotics are protective.

In the late 1960s clinical trials on antibiotic prophylaxis had proved their worth beyond question. Modern antibiotic prophylaxis gives empirical cover of the expected organisms encountered at the operation. This cover does not last longer than 24 hours and consists of one to three doses of the antibiotic. Therefore it is important not to confuse prophylaxis with therapy, which is the use of antibiotics beyond 24 hours.

Wounds are theoretically classified into four categories:
- clean
- clean contaminated
- contaminated
- dirty (or abscess)

In clean surgery without the insertion of a prosthesis, prophylaxis is probably not justified as the infection rate is likely to be between 1 and 2 per cent. However, if there is implantation of a prosthesis the patient's endogenous organisms (as well as his exogenous organisms) could cause prosthetic graft infection, which is a potential disaster in vascular or orthopaedic procedures. Prophylaxis is indicated for all clean contaminated and contaminated operations. In dirty operations or in the presence of abscess antibiotics should be given as therapy for a 3–5 days regimen. Wound infection rates should be audited with care and surveillance placed on the rate of infection.

Types of surgery

Antibiotics are only an adjunct to surgical care. They should be coupled to careful gentle meticulous surgery with perfect haemostasis. Theatre discipline must be constantly maintained. These criteria are well established, particularly in orthopaedic and prosthetic surgery where strict asepsis is critical.

Orthopaedic surgery also requires a superlative level of theatre ventilation which may incorporate the use of exhaust suits or laminar flow ventilation with many turnovers of theatre air.

Suggested regimes for antibiotic prophylaxis

Prophylaxis is not justified in clean surgery. However, in vascular and orthopaedic surgery patients may be at risk from endogenous skin organisms, particularly those related to slime-producing staphylococci. They may also be at risk from the multiple-resistant organisms such as the coagulase-negative staphylococcus and methicillin-resistant *Staphylococcus aureus*.

When the gastrointestinal tract is opened there is a risk of aerobic Gram-negative bacilli. Lower down the gastrointestinal tract, particularly beyond the small bowel, there is the added risk of anaerobes (predominantly Bacteroides) which can act in synergy.

Whenever patients have had rheumatic heart disease prophylaxis should be given, even for minor procedures such as ERCP or dental extraction. All urological instrumentations are at risk and a broad-spectrum second-generation cephalosporin or acylureide penicillin is recommended. Patients who have had a splenectomy in the past for any reason should be given penicillin cover. If splenectomy is about to proceed vaccination against pneumococcus should be given before the spleen is removed.

Prophylaxis of deep vein thrombosis and pulmonary embolus

DVT and PTE are both common in surgery and although often missed clinically are encountered in post-mortem examinations. DVTs are also linked with the post-phlebitic limb syndrome which causes significant morbidity in later years. It is now realized that DVT can be prevented in three-quarters of surgical patients and many regimes are available.

At risk cases
● Patients over 40 years old
● Smokers
● Patients with haematological problems such as polycythemia
● Dehydrated patients who need emergency surgery
● Patients undergoing orthopaedic (hip and knee) operations
● Patients with cancer who are about to undergo abdominal or pelvic surgery

If the patient has been investigated in a medical ward and then transferred for surgery, prophylaxis may not have been used and a DVT may already be established. These patients should also receive prophylaxis. Patients taking oral contraceptives who need elective surgery should be advised to stop 6 weeks before surgery and should also be given alternative contraceptive advice.

It is also possible to operate with anticoagulation. If patients are taking warfarin, the anticoagulation can be reversed slowly using blood factors and the patient can be transferred to heparin. If severe bleeding follows, heparin can be reversed much more easily using protamine.

Audit and surveillance of DVT and PTE prophylaxis are crucial. A high post-mortem rate of surgical deaths may reveal

Suggested prophylactic antibiotic regimes for representative surgical procedures

Type of surgery	Organisms encountered	Prophylactic regime suggested
Clean		
Clean general surgery non prosthetic	Endogenous skin organisms	Not justified
Vascular (prosthetic)	*Staph. epidermidis* (or MRCNS)	Three-dose flucloxacillin ± gentamicin
	Staph. aureus (or MRSA)	Vancomycin rifampin if MRCNS/MRSA a risk
	AGNB	(Alternative second generation cephalosporin or ureido penicillin)
Orthopaedic (prosthetic)	*Staph. aureus* and *Staph. epidermidis*	Three-dose second-generation cephalosporin ± gentamicin
	In hip surgery AGNB also a risk	Vancomycin if MRSA or MRCNS a risk
Clean contaminated		
Oesophagogastric	Enterobacteriaceae	One- to three-dose second-generation cephalosporin and metronidazole in severe contamination
	Enterococci (incl. anaerobic/viridans streptococci)	
Biliary	Enterobacteriaceae (mainly *E. coli*)	One-dose second-generation cephalosporin
	Enterococci (incl. *Strep. faecalis*)	
Small bowel	Enterobacteriaceae	One- to three-dose second-generation cephalosporin ± metronidazole
Contaminated		
Appendix	Enterobacteriaceae	Single-dose second generation cephalosporin (alternative gentamicin) with metronidazole (may be given rectally)
	Anaerobes (bacteroides, faecal streptococci)	
Colorectal	Enterobacteriaceae	Three-dose second-generation cephalosporin (alternative gentamicin) with metronidazole
	Anaerobes (bacteroides, faecal streptococci)	

MRCNS, Multiply resistant coagulase negative staphylococcus.
MRSA, Methicillin resistant *Staphylococcus aureus*.
AGB, aerobic Gram-negative bacilli.
All regimens are intravenous and should start preoperatively (at induction of anaesthesia). In emergency operations (or in gross contamination during elective surgery) antibiotics should be given at diagnosis and prolonged as therapy for 3–5 days if necessary.

higher incidence than was considered clinically, particularly in emergencies.

DVT prophylaxis

Early mobilization has always been considered as a method of preventing DVT, although there is no evidence to substantiate this. Antiembolism stockings have been shown to reduce DVTs in surgical patients and are very effective when combined with heparin. Subcutaneous heparin carries no increased risk of bleeding and appears to be particularly effective in the prevention of fatal pulmonary thromboembolism. The dose is 5000 units twice or three times daily. A special injection gun should be used to prevent bleeding at the injection sites. Soluble low-molecular-weight heparins are now available, and these need only be given once daily.

Low-molecular-weight dextran and oral warfarin have been used, but there is a risk of bleeding and allergy. Intermittent pneumatic compression during surgery is a further effective method, particularly when combined with antiembolism stockings.

DVTs may be recognized clinically, but only in about 50 per cent of cases. Detection should be by venography, although duplex Doppler imaging is now becoming much more accurate and has the advantage of being non-invasive.

Prevention of peri- and postoperative problems

When patients are under general anaesthesia several precautions need to be taken. These include the prevention of nerve injuries, which may cause prolonged disability and litigation. Pressure sores may be caused in only a few minutes or hours but often take many months to heal. Therefore any patient considered at risk, particularly those undergoing long surgical procedures or who are malnourished, should be considered for the appropriate pressure-relieving aids.

The prevention of chest infection involves early mobilization with pre- and postoperative physiotherapy and instruction. Patients with particularly poor respiratory reserve should have prophylactic antibiotics and if possible surgery should be avoided in patients who have chest infections. It is much safer to send the patient home with appropriate treatment (antibiotics and physiotherapy) and reoperate electively after 2–3 weeks.

HYPOTHERMIA

Hypothermia may become a problem during long operations, particularly cardiothoracic bypass procedures and those involving exposure of the viscera. In general surgery patients can be kept warm by increasing the ambient temperature or by using a warm circulating water device underneath the operating table. The use of space blankets and enclosing the limbs in plastic bags will also conserve heat. If hypothermia is thought to be a risk, the temperature can be monitored centrally by an oesophageal probe. Try to keep the abdominal viscera in the abdominal cavity as far as possible. When they are exposed for prolonged periods keep them covered with warm moist packs.

EVALUATION OF X-RAYS IN SURGERY

There is continuing controversy as to whether baseline pre-operative chest X-rays should be taken for all patients, and the policy will be dictated by common-sense and local hospital guidelines. The application of X-rays needs to be balanced against their usefulness as well as fears of litigation or mis-diagnosis. A useful example is the erect abdominal film in emergency gastrointestinal disease. This is rejected by many radiologists but is considered useful by surgeons who argue that both the erect and supine films should be used for diagnosing intestinal emergencies. Experienced radiologists claim that they are effective with the supine view only, but it has to be borne in mind that such experience may not be available at night.

It is nearly always worthwhile discussing the type of X-ray and its interpretation with the radiologist before operating. Surgeons in training can learn from doing this as well as improving their communication skills!

Always have the patient's X-rays in theatre. Specialized X-rays such as computed tomograms and angiograms should be on the X-ray viewing box in the operating theatre.

Good communication with radiologists and radiographers will provide the best on-table X-rays such as arteriograms and cholangiography. The surgeon must often interpret these X-rays himself and so specialized films such as angiography, cholangiography, ERCP, and ultrasound should not be taken by surgeons who are incapable of interpreting the results.

THEATRE DISCIPLINES

Theatre design and ventilation

Modern operating theatres work with positive (plenum) pressure. This involves approximately 20 changes of operation air per hour with flow being in a clean to dirty direction. In prosthetic surgery, laminar flow may be used with non-turbulent air flow and filters providing over 40 changes of theatre air per hour. Exhaust suits and modular theatres are also used in prosthetic surgery, but they do not decrease the risk of infection compared with the use of appropriate prophylactic antibiotics.

Microbiology should be checked in theatre to be sure that ventilation is adequate; this is done using settle plates. In the case of methicillin resistant *Staphylococcus aureus* (MRSA) outbreaks, nasal swabbing must be undertaken for all operating theatre personnel.

Theatre clothing

Vests, trousers, or skirts are usually made of comfortable light cotton and should be changed for each theatre session or if they become soiled. The use of masks and caps in general surgery remains controversial, and there is probably no added risk if they are omitted. Discipline is crucial, particularly in prosthetic surgery, and it has been argued that masks and caps should be used in all operations, particularly to provide adequate beard cover.

As theatre air flows from clean to dirty, the patient should also come into the anaesthetic room in the theatre through a clean entrance and leave after the operation by another route. Instruments should be brought into the theatre through a clean entrance and passed through a different exit after being used.

Modern scrubbing techniques include scrubbing the nails on the first scrub of an operating list using aqueous chlorhexidine or povidone iodine. The use of alcoholic skin antiseptics before gloving up is probably not necessary. After the nails have been scrubbed, the hands should be washed for a further 4–5 minutes. Unless there has been a particularly contaminated operation, further 'scrubs' should consist of hand washing only.

Linen drapes can be laundered and re-autoclaved after any repairs have been made. In many operating theatres there has been a move to disposable material which incorporates cellulose or man-made materials. These drapes and clothing do not permit the same degree of penetration of fluid as re-autoclaved linen. If the clothing is too small, this can lead to overheating so that it is uncomfortable to wear. Disposable materials, although expensive, may be justified in most prosthetic surgery. The use of incised drapes with adhesive thin polyurethane membranes and woundguards has not yet been shown to reduce infection rate. Surgeons should never operate if they know that they have a septic lesion. All instruments must be sterile. Most surgical instruments can be resterilized in an autoclave, but many materials used in surgery, such as the sutures, are disposable. These are usually sterilized with gamma irradiation or ethylene oxide during mass production. Some instruments are too delicate for the autoclave and immersion in agents such as gluteraldehyde is necessary. It should be remembered that this is a toxic material, and the unit policy for handling such materials should be followed.

Shaving before surgery is also controversial. It may be aesthetic but it is often inadequate, and if it is undertaken more than 24 hours before the operation skin wounds may well become infected. If shaving is necessary, it should be carried out immediately prior to surgery or be replaced by hair clipping or cream depilation. If adhesive dressings are used to cover an incision, it is kinder for the patient to ensure that the skin has been shaved so that the removal of the dressing 7–10 days later will not be so painful.

Correct patient

If you are going to perform the operation make sure that you talk to each patient beforehand. Do not allow the patient to be anaesthetized until you are satisfied. This is your sole responsibility.

Correct operation

Ensure that the correct procedure is going to be performed, marking the appropriate side in cases of hernias, varicose veins, lumps, etc. Use an indelible ink pen, see the patient in the anaesthetic room, and confirm both the site of the operation and his identity. Do not proceed if the mark has been washed off or the patient has had premedication and you are unable to speak to him. Again, this is your sole responsibility.

Swab counts

Always use large swabs and as few as possible at a time. Do not bury packs in the abdomen; rather, attach a clip to the tape outside the abdomen. Check the wound and the abdomen yourself once the procedure has been completed. Check that the count is correct. Remember that instruments may have been left in the wound and so check this assiduously before closure. There are no new mistakes. Try to avoid the time-honoured ones.

Consent

Ensure that consent is informed. In some operations specific points of consent have to be sought. Remember that parental or guardian consent is required if the patient is under 16 years old. Many consent forms are inadequate. If informed consent has been given with explanations, record this in the patient's notes.

90 Hepatitis and HIV precautions

Always ask yourself 'Is this operation really necessary?' if the patient has AIDS or hepatitis or is HIV-positive. Reduce the number of personnel in theatre and use disposable drapes. Always use the double-glove operating technique and protect your eyes with appropriate glasses or visors. As far as possible, all instruments should be disposable. Ensure that all instruments are passed to the operating table with eye contact to avoid 'stick' injuries. If any such injuries occur report them immediately. If a patient with AIDS is to be operated on, infection control will assist with AIDS precautions.

4 Tools of the trade

K. MARTIN

Introduction   94
General surgery   96
Orthopaedic surgery   116
Orthopaedic instruments and equipment   120
Urological instruments   126
Endoscopic instruments and sets   132
Laparoscopic surgery   136

INTRODUCTION

Instrument sets commonly used in surgical procedures are illustrated in this chapter. Although there are variations in the types of instruments used in different hospitals, you should attempt to become acquainted with their names and their use. It makes life much easier for the nursing staff if the surgeon actually knows which instrument he wants to use. Another reason for illustrating these packs is to provide a basis for those surgeons who may have to set up a field hospital or a hospital in the Third World.

GENERAL SURGERY

Abscess set

1 Green inner wrap
1 Blue outer wrap
1 Poly tray

1 B P handle no. 4
1 Sponge holder
1 Straight scissors
1 Toothed dissector
1 Alliss forceps
2 Mosquito artery forceps, curved
1 Sinus forcep
1 Volkman spoon

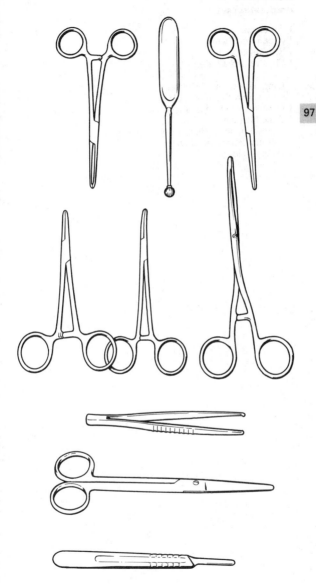

Abscess set.

Amputation set

1 Green tray liner
1 Green inner wrap
1 Blue outer wrap
1 Theatre tray 12 × 12

1 Amputation saw 9½ inches
1 Gigli saw with handles (2)
1 Ferguson's bone-holding forceps
1 Bone file rasp
1 Eckhoff bone-cutting forceps 8 inches
1 Medium periosteal elevator
1 Bone shields (set of two)

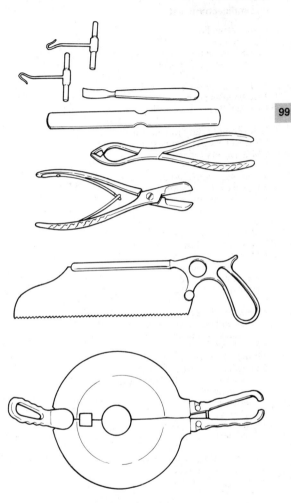

Amputation set.

GENERAL SURGERY (cont.)

Appendicectomy set

1 Green tray liner
1 Green inner wrap
1 Blue outer wrap
1 Theatre tray (12×23)

1 BP handle no. 5
2 BP handles no. 4
1 BP handle no. 3

10 Mosquito artery forceps, curved
5 Spencer Wells forceps, small straight   On pin
5 Mayo artery forceps

4 Rampley sponge-holding forceps
2 Laney cholecystectomy forceps   On pin
4 Alliss tissue forceps
4 Babcock tissue forceps } On pin

2 Mayo scissors, straight
2 Mayo scissors, curved on flat
1 McIndoe scissors, small
1 Kilner needle-holder } On pin
1 Hegar needle-holder
1 Hunt's needle holder

2 Debakey dissecting forceps, small
1 Fine-toothed dissecting forceps
1 Charnley dissecting forceps
1 Morris retractor
2 Langenbeck retractors, large
2 Langenbeck retractors, small
2 Langenbeck solid-handle retractors
1 Diathermy electrode
1 Diathermy cable
1 Sucker, medium
4 Cross-action towel clips
8 Bachaus towel clips

Towels and extras
6 Small green towels
3 Large green towels
1 Diathermy quiver
1 Disposable bag

1 Mayo cover
1 Large receiver
1 Medium receiver
2 Gallipots
1 Bowl (6 inch)

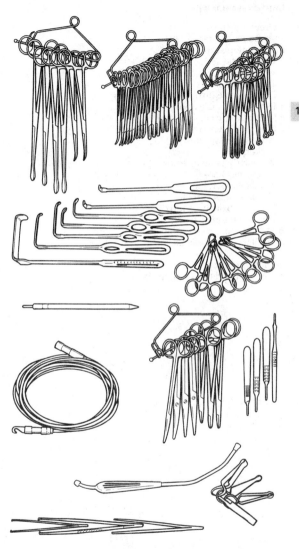

Appendicectomy set.

GENERAL SURGERY (cont.)

Cardiovascular set

1 Green tray liner
1 Green inner wrap
1 Blue outer wrap
1 Theatre tray (12 × 23)

2 Travers retractors
1 Debakey fine dissecting forceps, long
1 Debakey fine dissecting forceps, small
4 Multipurpose clamps, large
5 Mosquito artery forceps, shod
1 Potts angled scissors
1 Sucker, fine
2 Watson Cheyne dissectors
2 Strabismus hooks
1 Needle-holder, long
1 Needle-holder, small
1 Skin approximating forceps
1 Heparin flushing needle
6 Multipurpose clamps, small
12 Bulldog clamps, small

Supplementary
Right-angled cardiovascular clamps (packed single—3)

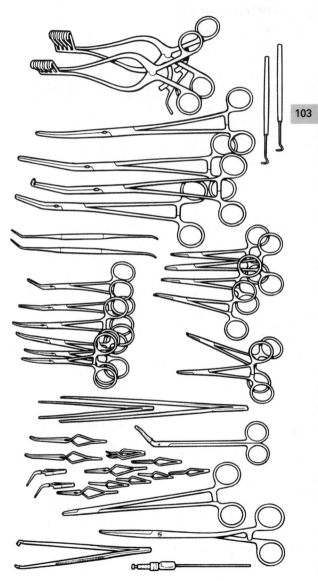

Cardiovascular set.

Cholecystectomy set

1 Green tray liner
1 Blue inner wrap
1 Blue outer wrap
1 Theatre tray (12×12)
1 Oschner's trocar and cannula (14F6)
1 Set of Bake's bile duct dilators (set of 9)
1 Set of Maingot's forceps, gall bladder (set of 3)
2 Heart-shaped frenulum probes

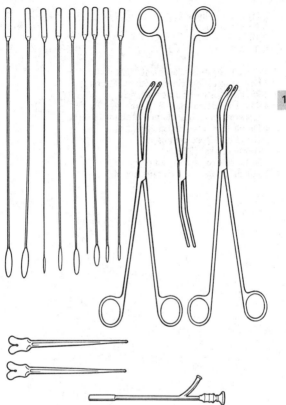

Cholecystectomy set.

GENERAL SURGERY (*cont.*)

Gastric set

1. Green tray liner
1. Green inner wrap
1. Blue outer wrap
1. Theatre tray (12 × 23)

4 Doyen intestinal clamps, straight 9 inch
2 Doyen intestinal clamps, curved 9 inch
2 Payr's intestinal clamps, 10 inch
4 Payr's intestinal clamps, 8 inch
2 Kocker's intestinal clamps, straight 11 inch
1 Demartel's intestinal clamp (set)
3 Duddfield Rose clamps
1 Nerve hooks, 10 inch
1 St Mark's retractors, set of 2
1 Hayes' cholectomy clamps, set of 2

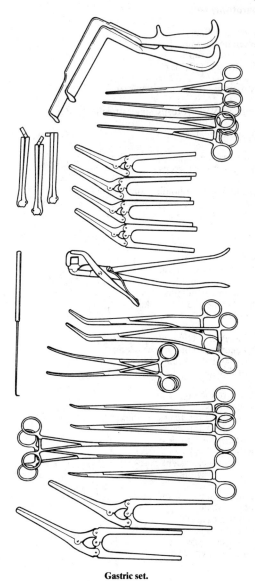

Gastric set.

GENERAL SURGERY (cont.)

Laparotomy set

1 Green tray liner
1 Green inner wrap
1 Blue outer wrap
1 Theatre tray (12×23)

20 Mosquito artery forceps, curved	On pin
10 Spencer Wells forceps, small straight	On pin
10 Mayo artery forceps	On pin
6 Alliss tissue forceps 4 Babcock tissue forceps	On pin
5 Rampley sponge-holding forceps 4 Laney cholecystectomy forceps 1 Haemoclip forceps	On pin
2 Mayo scissors, straight 1 Mayo scissors, curved on flat 1 McIndoe scissors, small 1 McIndoe scissors, large 2 Kilner needle-holders 2 Hegar needle-holders 1 Debakey needle-holder, long 1 Hunt's needle-holder	On pin

2 Debakey dissecting forceps, small
2 Debakey dissecting forceps, long
2 Fine-toothed dissecting forceps
1 Charnley toothed dissecting forceps

1 Morris retractor
2 Langenbeck retractors, large
2 Langenbeck retractors, medium
2 Langenbeck retractors, small
2 Diathermy electrodes
1 Diathermy cable
3 Suckers (fine, straight, rose)
3 Deaver retractors
1 Kelly retractor
1 Golligher retractor set
1 BP handle no. 7
2 BP handles no.4
1 BP handle no. 3
4 Cross-action towel clips
8 Bachaus towel clips

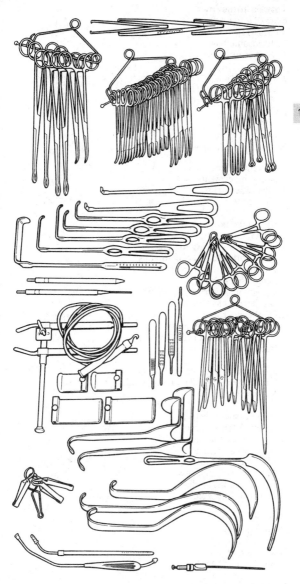

Laparotomy set.

Towels and extras
6 Small green towels
3 Large green towels
1 Disposable bag
1 Diathermy quiver

1 Mayo cover
1 Large receiver (10 inch)
1 Medium receiver (8 inch)
2 Gallipots
1 Bowl (6 inch)

Minor operations set

1 Green tray liner
1 Green inner wrap
1 Blue outer wrap
1 Theatre tray (22 × 23)

1 BP handle no. 3
1 BP handle no. 4
1 Debakey dissecting forceps
1 Fine-toothed dissecting forceps
1 Charnley toothed forceps
2 Langenbeck retractors, large
2 Langenbeck retractors, small
1 Diathermy electrode
1 Diathermy cable
2 Rampley sponge holders
2 Cross-action towel clips
4 Bachaus towel clips

5 Mosquito artery forceps, curved
3 Small Spencer Wells forceps, straight }On pin
5 Mayo artery forceps

3 Alliss tissue forceps
2 Babcock tissue forceps
2 Lane's tissue forceps
1 Mayo scissors, straight
1 Mayo scissors, curved on flat }On pin
1 McIndoe scissors, small
1 Kilner needle-holder
1 Hegar needle-holder

Towels and extras
1 Perineal towel
2 Gallipots
1 Medium receiver
5 Small green towels
1 Mayo cover
2 Abdo towels

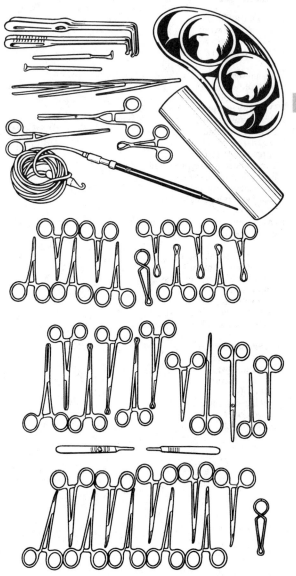

Minor operations set.

GENERAL SURGERY (cont.)

Paediatric set

1 Green tray liner
1 Green inner wrap
1 Blue outer wrap
1 Theatre tray (12×12)

1 BP handle no. 3
1 BP handle no. 4
1 Adson's toothed forceps
2 Debakey dissecting forceps
1 Diathermy electrode
1 Diathermy cable
2 Desmarres retractors
2 Langenbeck retractors, large
2 Langenbeck retractors, small
6 Bachaus towel clips
2 Cross-action towel clips
2 Rampley sponge-holding forceps

10 Mosquito artery forceps, curved
5 Baby mosquito forceps, curved   }On pin

4 Babcock's tissue forceps
2 Alliss tissue forceps
1 Gold-handled curved scissors
1 Small straight scissors   }On pin
1 Mayo straight scissors
1 McIndoe dissecting scissors
1 Small needle-holder

Towels and extras
1 Diathermy quiver
1 Perineal towel
1 Medium receiver
2 Gallipots
6 Small green towels
1 Mayo cover
1 Large towel

113

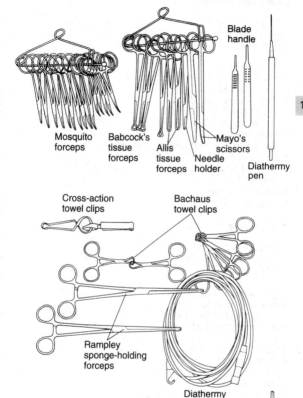

Mosquito forceps

Babcock's tissue forceps

Allis tissue forceps

Needle holder

Mayo's scissors

Blade handle

Diathermy pen

Cross-action towel clips

Bachaus towel clips

Rampley sponge-holding forceps

Diathermy cable

De Marr retractors

Langenbeck retractors

Toothed

Non-toothed

Adson's dissectors

Paediatric set.

GENERAL SURGERY (cont.)

Zadek instruments

1 Green inner wrap
1 Blue outer wrap
1 Poly tray

1 BP handle no. 3
1 Small non-toothed forceps
1 Small toothed forceps
1 Mayo scissors, small straight
1 McIndoe scissors
3 Mosquito artery forceps, curved.
1 Spencer wells artery forceps, small straight
1 Spencer wells artery forceps, large curved
1 Small needle-holder
1 Sponge-holder
2 Skin hooks
1 Volkman spoon
1 Jacques catheter

Toenail pack

1 Cardboard tray
1 Sterilwrap (600 × 600)
1 F bag

1 Fine-toothed forceps
1 Fine non-toothed forceps
1 Heavy toothed forceps
1 Heavy non-toothed forceps
1 Sponge-holder
1 Bard-Parker handle
1 Mayo scissors, straight
1 Mayo scissors, curved
1 Iris scissors
2 Spencer Wells artery forces, large
2 Mosquito artery forceps, small
1 Allis tissue forceps
1 Needle-holder
1 Volkman spoon
1 Tourniquet
2 Skin hooks

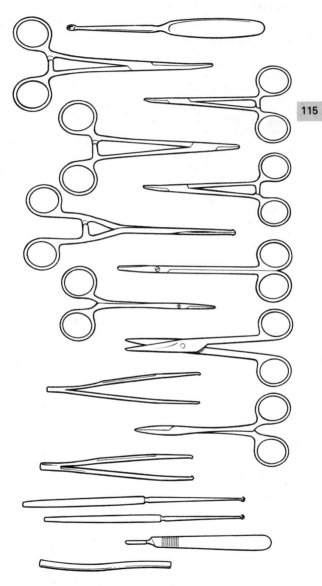

Some basic components of the toe-nail pack.

ORTHOPAEDIC SURGERY

Hip set

2 BP handles no. 3
1 large Charnley forceps
1 small Charnley forceps
1 large non-toothed forceps
1 Mayo straight scissors
1 Mayo curved scissors
2 Kochers
2 needle-holders—large
1 ligature carrier
5 lanes tissue forceps
5 small curved Spencer Wells
5 large curved Spencer Wells
1 Robert Jones elevator
2 Bristow levers
2 Trethowan levers
2 large Langenbeck retractors
2 Rampley sponge holders
10 towel clips
1 Volkman spoon
1 McDonald dissector
1 teaspoon
1 bag and clip

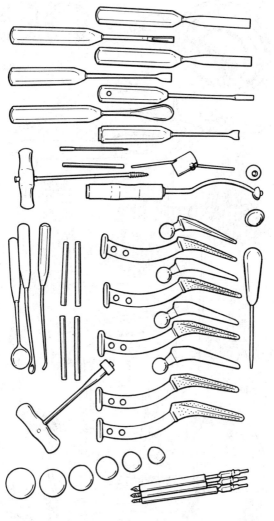

Hip set

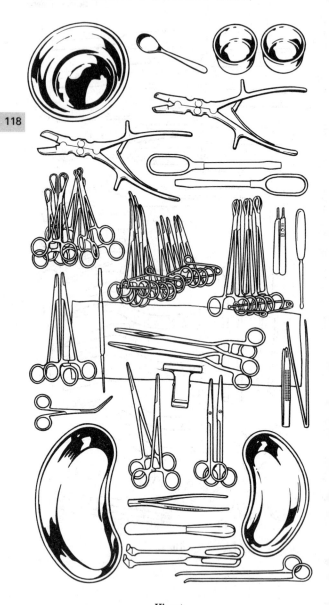

Hip set

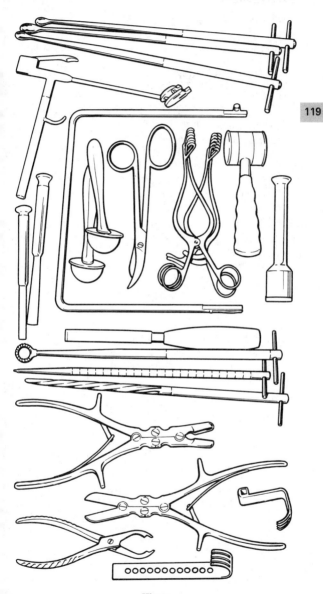

Hip set

ORTHOPAEDIC INSTRUMENTS AND EQUIPMENT

Knee sets

2 BP handles no. 3
1 large Charnley forceps
1 small Charnley forceps
1 small non-toothed forceps
1 Mayo straight – a curved scissors
2 Kochers
1 large – 1 small needle holder #1 ligature carrier
2 Lanes
2 Littlewoods   tissue forceps
5 small curved Spencer Wells
6 towel clips
2 large Langenbeck retractors
2 Trethavans
2 Bristows
1 McDonald
1 Volkman spoon
2 sponge-holders
1 bag and clip
1 large bone nibbler
1 small bone nibbler
1 large bone cutter

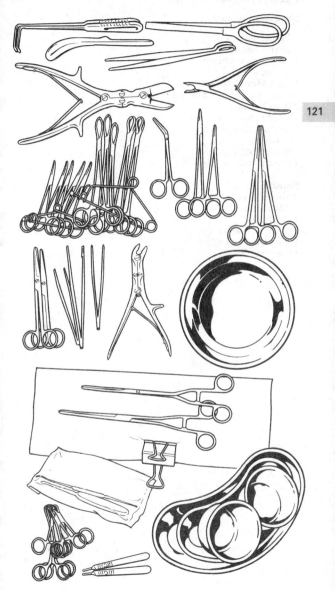

Knee set

Menisectomy set

2 BP handles no. 3
1 small Charnley forceps
1 fine toothed forceps
3 curved artery clips
1 large Mayo scissors
1 small black handled needle-holder
2 large Kochers
2 small Langenbeck
2 medium Langenbeck
5 towel clips
2 sponge holders
1 bag and bulldog clip

Bundle

2 Menisectomy clamps
1 blunt hook
1 McDonald
1 set of Smillies knives
1 solid handled knife
1 tenotomy knife

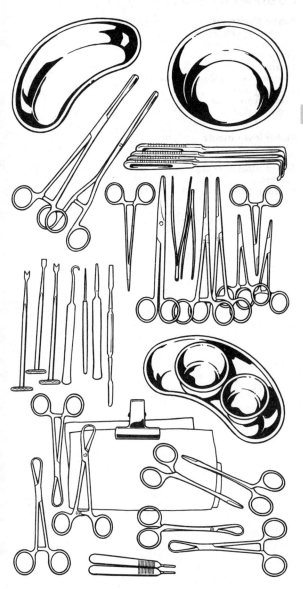

Menisectomy set

ORTHOPAEDIC INSTRUMENTS AND EQUIPMENT (*cont.*)

Austin Moore set
1 measuring gauge
1 punch # 1 impactor
1 corscrew
1 extractor
2 reamers—1 standard, 1 narrow
2 Tommy bars
1 gunbarrel reamer
1 murphy skid

Muller instruments

Prostheses
Test prosthesis
5 reamers
5 Tommy bars

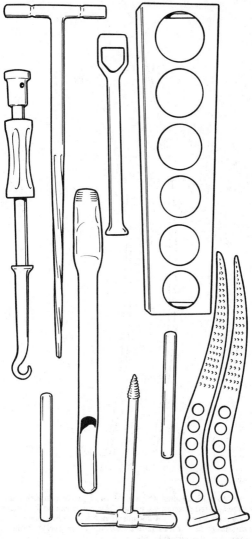

Austin Moore set

UROLOGICAL INSTRUMENTS

Turner–Warwick needles

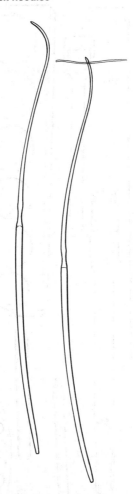

Turner–Warwick needles. The needle with a pre-loaded suture through the eye is passed through the tissues. The suture can ten be grasped by long dissectors or a narrow hacmostat and the needle withdrawn, leaving the suture *in situ* for ligation. Essential for posterior urethroplasty performed by the perineal route.

Dormia baskets

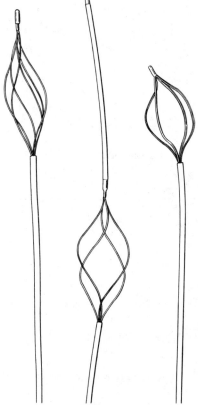

Dormia basket   Filiform tip   Segura basket

Dormia (bluntend and filiform tip) and Segura baskers. The Dormia
baskets have *round* wires and therefore have a tendency to collapse
and allow stones to slip through. The Segura has *flat* wires and can be
manipulated onto the stone without collapsing, but should only be
used under direct vision since the ureter can be trapped equally easy.

Irrigating resectoscope

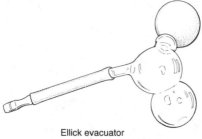

Ellick evacuator
(to wash out the bladder)

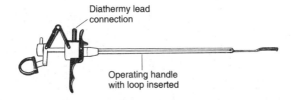

Diathermy lead
connection

Operating handle
with loop inserted

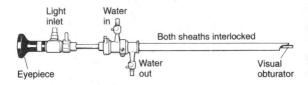

Light
inlet

Water
in

Both sheaths interlocked

Eyepiece

Water
out

Visual
obturator

Irrigating resectoscope (components).

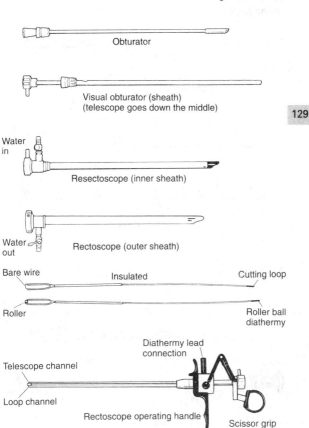

Obturator

Visual obturator (sheath)
(telescope goes down the middle)

129

Water in

Resectoscope (inner sheath)

Water out

Rectoscope (outer sheath)

Bare wire   Insulated   Cutting loop

Roller   Roller ball diathermy

Diathermy lead connection

Telescope channel

Loop channel

Rectoscope operating handle

Scissor grip to move loop back and forth

Irrigating resectoscope (assembled).

UROLOGICAL INSTRUMENTS (cont.)

Stone punch

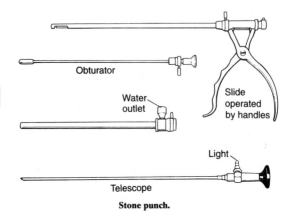

Obturator

Water outlet

Slide operated by handles

Light

Telescope

Stone punch.

Nephroscopes

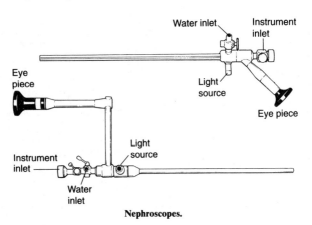

Water inlet

Instrument inlet

Eye piece

Light source

Eye piece

Instrument inlet

Light source

Water inlet

Nephroscopes.

Long and short ureteroscopes

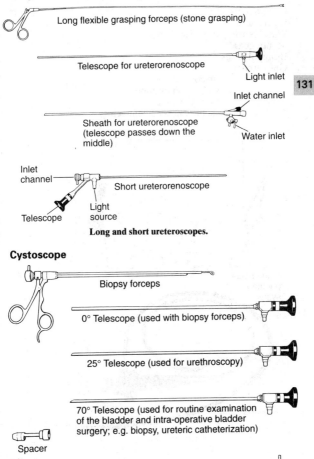

Long flexible grasping forceps (stone grasping)

Telescope for ureterorenoscope

Light inlet

Inlet channel

Sheath for ureterorenoscope
(telescope passes down the
middle)

Water inlet

Inlet channel

Short ureterorenoscope

Telescope

Light source

Long and short ureteroscopes.

Cystoscope

Biopsy forceps

0° Telescope (used with biopsy forceps)

25° Telescope (used for urethroscopy)

70° Telescope (used for routine examination
of the bladder and intra-operative bladder
surgery; e.g. biopsy, ureteric catheterization)

Spacer

Visual obdurator (for urethroscopy)

Cytoscope sheath with water inlets

Blind obturator

Cystoscope.

ENDOSCOPIC INSTRUMENTS AND SETS

Gastroscopy set

Components
Light source
Water bottle (air feed system)
Mouth guard
Biopsy forceps
Gastroscope—lens
　　　　　tip control
　　　　　air/suction buttons
　　　　　biopsy channel
　　　　　suction/air feed connectors

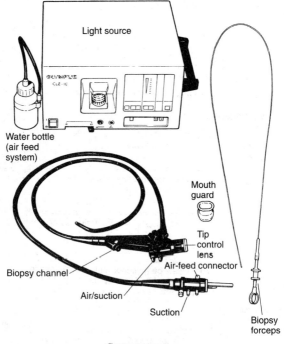

Gastroscopy set.

Proctoscopy/sigmoidoscopy set

Components
Light source
Light lead
Bellows and eyepiece
Biopsy forceps
Light attachment
Proctoscopes (adult and paediatric)
Sigmoidoscopes (rigid)

133

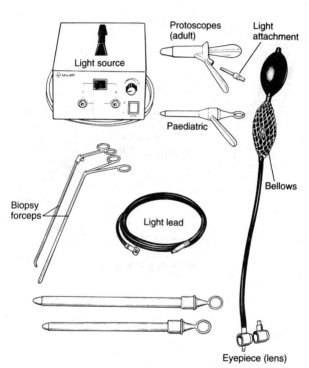

Proctoscopy/sigmoidoscopy set.

ENDOSCOPIC INSTRUMENTS AND SETS (*cont.*)

Flexible sigmoidoscope

Components
Light source
Light connection
Suction valve
Biopsy forceps
Flexible sigmoidoscope—tip control
                                  air/suction buttons
                                  biopsy channel

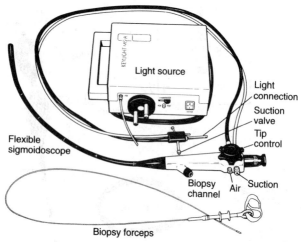

Flexible sigmoidoscope.

Colonoscope

Components
Light source
Light connection
Colonoscope—tip controls
     water/wash pipe
     suction valve
     light connection

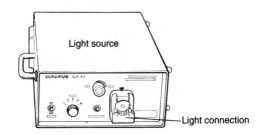

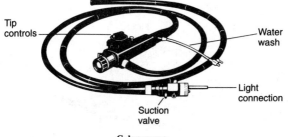

Colonoscope.

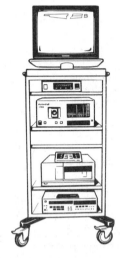

Laparoscope. Monitor (*top*), light source, Mavigraph (video printer), and VCR.

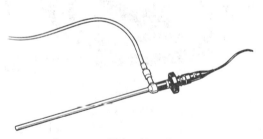

Laparoscope. Light cable and camera.

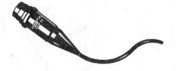

Camera.

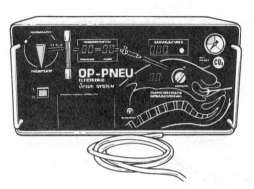

Insulator.

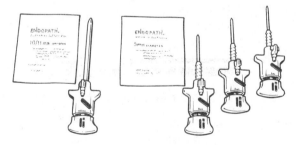

Endopath. Disposable surgical trochars.

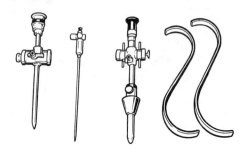

10 mm trochar, Veress needle, Hasson trochar, and 'S' refractors.

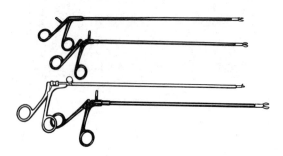

5 mm instruments.

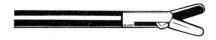

5 mm grasper.

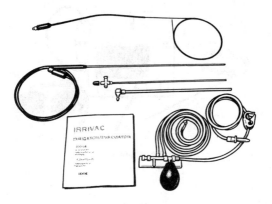

Laser fibre (*top*), laser scalpel, irrigator aspirator and Irrivac®.

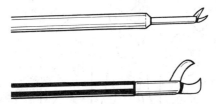

Laparoscopic scissors. Designed as either curved, hooked, or straight, there is a variety available.

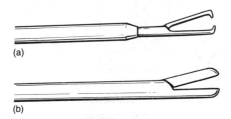

(a)

(b)

(a) 10 mm claw grasper; (b) 10 mm spoon forcep.

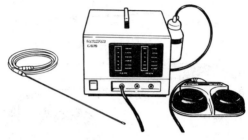

Heater probe.

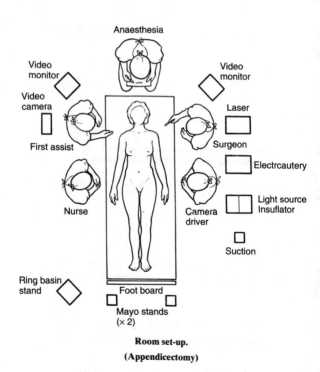

Room set-up.
(Appendicectomy)

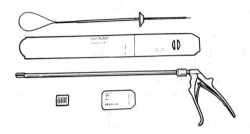

ENDOLOOP ligature with reducer (*top*), **LIGACLIP** endoscopic clip applier and clips.

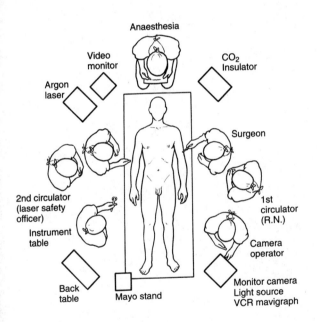

Room set-up.

(Cholecystectomy)

141

5 Surgical knots and basic skills

Suture materials	144
Knot tying	146
Surgical drains	158
Scrub-up technique	160
Vertical abdominal incisions	162
Transverse abdominal incisions	164
Oblique abdominal incisions	166
Upper gastrointestinal endoscopy	168
Examination of the anus and rectum	170
Sigmoidoscopy	172

5 Surgical knots and basic skills

SUTURE MATERIALS

Suture materials used in surgery are of two types—absorbable and non-absorbable. They may be constructed of organic or synthetic materials. Their gauge or calibre is expressed in numbers (British or US Pharmocopeia)

Metric gauge		British/US gauge
0.2	smallest	10/0
0.3		9/0
0.4		8/0
0.5		7/0
0.7		6/0
1		5/0
1.5		4/0
2		3/0
3		2/0
3.5		0
4		1
5		2
6	largest	4

Absorbable sutures

Organic
Catgut is the most common example of an organic absorbable suture. It consists of twisted collagen (from the intestines of sheep or cattle) and is absorbed by phagocytes over a variable period. When catgut is coated in a chromic solution the period of absorption is delayed. Absorption rates with both 'chromic' and 'plain' catgut are unpredictable, and inflammatory reaction is instigated and tensile strength is lost early. It is useful in intestinal anastomosis, closure of the peritoneum, and as a fat or subcutaneous tissue stitch. Predictable synthetic absorbables cause less reaction and are superior (see below).

Synthetic (Dexon, Vicryl, PDS)
These consist of braided fibres of polyglycolic acid, polyglactin, and polydioxanone. They are stronger than catgut, and since they are more slowly phagocytosed induce less tissue reaction. Tensile strength decreases linearly by about 50 per cent in two weeks. These sutures handle and tie better than catgut.

Non-absorbable sutures

Organic (silk, cotton)
These braided sutures tie and handle easily but may perpetuate infection by capillary action caused by the braiding. With the exception of silk, most have been replaced by synthetic sutures, although linen and cotton are still used in abdominal surgery. Synthetic sutures are superior (see below).

Synthetic (Prolene, Nylon, Surgilon)
These may be monofilament or braided. They are slightly

more difficult to handle and tie than silk, for example, but with experience handling becomes easier. They are relatively inert and therefore induce little tissue reaction. Their use is widespread for skin closure, abdominal wall closure, and repair of hernias. They are not absorbed and retain their tensile strength, but braided sutures show the same capillary action as silk and therefore are often coated with polytetrafluoroethylene (PTFE) which renders them smooth and reduces the capillary action (e.g. Ethiflex, Ticron).

Sinus formation is a recognized complication of non-absorbable sutures, but only when sepsis prophylaxis is inadequate.

145

Stainless steel wire

This suture is used for the closure of the sternum after splitting. It is very strong and may be mono- or multifilament. It rarely leads to sinus formation, but it handles poorly and makes re-exploration of a wound difficult.

Needle types

Cutting needles are usually triangular in cross-section with the apex of the triangle in the concavity of the needle. Reverse cutting needles have the apex on the convexity and are less traumatic. Both types are used for skin or tendons.

Round-bodied needles (taper point) are oval or round in cross-section. They are used for anastomosis of the GI tract and vascular work.

Needles may be straight, if the tissues are easily accessible, or curved. Half-circle needles are most commonly used. Deeper tissues require a larger circle arc.

KNOT TYING

Safe knot tying is elementary to good surgical practice. The surgical trainee can rapidly acquire competence by using a practice board. A typical example would include:
- A hook for superficial ties
- A hook with a cylinder for deep ties
- Rubber bands in parallel for tension ties

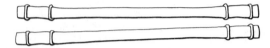

Parallel rubber bands for practising tension knot tying.

Guidelines for proper knot tying

1. Tie knots firmly.
2. Avoid friction between the strands when tying or the suture may weaken.
3. Carry the knot down to the tissues with the tips of the index fingers and make sure that the strands of the ligature are flat by drawing them in opposite directions. This prevents twisting.
4. Do not use undue force otherwise the knot will cut through the tissue.
5. Do not clamp the knot to complete your tie. This will weaken the suture.
6. Tie knots in anticipation of postoperative tissue swelling to prevent necrosis.
7. Do not add extra knots 'to make sure'. This also avoids unnecessary bulk.

Four basic knots are illustrated. Granny knots and twisted square knots are unreliable. They should be eliminated and replaced by flat square knots. These consist of two halves. If

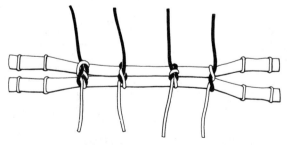

Adequately tied tension knots.

the first half is not flat, the ligature is weakened by twisting and the second half may then cause it to become loose and slip. Twisting can be eliminated if the ligature is crossed before tying each half. Examples of square knot tying are illustrated.

The 'one-hand tie' saves time by eliminating the need to change hands. There is frequently an opportunity in surgery to tie knots in the sagittal plane. The ligatures can be crossed before the knot is tied by simply moving the hands up and down in opposite directions. This 'passing manoeuvre' permits the knots to be tied very quickly. A further advantage of tying in the sagittal plane is that twisting is eliminated because the ligature is kept in one plane. The result is a reliable square knot which will not slip. The 'one-hand tie' should be practised until perfection is achieved because it is one of the most important basic techniques in surgery.

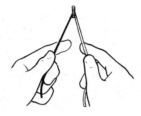

With the palms up and the strands running over the index fingers, hold the strands against your palms with the fourth and fifth fingers. Perform all manipulations with the thumb, index and third fingers.

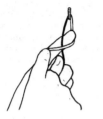

Bring the right-hand strand over to make a *loop* around the left index finger.

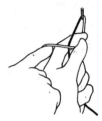

Form a *pinch* with the left thumb and index finger.

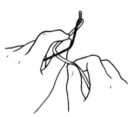

Push the left-hand pinch through the loop with the thumb.

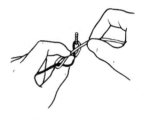

Bring the right-hand strand over and grasp it with the pinch.

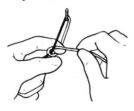

Push your pinch with the strand through the loop with index finger and grasp the strand on your side with the right thumb and index fingers.

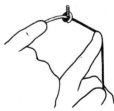

Draw the strands in opposite directions with right hand, crossing over the left side.

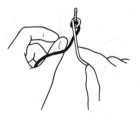

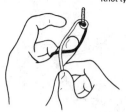

Hook left thumb pushing the left strand up over the thumb.

Form a loop around the left thumb by bringing the right-hand strand from left side to the right, over the left thumb and left-hand strand.

149

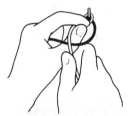

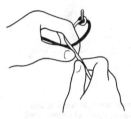

Form a pinch with the left thumb and index finger.

Push the pinch through the loop with the index finger and grasp the right-hand strand with the pinch.

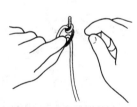

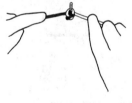

This time, push the pinch with the strand through the loop with the left thumb.

Again grasp the strand with the right thumb and third finger and carry the knot down with the index fingers to complete the square knot.

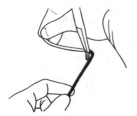

Swing the right-hand strand behind and around the clamp.

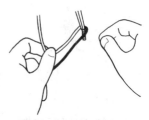

Grasp the right-hand strand with the left thumb and index finger.

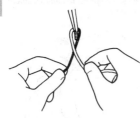

Catch the right-hand strand (black) again with right hand. Now the right-hand strand is crossing over the left-hand strand.

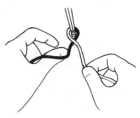

Push the left-hand strand with the left thumb, the tip riding over the left-hand strand.

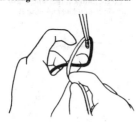

Make a loop by bringing the right-hand strand over the thumb, crossing over the left-hand strand.

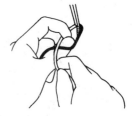

Make a pinch with the left index finger and the thumb.

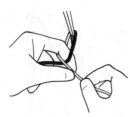
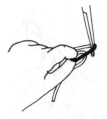
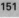

Push the pinch through the loop with the index finger and then grasp the right-hand strand with the pinch.

Push the pinch and the strands through the loop with the thumb.

151

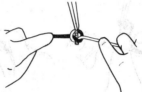

Regrasp the right-hand strand with the right hand and carry down the knot with the index fingers.

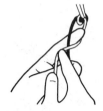

Make a loop around the left
index finger.

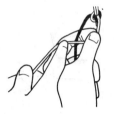

Make a pinch with thumb and
index finger.

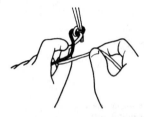

Push the pinch through the loop
with the thumb.

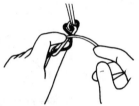

Grasp the right-hand strand by
the pinch.

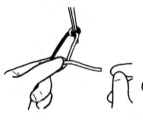

Push the pinch with the strand
through the loop.

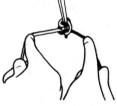

Regrasp the right-hand strand
and carry the knot down, with
the right hand crossing over the
left hand.

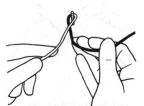

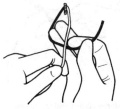

With the right-hand strand rossing *under* the left, hold the strands with the thumb and index finger. Tie around clamps, as on pages 18, 19, except that the right-hand strand is grasped from under the left.

Place the right third and fourth fingers over the right-hand strand and loop the left-hand strand around them. After mastering this, you need use only the third finger.

153

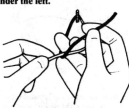

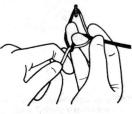

Flex the distal phalanx of the right third finger over the black left strand of the loop.

Swing the white right strand through the loop with the back of the third finger.

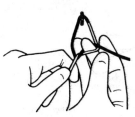

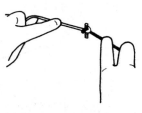

Pull the white strand through the loop with the right third and fourth fingers.

Carry the knot down with the index fingers and lay the knot flat.

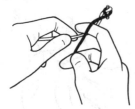

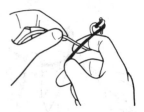

Push the right-hand strand up and over the right index finger and bring it over to form a *loop* over the left-hand strand.

Flex the right index finger around the left black strand of the loop.

154

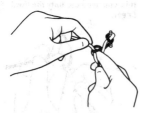

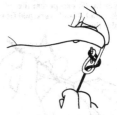

Swing the right-hand strand with the back of the right index finger and pull it through the loop with the help of the third finger.

Cross the left-hand strand up and over to the right while right hand pulls towards the left.

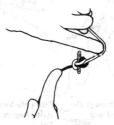

Carry the knot down with the index fingers and lay it flat.

Surgeon's or friction knot

This knot is used as a tension tie, usually in repairing tendons or approximating the fascial planes. It can also be used when closing skin incisions. The steps are described in the illustrations.

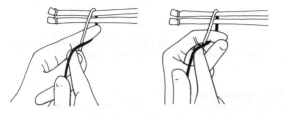

A loop is formed around the left index-thumb pinch.

155

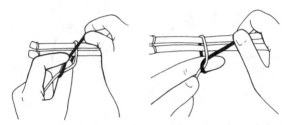

The pinch is put through the loop and the right-hand strand is grasped by the pinch and pushed through with the left index finger.

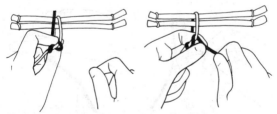

The index-thumb pinch is once again put through the loop and the right-hand strand is again grasped by the pinch and pushed through the loop with the index finger for the second time.

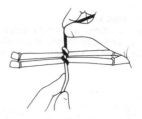

The knot is carried down by the index fingers and kept flat. The knot can be completed with the second half of the two-hand tie.

156

The instrument tie

This is frequently used when closing skin incisions and also during GI or vascular anastomosis.

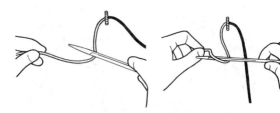

With the needleholder in the right hand, hold one end of the string with the left hand.

Form the first loop around the needleholder by passing it over and then under the left strand.

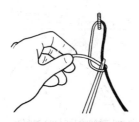

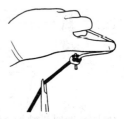

Pick up the free end with the needleholder and pull it through the loop.

Lay the knot flat by crossing the left hand over the right.

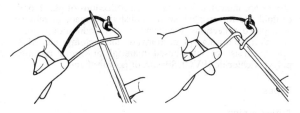

Make a loop around the needleholder, this time, by pushing it under
and then over the left-hand strand.

157

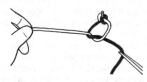

Pick up the free end with the needleholder and pull it through the
loop. Lay the knot flat by pulling on the strands in opposite directions.

Sutures

The following sutures are illustrated: simple; vertical mattress;
horizontal mattress; half-buried horizontal mattress; subcuticular continuous; over-and-over; continuous locking;
continuous mattress; purse-string; continuous Lembert; figure-
of-eight; Lembert; Halsted.

Guidelines for obtaining a fine scar

Try to place the incision in contour lines. Use atraumatic tech-
niques and avoid tension. Remove sutures as follows.
- Face and neck: 3–4 days
- Scalp: 5–7 days
- Abdomen and chest: 7–10 days (up to 14 days after aortic
  surgery)
- Limbs: 5–7 days
- Feet: 10–14 days

Sutures can be removed earlier than these times for cosmetic
reasons. Once removed, they should be replaced with Steri-
strip adhesive skin strips. These may also be used as an alternative to skin sutures, particularly in children.

Skin clips are another alternative to skin sutures. They do
not penetrate the skin and have the advantage of a lower
infection rate. However, they are more expensive than sutures
if disposable stapling sets are used.

SURGICAL DRAINS

Drains are indicated for established collections of pus, blood, or fluid and for prophylaxis to abolish dead space or remove anticipated collections, for example after abdomino-perineal resection, following splenectomy or mastectomy, etc. Most drains consist of latex-based material or, more recently, polyvinylchloride (PVC), Silastic, or polyurethane.

Types

Active drains

Closed systems   These comprise either reusable or disposable systems. The reusable system provides high pressure suction (500 mmHg) with a reservoir capacity of around 300 ml. The bottles can be autoclaved and hence exchanged for a sterile system after use.

Disposable drains provide low pressure suction (100 mmHg) by way of a compressible bottle. The system can be recharged by emptying the bottle, compressing, and reconnecting the drainage tube. Non-return valves should be used to prevent reflux. Since these drainage systems are never entirely empty, colonization of the reservoir contents by bacteria can occur.

Sump drains contain an air inlet lumen which prevents blockage by soft tissue. Although more efficient than closed suction systems, they have the disadvantage of requiring a non-portable suction system and may permit the entry of bacteria although this can be reduced by filters.

Passive drains

These may also be open or closed. Closed systems drain into bags by low pressure suction working on the siphon principle. Open systems drain by capillary action or gravity into dressings or stoma bags. Therefore their efficiency depends on the position of the patient and the volume and site of the collection.

Complications

- Infection (more common with open drains): this can be reduced by the presence of non-return valves.
- Haemorrhage at the site of insertion of the drain.
- Pressure or suction necrosis of bowel leading to leakage of contents.

For those reasons most drains should be removed within 5 days unless the daily volume is large. If a track is necessary to provide a long period of drainage an inert material like PVC or Silastic should not be used. Rubber drains stimulate fibrosis and are better in this situation.

Reference

Broome, A. E., Hanson, L. C., and Tyger, J. F. (1983). Efficiency of various types of drainage of the peritoneal cavity—an experimental study in man. *Acta Chirurgica Scandinavica*, **149**, 53–5.

SCRUB-UP TECHNIQUE

The aim of the preoperative scrub-up is to remove surface organisms from the hands and forearms. The technique does not remove deeper organisms from the hair follicles or sweat glands, and recolonization usually occurs within 20–30 minutes. However, modern washing agents such as povidone iodine (Betadine) and chlorhexidine (Hibiscrub) will kill organisms for up to 2 hours after scrubbing. There is no advantage to excessive and lengthy scrubbing, and there is some evidence that only the nails need scrubbing. Hand and wrist jewellery should be removed. Three to four minutes is adequate for the first scrub of the morning. The hands should be washed between cases with a spirit solution or rescrubbed for 1–2 minutes. Staff with boils of the skin or other infective foci should not be in theatre until recovery is complete.

1. Turn on the water and adjust the temperature until it is acceptable. Give the hands and forearms a light wash. Rinse and take a sterile brush from the dispenser. Apply some Betadine or Hibiscrub to the brush and scrub the fingernails carefully. Rinse.
2. Wash the forearms and hands for about 2 minutes. Rinse and allow the water to run downwards towards the elbows.
3. Dry each hand and forearm separately with the disposable towels provided, using half of each of the towels for each hand and forearm. Dry from distal to proximal, e.g. wrist to elbow.
4. Avoid the use of glove powder if possible. (Dry hands do not need powder. Biogel gloves need no powder.) Put your gown on and then put the gloves on left hand first. Pick the folded glove up with the fingers of the right hand on the inside and apply it to the left hand. Now pick the right-hand glove up by passing the fingers of the left hand under the fold (i.e. to the outside) of the right-hand glove. Slip the right hand into the folded glove. Now fold your gown cuffs and complete gloving by straightening the glove folds over your wrists with your gloved fingers on the outside of the folds. An alternative is to have your surgical gloves put on by a nurse (USA) or to use the nurses' method (the 'closed' technique). After donning the gown, pick up the left glove with the left hand still enclosed in the gown cuff and apply over the left cuff and hand. The left cuff is gently pulled down to let the fingers enter the glove and the process is repeated on the right side. This method is usually not acceptable to the surgeon as the cuff ends up on the palms.

Punctured gloves

Sixty to seventy per cent of gloves will become punctured during surgery and should be replaced, as should gowns with soiled sleeves.

Shaving

The operative field should be shaved, allowing ample room to apply dressings. This is best done by an orderly, a nurse, or the surgeon on the morning of surgery or on the table itself. Do not carry out shaving on the day before because folliculitis may follow, leading to postponement of the procedure, due to increased risk of infection.

Skin preparation

In theatre the operative field will be prepared with aqueous Betadine or 0.5 chlorhexidine in alcohol. Two applications are usually made. When operating on mucus membranes use normal saline but remove all debris first. In procedures on the head protect the eyes with adhesive tapes to keep them closed.

VERTICAL ABDOMINAL INCISIONS

Abdominal incisions should be large enough to permit the intended procedure to be performed safely and efficiently. They should be closed as cosmetically as possible without compromising their strength.

Upper midline
This permits access to the stomach, duodenum, gall bladder, liver, and transverse colon. The incision extends from the xiphisternum to the umbilicus but can be extended distally if necessary. It is continued through the linea alba to the peritoneum, which is held between artery forceps away from the abdominal contents and then incised with a scalpel. Two fingers are then inserted to allow safe division of the peritoneum upwards and downwards. After the procedure the wound is closed in layers with a non-absorbable suture to the linea alba and with interrupted Nylon, or subcuticular Dexon, Nylon or prolene with or without beads (easier), to skin.

Mass closure
This is closure of all layers of the wound except skin with a single suture which may be an over-and-over technique or a far-and-near figure-of-eight continuous suture. Wide bites greater than 1 cm are taken with alternate more superficial bites to form the figure-of-eight.

Lower midline
This permits access to the pelvic organs. The incision extends from the umbilicus to the symphysis pubis. Ensure that the bladder is empty because of its relationship to the anterior abdominal wall when full. Close the peritoneum with Vicryl or Dexon, the linea alba with non-absorbable sutures, and the skin with Nylon or Dexon.

Full-length midline
This incision skirts the umbilicus and is useful when wide exposure is required, as in aortic surgery.

Paramedian incision
This incision is in the upper or lower abdomen parellel to and 2 cm from the midline. It permits access to the organs of each quadrant of the abdomen according to its site but tends to have been replaced by the faster open–close midlines.
  The anterior rectus sheath is divided and the muscle dissected laterally to expose the posterior sheath. This is divided vertically, together with the transversalis fascia and peritoneum. The peritoneum and posterior rectus sheath are closed together in one layer of non-absorbable sutures followed by the anterior sheath and skin.

Lateral paramedian incision
This is a modification of the paramedian. It is a vertical inci-

sion over the junction of the middle and outer thirds of the width of the rectus muscle. The sheath is opened vertically and the muscle reflected laterally. The posterior sheath and peritoneum are opened in the same vertical plane as the anterior sheath. There is a lower risk of wound dehiscence or incisional hernia because of the overlying rectus muscle when the wound is closed.

TRANSVERSE ABDOMINAL INCISIONS

Skin crease incisions
True skin crease incisions can be made in Langer's lines in the upper or lower abdomen. They can be used to approach the gall bladder, stomach, duodenum, aorta, etc. Exposure and drainage are better. Chest complications and postoperative pain are less common and incisional herniation is seldom seen.

Upper abdominal transverse incision
This exposure allows access to the upper abdomen and can be modified into a 'roof-top' incision (bilateral subcostal incisions confluent transversely below the xiphisternum) to permit access to the pancreas and classically the adrenal glands. Closure is in layers with Vicryl to the peritoneum, interrupted or continuous PDS or Nylon to the rectus muscles, and Nylon (subcuticular with beads) to skin.

The wound offers two advantages:
- A sound scar
- Less postoperative pain

Pfannenstiel incision
This suprapubic transverse incision allows access to the pelvic cavity. The incision is 8–12 cm long and skirts the upper border of the pubis. It divides skin, fat, external oblique, internal oblique, and transversalis fascia from one inferior epigastric artery to the other. The rectus abdominis muscles are split vertically in the midline for several centimetres to expose the peritoneum, which is then opened between artery forceps. If greater access is required, the rectus may also be divided transversely and retracted cranially (Czermy incision).

Selection of needles used with various types of suture materials

Cutting	Round-bodied
Slim-blade curved cutting	Half-circle round-bodied
Curved reverse cutting	Round-bodied heavy Mayo
Half-circle tapercut	Curved round-bodied
Curved super cutting	Five-eighths circle round-bodied
Tapercut fish hook, heavy	Straight round-bodied
Half-circle cutting	Blunt-point curved round-bodied
Precision point reverse cutting, curved	
Straight cutting	
Trocar point half-circle, heavy	

OBLIQUE ABDOMINAL INCISIONS

Kocher's (subcostal) incision

This allows access to the contents of the right and left upper quadrants and is particularly indicated for operations on the gall bladder and spleen in patients with a wide costal angle. The incision extends from the midline to the lateral edge of the rectus muscle. It lies parallel to and about 2–2.5 cm below the costal margin. All tissues are divided in the line of the incision. Closure is by the mass technique or in layers in the following order: peritoneum and posterior sheath together, and then anterior sheath (with non-absorbable or delayed absorption sutures, e.g. Nylon, PDS) and Nylon (preferable), or Dexon to skin.

Rutherford–Morrison incision

This allows access to the lower ureter, the colon, and the iliac arteries. The approach can be trans- or extraperitoneal. The incision extends laterally from just above the anterior superior iliac spine to a point about 2.5 cm above the pubic tubercle medially. All tissues are divided in the same line and the inferior epigastric vessels are ligated. The peritoneum can then be reflected anterially to approach the ureter, inferior vena cava, or lumbar sympathetic chain.

Gridiron incision

This is a classic appendicectomy incision extending obliquely from a point two-thirds of the way along the imaginary line drawn from the anterior superior iliac spine to the umbilicus. The incision is made at right angles to this line. Skin, subcutaneous fat, and fascia are divided in the same line, but the external oblique, internal oblique, and transversus abdominis are all split in the line of their fibres to expose the peritoneum, which is then opened between artery forceps. Closure is in layers, with catgut to peritoneum and loose catgut muscle closure. The external oblique aponeurosis is closed with Vicryl. Use Nylon or Dexon for skin.

This incision has disadvantages in that, although providing strong healing, it is limited medially by the rectus sheath and inferior epigastric vessels. However, it can be extended laterally and upwards.

If the preoperative diagnosis of appendicectomy is found to be wrong, this incision should be closed and a right lower paramedian performed. For this reason it has been condemned as the incision of the 'Cocksure'. Its real value is to provide access to the appendix, but it can be extended to permit a right hemicolectomy. It affords poor access to the gall bladder and duodenum.

Lanz incision

This is a right lower-quadrant transverse incision which gives a cosmetic scar. It is similar to the gridiron.

UPPER GASTROINTESTINAL ENDOSCOPY

Check list

- Ensure that the patient is fully prepared, has received an adequate explanation, and has given consent.
- Ensure that the endoscope is working properly.
- Ensure that the endoscope has been cleaned.

Insertion technique

Insert a butterfly needle into a vein on the dorsum of the hand. Spray the fauces with anaesthetic. Ask the patient to lie in the left lateral position. Insert a mouth guard if he has teeth. Give the patient sedation. This varies according to preference, but often diazepam 10 mg IV slowly is adequate (large dose midazolam is an alternative, but patients need care after sedation). Buscopan may also be given (20 mg IV) to provide smooth-muscle relaxation. Wear gloves during the procedure. Hold the instrument controls in the left hand. Insert the index finger of the right hand into the mouth and pass the tip of the endoscope under the finger. Now gently pull the tongue and the tip of the endoscope forwards. Gently advance the endoscope asking the patient to swallow. *Do not use force to pass the instrument.*

An alternative method is to insert the instrument without directing it with the right index. The instrument is inserted into the mouth and aligned with the pharynx under direct vision. It is passed over the tongue with the tip flexed. As it passes down, the tip is returned to neutral and the patient is asked to swallow.

Inspection of upper GI tract

Oesophagus

Look for webs or carcinoma in the upper third. Gently inflate after clearing mucus by suction. The gullet usually distends so that a clear view can be obtained. Look for landmarks like the cardiac impulse. In the lower oesophagus check the mucosal folds for inflammation due to oesophagitis and note the distance from the incisor teeth. Check also for hiatus hernia. Deep inspiration by the patient helps to identify the position of the diaphragm. If there is an obvious lesion, pass the biopsy forceps down the biopsy channel and take a specimen for histology (preferably brushings for cytology, which is safer).

Stomach

Follow the lumen at all times. Inflate as required. On entry note obvious abnormalities like abnormal folds, tumours, blood, bile, retained fluids, or foods. Aspirate excessive fluid to prevent inhalation. Now inspect in turn the whole lumen, the greater and lesser curves, the roof of the pyloric antrum (by flexing the tip), and the fundus by increasing flexion of the tip and rotating the instrument over more than 90°. Carry out biopsy or brushings if indicated. You will be able to see the proximal part of the endoscope entering the cardia. This is a useful point for orientation. Now advance the endoscope to inspect the pylorus. Note its mobility and the presence of deformity or inflammation.

Duodenum

Enter the duodenum by keeping the pylorus in the centre of your view. The 'up-and-down' control with the left hand assists advancement. Once inside the duodenal cap carry out a full inspection, withdrawing the tip and depressing it to achieve this. To examine the remainder of the duodenum the endoscope usually has to be rotated 90° to the right using the up-and-down control to see the lumen.

169

Withdrawal

Re-inspect the lumina of the duodenum, stomach, and oesophagus on withdrawal by rotating the tip. Aspirate excessive air from each area once you are satisfied with the examination.

EXAMINATION OF THE ANUS AND RECTUM

Tell the patient what you intend to do. Ask him to lie on his left side with his knees drawn up towards his abdomen and his buttocks at the edge of the bed. Raising the buttocks on a sandbag facilitates sigmoidoscopy. Stand with your left side next to the patient's back.

Action

Separate the buttocks and inspect the anus. Note whether there are changes of excoriation, erythema, or moistness of the perianal skin. Are there anal skin tags? Is there a prolapsed haemorrhoid? Are there perianal warts?

Digital examination

Put a rubber glove on your right hand. Apply some KY Jelly (Johnson & Johnson) to the tip of the index finger. Place the pad of your index finger on the anal orifice posteriorly and apply enough pressure to permit entry. At this stage the patient may complain of pain and discomfort, and you may note spasm of the sphincter. This suggests an anal fissure. Do not persist with digital rectal examination, but gently separate the buttocks to expose the anal verge, the lower end of the fissure, and a sentinel pile, usually situated posteriorly. Lubrication of the finger with lignocaine gel may permit digital examination. However, if there is spasm and pain it is better to examine the patient under anaesthetic.

Once the finger is in the anus, change its direction so that the tip 'points' into the rectum. With the pad of the finger feel the posterior and lateral walls. Are there any abnormalities—mass, ulcer, polyp?

Now bend your knees and rotate the finger so that you can feel the anterior rectal wall. Is there a mucosal abnormality? Can you feel the prostate anteriorly in a male patient? Note its consistency. In female patients you can feel the cervix through the anterior wall as a knob-like projection. The os is usually palpable as a slit. Note whether movement of the cervix leads to pain or discomfort.

Proctoscopy

The proctoscope is a short instrument consisting of an obturator enclosed in a viewing barrel with a handle and a light source.

Action

Apply KY Jelly to the tip of the obturator and press it on to the anal orifice until it has penetrated. Once the instrument has been completely inserted, remove the obturator, attach the light source, and gently but slowly withdraw the instrument. Note the state of the rectal mucosa. Is it pink (normal)?

Does it bleed easily? Does it completely fill the barrel (prolapse)? As you withdraw the instrument, note whether there are haemorrhoids. They appear as purple cushions at positions 3, 7, and 11. Band or ligate them if indicated. Note also whether there are polyps or an anal fissure anteriorly or posteriorly (proctoscopy is usually painful in the presence of a fissure but it may be made possible by applying lubricating jelly containing a local anaesthetic).

SIGMOIDOSCOPY

The sigmoidoscope is a rigid steel or plastic hollow tube about 25–30 cm in length and up to 2 cm in diameter. It comprises an outer hollow tube, an obturator which is withdrawn after the instrument has been inserted, and a light source which is fibre-optic in modern instruments. There is an attachment on the lens piece for the insufflation of air to open up the lumen ahead of the instrument.

Preparation of patient

The patient should have the procedure explained fully and give consent. Preparation of the bowel is often unnecessary. A disposable enema may help in cases of difficulty, but sometimes may have the reverse effect.

Position of patient

The patient lies in the left lateral position with the hips flexed and the buttocks raised on a sandbag or pillow.

Procedure

Carry out a digital examination of the rectum. If it is loaded, defer sigmoidoscopy until the bowel has been prepared with a disposable enema.

Lubricate the sigmoidoscope with KY Jelly. Disposable plastic sigmoidoscopes are lubricated under running warm tap-water. With the obturator in place, introduce the sigmoidoscope gently through the sphincter to about 5 cm by pointing it towards the umbilicus. Remove the obturator and advance under direct vision after attaching the eyepiece, insufflator, and light source. Keep the lumen in view at all times as you pass the instrument upwards to its full length. Negotiation of the rectosigmoid junction requires considerable experience and skill. If the patient suffers discomfort, do not persist.

Note the appearance of the mucosa, and the presence of contact bleeding, ulceration, or neoplasm. Take biopsies of suspected abnormalities for histological examination using the specialized biopsy forceps provided. Polyps can be removed by snaring and diathermy. It requires considerable experience to interpret what you see.

NB If a biopsy has been taken the patient should not have any type of enema for at least a week because of the risk of perforation of the bowel or air embolus. Carry out proctoscopy last; this is best for banding and injection procedures.

Flexible sigmoidoscopy

This fibre-optic instrument is now in routine use. It is longer than the rigid sigmoidoscope (up to 40 cm) and good bowel preparation is required. As with OGD, considerable training is required to become skilful.

Colonoscopy

The colonoscope is even longer than the flexible sigmoidoscope and can be passed through the anus or through a terminal or loop colostomy or ileostomy. It is particularly useful for assessing the sigmoid and descending colon which may present difficulties radiologically because the two segments overly each other.

Indications

- Assessment of the colon in patients with suspected malignant disease (can be passed to the caecum).
- Follow-up assessment of patients with resected malignancy.
- Assessment and biopsy of inflammatory bowel disease.
- Screening of patients with adenomas (and their removal).
- Assessment and biopsy of diverticular disease (which may mimic carcinoma on occasions).
- Removal of polyps.
- Decompression of sigmoid volvulus.
- Investigation and decompression of pseudo-obstruction.

6 General and gastrointestinal surgery

Introduction	176
Tracheostomy	178
Excision of the submandibular gland	182
Excision of a pharyngeal pouch	186
Superficial parotidectomy	188
Excision of branchial cyst, sinus, or fistula	190
Heller's oesophageal cardiomyotomy (thoracic approach)	192
Heller's oesophageal cardiomyotomy (abdominal approach)	194
Truncal vagotomy and drainage	196
Highly selective vagotomy	200
Perforated duodenal ulcer	204
Insertion of an Angelchik prosthesis	206
Oesophagectomy	208
Oesophagogastrectomy for lower-third carcinomas	212
Total oesophagectomy	214
Celestin intubation of inoperable oesophageal cancer	218
Hiatus hernia	220
Gastrectomy	222
Cholecystectomy	226
Exploration of the common bile duct	230
Transduodenal sphincteroplasty	232
Cholecystotomy	234
Biliary bypass procedures	236
Small bowel resection and anastomosis	240
Ileostomy	244
Excision of Meckel's diverticulum	246
Splenectomy	248
Appendicectomy	250
Large bowel resection and anastomosis	254
Right hemicolectomy	258
Transverse colectomy	262
Left hemicolectomy	264
Sigmoid colectomy	266

Total colectomy	268
Colostomy	270
Anterior resection	278
Procedures for dealing with colonic obstructive lesions	282
Abdominoperineal excision of the rectum	284
Haemorrhoids	286
Anal warts	290
Anorectal polyps	292
Rectal cancer	294
Fissure in ano	296
Perianal abscess	298
Fistula in ano	300
Ingrowing toenail	304
Inguinal hernia	306
Repair of femoral hernia	310
Repair of incisional hernia	312
Thyroidectomy	314
Parathyroidectomy	320
Adrenalectomy	322

INTRODUCTION

In each of the procedures described it should be assumed, unless otherwise stated, that the patient will have given informed consent and that the operation will be under general anaesthetic with the patient lying supine on the table. Appropriate DVT prophylaxis and antibiotics will also have been given.

TRACHEOSTOMY

This procedure is usually performed under general anaesthetic and may be resorted to after an appropriate period of ventilation with an endotracheal tube. It may also be decided upon for patients undergoing head and neck surgery or for managing those with severe head or spinal injuries. It can be performed electively or as an emergency.

Indications

- Severe respiratory or cardiac disease in infants and children.
- Long-term care of patients with chest trauma.
- Pulmonary insufficiency in the elderly when other treatments are ineffective.
- Neurological problems, e.g. coma, stroke, poliomyelitis, bulbar palsy, etc.

Equipment required

The patient will already have an endotracheal tube in place. If he is conscious, a full explanation of the procedure must be given. Ensure good lighting and a range of sizes of tracheostomy tubes which may be silver or PVC (ideal as the first tube), ranging from 24 to 42 French gauge (36 to 39 for men, 33 to 36 for women). Ideally, they should be double-cuffed so that the cuffs can be inflated alternately to reduce the risk of tracheal trauma. Remember that an aseptic technique is required.

Site of incision

Transverse, about 5 cm long, midway between the cricoid cartilage and the sternal notch.

Procedure

Make the incision and deepen it by dividing the platysma transversely to the pretracheal fascia. Identify the midline. Split and retract the strap muscles in this line to expose the trachea. Secure haemostasis and identify first the cricoid cartilage and then the first tracheal ring. From this point the second to fifth rings may be covered by thyroid tissue. It may be necessary to divide the thyroid isthmus to expose them.

The removal of large discs of trachea is unnecessary, as is the use of tracheal flaps sutured to the skin. A longitudinal incision from the second to the fourth tracheal ring permits the insertion of an appropriately sized tracheostomy tube. This is done by retracting the edges of the tracheostomy, asking the anaesthetist to remove the endotracheal tube, and inserting the tracheostomy tube. Remember that the endotracheal tube cuff is usually damaged; therefore rapid insertion of the tracheostomy tube is needed. Inflate the balloon,

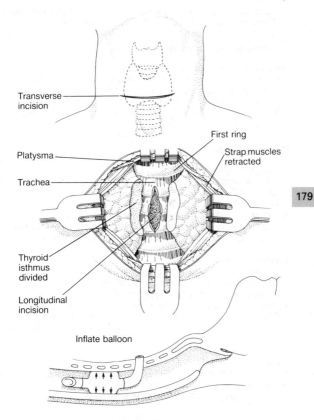

Tracheostomy.

suture the wound loosely, place swabs under the tracheostomy tube, and tie the tapes behind the patient's neck using tight knots to avoid inadvertent loosening by well-intentioned staff in mistake for the patient's night-gown ties. The tube may be changed after 24 hours.

Care of the tracheostomy

All procedures should be performed under sterile conditions. Patients require removal of retained secretion by sterile suction every 15–30 minutes. The cuff may also be deflated for 5 minutes in every hour (although this may be unnecessary with the more modern tracheostomy tubes). The inspired gases should be humidified and the patient's hydration well maintained.

Removal of the tracheostomy

As a preliminary the tube can be exchanged for a smaller silver non-cuffed tube so that the patient can breathe through the tube and normally. A speaking tube may also be used, enabling the patient to cough and speak. After a period of a few days the tube can be removed and the wound covered after closure with a few stitches.

Complications

Early (postoperative)
● Displacement of tube: if this occurs the patient should have an endotracheal tube reinserted until a new tracheostomy tube can be reintroduced.
● Infection with *Pseudomonas* spp., *Escherichia coli*, and *Staphylococcus aureus* increases the risk of local necrosis and stenosis. It can be avoided by using sterile technique.

Intermediate
● Haemorrhage: from the wound, from erosion of the innominate artery. This is a terminal event and is usually preceded by small bleeds. Further surgery may prevent disaster.
● Acquired tracheo-oesophageal fistula: this is due to overinflation of the tube. Suspect this complication when gastric juice or feeds appear around the tube. Further surgery is indicated.

Late
● Stricture formation.
● Failure of spontaneous closure of tracheostomy.
Further surgery is indicated in both situations.

EXCISION OF THE SUBMANDIBULAR GLAND (intermediate)

Surgical anatomy

The submandibular gland lies under cover of the medial border of the mandible below the mucous membrane of the mouth on the hyoglossus and mylohyoid muscles. It is supported inferiorly by skin, platysma, and fascia. It has superficial and deep lobes continuous behind the posterior edge of the mylohyoid. The duct originates from the anterior pole of the deep lobe and passes forward to open near the midline on each side. The facial artery and vein pass deep to the posterior pole of the superficial lobe. The lingual nerve loops around the duct from above and returns to lie medial to it.

Special anatomy

- The mandibular branch of the facial nerve at the angle of the jaw; it may be damaged if the incision is too high.
- The lingual nerve during forward dissection of the duct.

Special consent

Warn the patient of potential mandibular nerve damage (drooping angle of lip) and lingual nerve damage (sensory to the anterior two-thirds of the tongue).

Position of patient

Use a head ring. Extend the neck. Turn the face away so that the gland presents. Tilt the head up to empty the external jugular vein. Expose a rectangular area of the face with the gland at its centre.

Incision

Transverse, skin crease, 5 cm below the lower border of the mandible. Divide platysma. Insert a self retainer. Make the skin incision at least two finger breadths below the angle of the jaw. Stay as close to the gland as possible. Use retraction widely.

Procedure

Deepen the incision. Expose the lower border of the superficial lobe. Stay close to the gland anteriorly. Identify where the two lobes are continuous. Expose the facial artery and vein above and below. Ligate and divide them at these sites.

Apply tissue forceps to the anterior pole of the superficial lobe. Ask your assistant to retract it laterally and the border of mylohyoid medially. Free the deep lobe from the undersurface of the mylohyoid.

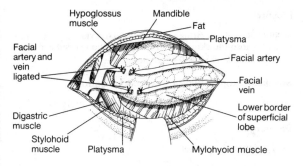

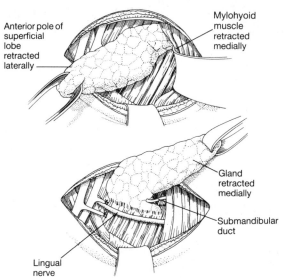

Excision of the submandibular gland.

Now retract the gland medially. Free the deep surface of the deep lobe from hyoglossus. Dissect along the duct as far as possible. Identify the lingual nerve running forwards and medially. Ligate the duct with Vicryl and divide it.

EXCISION OF THE SUBMANDIBULAR GLAND (intermediate) (cont.)

Closure

Secure haemostasis. Bring a suction drain out via a separate stab wound. Close the skin with interrupted nylon or subcuticular prolene. Apply an Opsite dressing.

Special postoperative care and complications

Observe for haematoma, infection, and nerve injury.

Discharge

Two to four days after operation.

EXCISION OF A PHARYNGEAL POUCH (major)

Aim

- To deal with the pouch—excise or reduce
- Cricopharyngeal myotomy

Special anatomy

The pouch herniates between the fibres of the inferior constrictor. Avoid recurrent laryngeal nerve damage and causing an iatrogenic post-cricoid oesophageal stricture.

Special consent

Warn the patient of the risks. Obtain informed consent.

Position of patient

Supine with the head rotated to the right, left arm by the side, and sandbag or pillow between the shoulder blades.

Incision

10–15 cm long parallel to the anterior border of left sternomastoid centred on the cricoid cartilage.

Procedure

Incise platysma and deep fascia. Retract sternomastoid, internal jugular vein, and carotid sheath posteriorly (carefully!). Retract the thyroid gland and the larynx anteriorly. Use blunt (pledget) dissection to identify the sac. Clean it down to its neck, grasping its fundus with tissue forceps to provide gentle traction.

The pouch

Small pouches may be left alone. Larger sacs should be excised. Ask the anaesthetist to pass a 28–30 French gauge bougie into the upper oesophagus. This procedure avoids narrowing. Apply a vascular clamp across the neck of the sac and excise it. Suture the sac with interrupted catgut sutures and tie them after releasing the clamp.

Cricopharyngeal myotomy

This is done to prevent postoperative fistula or late recurrence. Gently insert curved artery forceps between the cricopharyngeus muscle and the oesophageal mucosa. Open and close them to free the two layers. Incise the muscle between the open forceps for a length of 2–4 cm distally. When this is done small or moderate sacs may be suspended to the prevertebral fascia and their contents emptied into the gullet.

Closure

Suction or corrugated drain to site. Close platysma and skin in separate layers.

Special postoperative care

Limit oral fluids on the first 2 days to 30 ml/hour and 60 ml/hour respectively. Start free fluids on the third day and graduate to diet thereafter.

Complications

Fistula formation, mediastinitis, inhalational pneumonia.

Discharge

Seven to ten days after operation.

SUPERFICIAL PAROTIDECTOMY (complex)

Indications

Recurrent parotitis due to inaccessible stone disease and keratoconjunctivitis (Sjögren's syndrome), salivary adenomas.

Special anatomy

The parotid gland lies in the hollow between the sternomastoid and the ramus of the mandible. It extends anteriorly to overlie the masseter. Its duct emerges from the anterior extension, runs across the masseter, turns medially to pierce the buccinator, and opens into the mouth opposite the second molar tooth of the upper jaw. Several structures penetrate the gland. The external carotid artery is at first posteromedial and then pierces the gland, emerges level with the neck of the mandible, and divides into superficial temporal and maxillary arteries. It is accompanied by the posterior facial vein. The facial nerve emerges from the stylomastoid foramen, pierces the posteromedial part of the gland, and runs forwards in the substance of the gland where it divides into its five terminal branches: temporal, zygomatic, buccal, mandibular, and cervical. The carotid artery and posterior facial vein lie deep to the gland.

Special consent

The facial nerve and its five branches must be identified and protected early in the procedure. Informed consent must be obtained.

Position of patient

Use a head ring, head-up tilt, and turn the patient's face away from you with the neck extended. Clean the skin. Apply gowns with the parotid and mandible clearly exposed. Put a swab or cotton-wool bud in the external auditory meatus.

Incision

S-shaped in front of the pinna extending towards the mastoid process and then into the upper skin crease of the neck. Make the incision in three parts, securing haemostasis at each before proceeding to the next. Deepen the cervical part of the incision, removing the anterior branch of the greater auricular nerve and retaining in saline until the end of the procedure. Now deepen the facial part until you can identify the junction of the cartilaginous and bony external auditory meatus.

Procedure

Concentrate on the mastoid part of the incision. Dissect the tissue carefully to identify the insertion of sternomastoid. You are approaching the facial nerve. Identify and ligate the stylo-mastoid artery. The facial nerve runs in much the same direction but a few millimetres deeper. Identify the main trunk. The aim is now to dissect the parotid tissue superficial to the trunk and its branches. Pass fine artery forceps, convex surface down, along the nerve and in contact with it. Allow the tips to protrude through the parotid tissue and divide the area so identified with scissors. Repeat this process with each branch until the parotid is reflected. Reflect the skin off the anterior flap and identify the parotid duct at the anterior margin. Dissect and ligate it at the anterior border of the masseter.

Closure

Close the wound with fine interrupted Nylon sutures (4/0 or 5/0). Bring a suction drain through a separate stab wound.

189

NB Superficial parotidectomy may also be performed for lumps superficial to the facial nerve. This cannot be established clinically. If the lump is deep to the facial nerve, a conservative or radical parotidectomy may be indicated. In conservative parotidectomy the facial nerve is preserved and the lump dissected from below it. In radical parotidectomy the nerve is sacrificed.

Special postoperative care/complications

Observe for haematoma, infection, and nerve injury.

DISCHARGE

Two to four days postoperation.

EXCISION OF BRANCHIAL CYST, SINUS, OR FISTULA (major)

Aim

Excision of all vestigial remnants. Make sure that a large branchial cyst is not a swelling of the lower pole of the parotid or encroaching upon it. If there is doubt, proceed as for formal parotidectomy.

Small cyst

Special anatomy
- The external and internal carotid arteries and vagus nerve lie deep to the cyst.
- The hypoglossal and glossopharyngeal nerves lie deep to the cyst above and below the posterior belly of the digastric.

Position of patient
Supine. Head turned to the opposite side with upward tilt of the table to collapse the external jugular vein.

Incision
Transverse over the lesion for a length of about 7 cm. Raise subplatysmal flaps above and below.

Procedure
Divide the fascia over the anterior border of sternomastoid. Retract it laterally. Free the cyst on all sides until its track can be seen. Divide this between two pairs of artery forceps. Often there is no track and the cyst can be removed by blunt dissection.

Closure
See below.

Large cyst

It is best to perform a superficial parotidectomy if the parotid gland is pushed outwards. Define the facial nerve and proceed.

Branchial sinus and fistula

Incision
Elliptical over external opening.

Procedure
Deepen the incision through the platysma. Apply traction to the ellipse. The track may be felt running upwards between the carotid arteries and above the hypoglossal and glosso-pharyngeal nerves. It may also proceed towards the ear or parotid region, when a superficial parotidectomy may again be necessary.

In most cases it runs towards the mouth. Excise it by dissection, traction and multiple step-ladder incisions. Divide the posterior belly of the digastric and follow the track to the middle constrictor where it blends with the muscle. Excise it with an ellipse of muscle.

Closure
Secure haemostasis. Bring out a single suction drain through a separate stab wound. Close skin with interrupted nylon.

Special postoperative care
Remove the drain in 3–5 days, sutures in 7 days.

Discharge
Two to four days postoperation.

HELLER'S OESOPHAGEAL CARDIOMYOTOMY (thoracic approach) (major)

Aim

To restore normal swallowing by division of the lower oesophageal musculature without breaching the mucosa.

Special consent

Informed.

Position of patient

Right lateral position with left side uppermost.

Incision

In the line of the seventh rib to the costal margin.

Procedure

Approach the oesophagus through the bed of the seventh rib. Divide the pleura; retract the lung forwards, and the diaphragm downwards. Free the oesophagus from the hiatus to the inferior pulmonary vein. Pass a rubber sling around it. Ask your assistant to apply gentle traction. Pass the index around the lower oesophagus and gently incise the muscle layer longitudinally. Separate the divided muscle with artery forceps or right-angled vascular clamps until the mucosa pouts outwards. Apply tissue forceps to the edge of the divided muscles and continue this process until the lower 10–12 cm of the muscle has been divided to the cardia. Take extreme care not to breach the mucosa. Ligate small vessels to apply gentle pressure until haemostasis is secure.

If perforation does occur, repair it with fine sutures (Vicryl). If this is unsuccessful it may be necessary to resuture the muscle layer to avoid fistula formation. In such cases consider oesophagectomy with either oesophagogastric anastomosis at the aortic arch or short-segment colon replacement.

Closure

Bring a chest drain through a separate stab wound. Approximate the ribs with a rib approximator. Close the rib bed with continuous nylon and the muscle layers separately with continuous Dexon. Close the skin with continuous nylon or Dexon.

Complications

- Leaking from unnoticed mucosal perforation. If this happens re-exploration should be carried out, with repair if possible. Oesophagogastrectomy may have to be considered.
- Dysphagia due to failure of the procedure. A further myotomy is necessary.
- Peptic stricture due to reflux. Prevent by the use of oral H_2-receptor antagonists or an antireflux procedure at the time of myotomy.
- Carcinoma of oesophagus. Patients should be screened on a regular basis by endoscopy or barium swallow. Achalasia is a premalignant condition.

HELLER'S OESOPHAGEAL CARDIOMYOTOMY (abdominal approach) (major)

Aim

To restore normal swallowing by longitudinal division of the lower oesophageal musculature.

Incision

Left upper paramedian.

Procedure

Mobilize the left lobe of the liver by division of the left triangular ligament. Fold the lobe to the right. Explore the abdomen and confirm the diagnosis.

Identify the oesophagus by palpation of the nasogastric tube. Divide the peritoneum and phreno-oesophageal ligament in front of the oesophagus. Preserve the vagus nerves. Now encircle the oesophagus with the index and thumb so that they meet behind. Pass a rubber tube around the gullet to provide traction.

Divide the muscle on the anterior wall of the stomach 1 cm below the cardia until *intact* mucosa bulges through. Extend this upwards for about 8–10 cm so that tissue forceps can be applied to the edges of the muscle.

NB The oesophageal mucosa is like wet blotting paper when isolated. Take care *not* to perforate it as it takes sutures poorly.

Identify the plane between muscle and mucosa with artery or vascular forceps alternately opening and closing them to split the muscle longitudinally and allowing mucosa to bulge through.

Check that there are no leaks. Stop bleeding.

Closure

Close the wound in layers with a suction drain brought out through a separate stab wound. Suture skin with interrupted sutures.

Discharge

Seven to ten days after operation for both thoracic and abdominal approaches.

195

TRUNCAL VAGOTOMY AND DRAINAGE (major)

Aim

To divide the vagus nerves to the stomach and so reduce the output of hydrochloric acid. It leads to a considerable degree of gastric stasis, and so a drainage procedure such as a gastro-enterostomy or pyloroplasty is carried out to prevent gastric stasis.

Special consent

Warn the patient of the possible postoperative complications, particularly dumping and diarrhoea, and obtain informed consent.

Preoperative preparation

This procedure is most commonly performed now for perforated or bleeding duodenal or gastric ulcers. However, it is still carried out in some hospitals for patients who fail to respond to H_2-receptor antagonist therapy. The diagnosis will have been established by endoscopy or barium studies. Patients with bleeding duodenal or gastric ulcers may need preoperative resuscitation with blood and IV fluids.

Routine haematological and biochemical parameters should be established before theatre and antibiotics prophylaxis should be given in emergencies, particularly after H_2-receptor antagonist therapy which leads to changes in the gastric and duodenal flora.

Incision

Upper midline.

Procedure

The peritoneal cavity is opened between artery forceps. The contents of the abdomen are examined. The size of the diaphragmatic hiatus is established, and the presence or absence of gallstones or diverticular disease is particularly noted. Insert a self-retaining retractor. Instruct your assistant to hold the retractor under the xiphisternum so that the left coronary ligament of the liver can easily be identified. Divide this ligament and fold the left lobe of the liver towards the midline. The peritoneum overlying the gastro-oesophageal junction can now be seen and identified as a fine white line. Gently incise this peritoneum and enlarge the opening so that the index finger of the right hand can be gently insinuated around the oesophagus to encircle it so that a length of red tubing can be passed around the lower end of the oesophagus to control it and so perform the vagotomy. Apply an artery forceps to the two ends of the rubber tubing.

Vagotomy technique

Apply gentle traction to the rubber tubing and, using the right index finger, carefully identify the anterior (which may be in multiple strands) and posterior vagus nerves. Clamp and divide them. They can be felt as tight bands on the anterior and posterior surfaces of the oesophagus. Ensure that haemostasis is secured. When the vagotomy has been performed, the oesophagus will appear to descend for some distance into the abdomen.

Drainage procedure

Either a pyloroplasty (preferable) or a gastroenterostomy can be performed.

Pyloroplasty (Heineke–Mikulicz) Identify the pylorus. Insert non-absorbable stay sutures at its upper and lower aspects. Using a knife divide the circular muscle longitudinally in line with the duodenum for a distance of only about 1–2 cm. Aspirate any contents, and suture the pylorus transversely to increase the size of its lumen using interrupted fine Dexon or Vicryl (more popular) sutures. If necessary, place an omental tag over the pyloroplasty.

Gastroenterostomy This procedure involves a gastro-jejunal anastomosis between the most dependent part of the stomach and the proximal jejunum. This can be performed in antecolic or retrocolic (better because it drains more easily).

Retrocolic isoperistaltic gastroenterostomy Identify the duodenojejunal flexure and select a portion of jejunum which is mobile enough to reach the most dependent part of the stomach. Ask your assistant to lift the transverse colon vertically. Make an incision on the lower aspect of the transverse mesocolon well clear of the middle colic artery. Enlarge this opening so that the most dependent part of the stomach can be pulled through it using Babcock's forceps. Apply soft gastro-intestinal clamps or gastroenterostomy clamps (Lane's) to the stomach border and the portion of jejunum selected for anastomosis. Carry out a gastrojejunal anastomosis in two layers with continuous absorbable sutures. Fix the edges of the gastroenterostomy to the mesocolon with interrupted absorbable sutures to prevent intussusception or herniation by a loop of small bowel.

Closure

Unless mass closure is used, close the wound in layers with absorbable suture to the peritoneum, non-absorbable to the midline, and interrupted Nylon or subcuticular Prolene to skin.

TRUNCAL VAGOTOMY AND DRAINAGE (major) (*cont.*)

Special postoperative care

Aspirate the nasogastric tube hourly for the first 12 hours and then remove it. (Some surgeons remove it at the end of the operation.) Give ice on the first postoperative and then 30 ml hourly by mouth on the second day. Encourage the patient to sit up to improve drainage. Increase fluids on the third day and graduate to light diet.

HIGHLY SELECTIVE VAGOTOMY
(parietal cell vagotomy, proximal gastric vagotomy) (major)

Aim

To denervate the acid-secreting portion of the stomach. The anterior and posterior nerves of Latarjet are preserved, but the branches which they give to the parietal cell area are divided. Thus the vagus nerve remains intact to supply the alkali-secreting cells of the gastric antrum and the vagal branches to the other abdominal viscera are preserved.

Special anatomy

The anterior and posterior nerves of Latarjet pass down the lesser curvature, giving off branches to the parietal cell area of the stomach. At the angulus they spread out in a 'crow's foot' to supply the antrum.

Preoperative preparation

As for truncal vagotomy and drainage. Cefuroxime prophylaxis is warranted in case of inadvertent gastrostomy and should always be used in emergencies.

Incision

Upper midline or left upper paramedian.

Procedure

After carrying out a laparotomy, open the gastrocolic omentum through an avascular area. Lift the stomach forwards and carefully separate its attachments posteriorly from the pancreas. Pass the right index finger through the defect in the gastrocolic omentum and grasp the gastric antrum, pulling it downwards. Stretch the lesser curvature of the stomach and so identify the anterior nerve of Latarjet. This nerve runs parallel to the lesser curve of the stomach and separates into branches over it. When the nerve has been identified, make a hole through the lesser omentum. Pass a tape around the angulus of the stomach to keep it on the stretch. Now, keeping close to the gastric wall, proceed proximally along the lesser curve, doubly clamping, dividing, and ligating the vessels and accompanying nerve filaments so as to strip the lesser omentum from the lesser curve. Continue this process along the anterior surface of the stomach and the gastro-oesophageal junction. Identify the angle of His between the fundus and the left edge of the lower oesophagus. Carefully incise the peritoneum and the angle and use finger dissection to encircle the cardia completely. Divide all loose tissue overlying the oesophagus and anteriorly and posteriorly, but keep the oesophageal muscle wall intact.

Now complete the mobilization of the greater curve of the stomach with division of the gastrocolic omentum to show the posterior nerve of Latarjet which terminates in the antrum distal to the incisura. Preserve the terminal fork of the nerve, and divide all other branches to the stomach. The objective of this operation is to separate the lesser omentum from the lesser curvature from the incisura to the cardia by dividing all

201

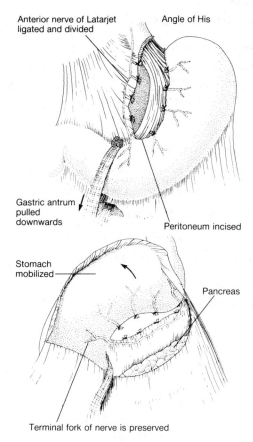

Highly selective vagotomy.

HIGHLY SELECTIVE VAGOTOMY
(parietal cell vagotomy, proximal gastric
vagotomy) (major) *(cont.)*

blood vessels and nerves that enter the lesser curvature from the lesser omentum. Vessels and nerves should be divided individually, and it is important to have early access to the posterior aspect of the stomach since the blood vessels run in two distinct bands, one to the anterior aspect and the other to the posterior aspect of the stomach.

Closure

Layers with interrupted Nylon or subcuticular Prolene to skin.

Special postoperative care

Withdraw the nasogastric tube and remove the IV infusion at the end of the procedure. Give ice only on the first postoperative day, graduating to 30 ml and 60–90 ml of water hourly by mouth on the second and third days respectively. Free fluids can commence on the fourth day, graduating to light diet thereafter.

Postoperative complications

- Necrosis of the lesser curvature of the stomach can occur owing to ischaemia or trauma to the gastric wall by diathermy or instrumental damage. It may cause death in one in 1000 highly selective vagotomy operations.
- Splenectomy may be necessary because of operative damage to the splenic capsule. If the organ cannot be repaired by suture or patched, it should be removed. Operative mortality, 0.3 per cent
- Recurrence in up to 15 per cent of patients.

Discharge

Seven to ten days after operation.

PERFORATED DUODENAL ULCER (major)

The gastric contents spill through the perforation leading to chemical peritonitis. Patients who undergo early surgery have an excellent prognosis. Conservative treatment should only be considered in patients who have had a long-standing perforation or who are too old or infirm to survive surgery.

Preoperative preparation

Establish urea and electrolyte status, and start an IV infusion. Exclude the possibility of acute pancreatitis by serum amylase estimation. In elderly patients or those with chronic obstructive airways disease take arterial samples for blood gas estimation.

Incision

Upper midline (preferable) or right paramedian.

Procedure

On opening the peritoneal cavity, a variable quantity of gastric fluid intermingled with bile will be encountered. Aspirate this with suction and retain a specimen for bacteriology. Identify the perforation. It is usually on the first part of the duodenum on its anterior wall. If not, check the posterior and superior aspects and the stomach. Perforations can also occur into the lesser sac. Oversew the perforation with one, two, or three Vicryl sutures (1/0, 2/0) placed some way (0.5 cm) proximal and distal to the ulcer. Tie them to close the perforation. Leave the ends long and bring an omental tag over the perforation. Lightly tie it in place. If it necroses, it falls off.

Now aspirate all four quadrants of the abdomen, the paracolic gutters, and the pelvis. There is usually no need to drain the abdomen unless the perforation is long-standing, but lavage with warm saline with or without antiseptics is valuable.

Closure

Layers with non-absorbable or absorbable sutures to rectus sheath and Nylon to skin.

Complications

Infection, abscess formation. Twenty-five per cent will relapse and may need definitive surgery, which should always be considered in fit patients, those with a proven chronic ulcer, those with a history of previous complications, and those with NSAID-induced perforation.

Discharge

Seven to ten days after operation.

INSERTION OF AN ANGELCHIK PROSTHESIS (major)

The Angelchik prosthesis is an anti-reflux device which is indicated in patients who have severe unremitting gastro-oesophageal reflux symptoms usually due to hiatus hernia.

Preoperative assessment

As for vagotomy procedures. Ask the anaesthetist to pass a nasogastric tube to facilitate identification of the oesophagus once the patient has been anaesthetized. Give prophylactic antibiotics (cefuroxime and metronidazole) on induction and 8 and 16 hours postoperatively.

Incision

Upper midline or left upper paramedian.

Procedure

Insert a self-retaining retractor. Mobilize the left lobe of the liver by dividing the left triangular ligament as in truncal vagotomy procedures. Divide the peritoneum overlying the oesophagus and encircle it. At this stage assess the extent of any hiatus hernia and attempt to reduce it gently into the abdomen.

When the oesophagus has been encircled pass the C-shaped Angelchik prosthesis around the gullet so that it sits at the cardio-oesophageal junction. Use Ligaclips to clamp its tapes together at two or three sites. Cut the redundant tape.

Closure

Mass or close in layers with interrupted Nylon to skin. No drain is required.

Special postoperative care

As for vagotomy and drainage.

Complications

- Infection. When this occurs the prosthesis must be removed. Therefore the operative technique must be as aseptic as possible and prophylactic antibiotics must be used.
- Migration of the device proximally. This may occur when there is a large diaphragmatic defect. Often it produces no symptoms.
- Ulceration of the prosthesis through the oesophagus or stomach.
- Oesophageal stricture. If stricture or ulceration of the prosthesis occurs it may be necessary to remove it. The patient

should be reassessed both endoscopically and radiologically, and full account taken of symptoms.

Discharge

Seven to ten days after operation.

OESOPHAGECTOMY (complex)

Indications

- Carcinoma
- Benign stricture due to caustic ingestion or trauma (not responsive to dilatation).
- Congenital disease

Preoperative investigations in carcinoma include endoscopy, barium studies, ultrasound, and CT scanning to determine both the size and length of the oesophageal lesion and to exclude hepatic metastases. Laparoscopy can assist in this.

Ivor Lewis oesophagectomy

This allows access to the oesophagus up to the aortic arch. It is a useful procedure to resect carcinomas of the middle and lower thirds of the oesophagus.

Position of patient

Initially supine for the abdominal part. Then in the left lateral position with pelvic and shoulder support for the thoracotomy.

Incision

Abdominal: upper midline

Thoracic (if resectable): right thoracotomy in the fifth or sixth rib space.

Procedure

Abdominal Exposure can be improved with a sternal retractor. Divide the left triangular ligament and retract the left lobe of the liver. Mobilize the stomach as for total gastrectomy. Preserve the spleen. Ligate and divide the left gastric artery last from behind the stomach but preserve the right gastric and right gastro-epiploic arteries. Divide the gastro-epiploic omentum but preserve the gastric arcades near the short gastrics proximally to maintain gastric viability. Make a 3–4 cm pyloroplasty, closing it with one or two layers of 3/0 Vicryl. Kocherize the duodenum to make it capable of being brought up virtually to the hiatus. Free the stomach from the diaphragm and dilate the oesophageal hiatus. Next divide the phreno-oesophageal ligament and begin the oesophageal dissection from below for as far as you can within the chest oesophageal hiatus. Divide the phreno-oesophageal ligament and begin the oesophageal dissection from below as far as you can within the chest.

Closure Close the abdomen with mass Nylon, with Prolene or nylon to skin. Insert a suction drain if you feel it necessary (not usually required).

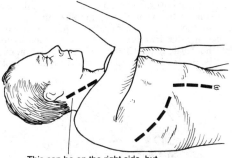

This can be on the right side, but
it is more usual on the left, as shown below.

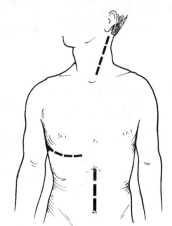

Abdominal and thoracic incisions are used
in Ivor Lewis's procedure.
Neck incision is for three-stage procedure.

Incisions for Ivor Lewis oesophagectomy. *Top*: **Three incisions for three-stage oesophagectomy.** *Below*: **Two incisions for Ivor Lewis oesophagectomy.**

Right thoracotomy Now place the patient in the left lateral position. Through the right thoracotomy assess the extent of the oesophageal tumour. The aim is to achieve 10 cm clearance above the tumour and at least 5 cm below, including the subcarinal and hilar lymph nodes. Divide and ligate the azygos vein and then dissect between the oesophagus and trachea anteriorly and the aorta posteriorly. Retract the lung forward and divide the pleura over the dorsal spine and the pulmonary ligament to the hiatus. Continue to mobilize the specimen downwards to the hiatus and, once free, pull the stomach through, checking that it will reach the proposed anastomotic site under the aortic arch. Clamp and divide the stomach about 5 cm below the tumour. Oversew the proximal end of

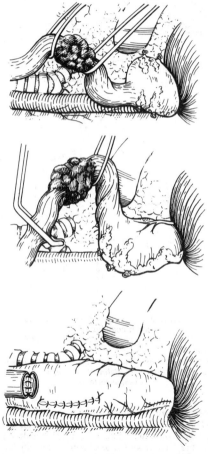

Thoracic mobilization via the right thorax (Ivor Lewis oesophagectomy).

the stomach with 3/0 Vicryl. Alternatively, use a linear stapler. Apply Babcock's forceps and a paediatric Doyen soft bowel clamp to the site of proximal division of the oesophagus to prevent retraction superiorly or spillage of oesophageal contents.

Now fashion the anastomosis between the gastric remnant (usually the cardia) and the proximal oesophagus either by hand with 3/0 Vicryl or by using a curved stapling gun passed through an anteriorly placed gastrostomy. A purse-string suture is only required on the oesophageal end.

In a hand-sewn anastomosis place two 4/0 sutures through the mucosa and muscle proximally to keep the mucosa in place. Insert 3/0 Vicryl interrupted sutures, taking good bites and tying the knots on the inside on the posterior wall. A seromuscular lay can also be inserted. If it is difficult to insert and tie the sutures, use the 'parachute' technique where the sutures are first inserted and the stomach is run up to the oesophagus. Keep the nasogastric tube through the anastomosis throughout.

211

Closure Use a rub approximator and close the thoracotomy with 1/0 or 2/0 Nylon, leaving a basal under water chest drain. Insert Nylon or Prolene to skin.

OESOPHAGOGASTRECTOMY FOR LOWER-THIRD CARCINOMAS (complex)

Position of patient

Right semi-lateral position with right knee flexed and a soft pad between the legs. Pelvic and shoulder–arm stabilization. Both arms are flexed.

Incision

Oblique midway between the umbilicus and xiphisternum in the line of the seventh or eighth left interspace. Divide the costal cartilage for the thoracotomy after first assessing the tumour for operability in the abdomen.

Procedure

Mobilize the stomach. Kocherize the duodenum. Make a pyloroplasty. Preserve the right gastric and right gastro-epiploic arcades. Detach the omentum with the specimen. Make a radial incision in the diaphragm from costal margin to right crus, leaving it intact so that it can be removed with the specimen.

Insert a self-retaining rib retractor. If there is not enough access excise 3–4 cm of exposed rib. Mobilize the oesophagus to the aortic arch behind the pulmonary hilum by freeing the lower lobe of the left lung and dividing the pulmonary ligament. Divide the mediastinal pleura anterior to the thoracic aorta. Retract the lower lung lobe forwards to display the posterior mediastinum.

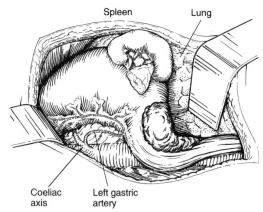

Thoraco-abdominal approach for lower-third oesophageal carcinoma.

Apply Babcock's forceps on each side of the oesophagus to prevent retraction and place Doyen paediatric soft bowel clamps across the proposed resection site which should be at least 5 cm above the growth. Transect the upper oesophagus and stomach (ow lower oesophagus) at least 5 cm below the growth. Transect the upper oesophagus and stomach (or lower oesophagus) at least 5 cm below the growth.

The anastomosis can be made either with a curved end-to-end stapler or by hand. In a hand-sewn anastomosis, make a gastrostomy underneath the stapled or sutured proximal stomach defect. Tuck the upper fundus behind the anastomosis and use 2/0 or 3/0 interrupted Vicryl through all coats. Pass a nasogastric tube through the anastomosis before completing this layer. Insert a second layer of sutures to draw the stomach over the anastomotic line.

Closure

213

Close the thorax in layers with a left basal underwater seal drain. Use mass closure for the abdomen with Nylon and Prolene to skin.

TOTAL OESOPHAGECTOMY (complex)

Incision

Abdominal: upper midline

Thoracic: right at the level of the fifth or sixth rib. This is not necessary if transhiatal dissection is successful.

Cervical: Right in line with the anterior border of sternomastoid.

Procedure

Abdominal

In the abdomen mobilize the stomach and begin transhiatal dissection using the fingers under direct vision as far as possible.

Through the cervical incision free the oesophagus from the trachea. Preserve the recurrent laryngeal nerve and continue finger dissection to meet below with the transhiatal dissection. If the tumour is bulky, it needs to be mobilized through the right thoracotomy (McKeown's three-stage procedure). Transhiatal resection is a blind procedure and must be undertaken very gently. The mobilized stomach and oesophagus is then drawn up through the thorax to the neck where, after resection of the specimen, an anastomosis can be fashioned between the pharynx and upper stomach in two layers of Vicryl. The stomach can be sutured to the anterior longitudinal ligament to relieve tension.

If the stomach cannot be mobilized to reach the neck or the patient has had previous gastric surgery, the right or left colon

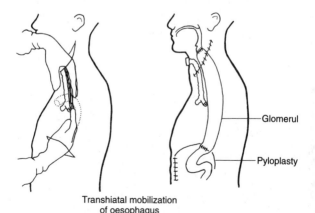

Transhiatal mobilization
of oesophagus

Pharangogastric anastomosis after three-stage or transhiatal oesophagectomy.

or jejunum can be used as a conduit mobilized on its mesentery or by microvascular anastomosis. A further alternative is to use a reversed gastric tube. Any pharyngeal defect can be closed with myocutaneous flaps and skin grafts.

Total oesophagectomy can be combined with laryngeal resection and pharyngogastric reconstruction (pharyngo-laryngo-oesophagectomy).

Right thoracotomy

Assess the oesophageal tumour. Divide adhesions. Ideally there should be 10 cm clearance of the oesophagus proximal to the tumour with at least a 5 cm clearance below. Include all subcarinal and hilar lymph nodes with the dissection of the specimen. Dissect between the oesophagus and the trachea anteriorly and the aorta posteriorly. The lung can be retracted forward. Divide the pleura over the dorsal spine and the pulmonary ligament to the hiatus. Mobilize the specimen downwards towards the oesophageal hiatus and, once it is free, pull the stomach through and ensure that it reaches the proposed anastomotic site under the aortic arch. Check its viability. Oversew the cardia. This can also be done with a linear stapler. Before dividing the oesophagus, apply Babcock's forceps to its proximal aspect to prevent retraction of it superiorly. Paediatric Doyen soft bowel clamps may also be used to avoid spillage of oesophageal contents.

When the cardia and the proximal oesophagus have been divided remove the specimen. Avoid retraction of the oesophageal mucosa on the proximal end by inserting some 4/0 sutures to pin the mucosa to the muscle layer. Good bites of the mucosa are the key to success with the anastomosis. The oesophagogastric anastomosis can be fashioned using a curved end-to-end anastomosis stapler passed through a gastrostomy. A purse-string suture is required at the oesophageal end. Hand-sewn anastomosis with an end-to-side oesophagogastric anastomosis can be fashioned using interrupted or continuous sutures in one or two layers. 3/0 Vicryl is ideal but the outer seromuscular layer can be fashioned with silk. Make the gastrostomy for the anastomosis in the anterior part of the pulled through stomach to tag some stomach behind the anastomosis, ensuring that there is no tension. When the anastomosis is being made, the posterior inner-layer (interrupted sutures) has the knots tied on the inside. A mattress suture may allow accurate interposition of the two mucosal edges. The 'parachute' technique can be employed where the sutures are placed first and then the stomach run up to the oesophagus. Remember to place a nasogastric tube through the anastomosis under vision and with digital control.

The azygos and hemiazygos veins can be divided if a further few centimetres are needed for clearance. This can be achieved by dividing the azygos anteriorly at the superior

215

TOTAL OESOPHAGECTOMY (complex)
(*cont.*)

vena cava and posteriorly over the dorsal vertebral bodies. Be sure not to damage the intercostal veins.

Closure
The thoracotomy is closed in layers using a rib approximator. 2/0 or 1/0 Nylon is ideal, leaving a basal underwater chest drain. Insert Prolene to skin.

Complications
- Anastomotic breakdown. Suspect if there is fever, leucocytosis, or pleural effusion. Investigate with Gastrografin swallow. Manage with nil by mouth, intercostal drainage, antibiotics, and parenteral nutrition.
- Aspiration pneumonia.
- Reflex or dumping type syndromes.
- Dysphagia from tumour recurrence or anastomotic stricture.
- Venous thromboembolism.
- Hiatus and diaphragmatic herniation.

CELESTIN INTUBATION OF INOPERABLE OESOPHAGEAL CANCER

This is a palliative procedure which should be considered in patients with advanced disease or who are too frail to undergo major oesophageal resection. It can also be performed as a preliminary to radiotherapy in patients with squamous carcinoma to ensure patency and to maintain swallowing.

Preoperative preparation

The patient may need a short period of IV feeding or IV fluid and electrolyte replacement, but there is no evidence that prolonged attempts at nutrition change the outcome (2–3 weeks). If the obstruction is complete, nasogastric aspiration of the oesophageal contents will prevent inhalation.

Incision

Upper midline.

Procedure

Identify the tumour. It usually lies at the oesophagogastric junction, the lower third of the oesophagus, or the proximal stomach. Confirm that it is not operable. Give the patient cefuroxime 500 mg IV at induction and 8 and 16 hours after operation.

Make a gastrostomy distal to the tumour. Aspirate the stomach contents. Insert the index finger proximally. Can you pass it into the oesophageal lumen? Is the nasogastric tube in the stomach? If so, ask the anaesthetist to attach the Celestin introducer to the nasogastric tube by passing a suture through both after removing the funnel of the nasogastric tube. Railroad the introducer into the stomach. The anaesthetist now ties the Celestin tube to the introducer using the special groove provided and the introducer is gently pulled downwards by the surgeon, with the tube being guided into the gullet at the mouth by the anaesthetist. Continue traction on the tube until its 'thistle-funnel' impacts against the shoulders of the tumour. Suture the tube in place with two 2/0 black silk sutures tied loosely and passing from outside the stomach through the lumen of the tube. Remove the redundant tubing by bevelling the end of the tube. Close the gastrostomy with two layers of continuous 2/0 catgut or Vicryl.

Closure

The peritoneum and linea alba can be closed together with continuous non-absorbable sutures. The skin can be closed with interrupted Nylon.

Special postoperative care

Take a chest X-ray to exclude perforation. Give ice on the first postoperative day and then graded fluids on the second and third days (as in vagotomy and drainage).

Complications

Since the procedure is not completely aseptic and the patient is often ill, wound infection is a potential risk. Be prepared to remove one or two sutures to allow drainage of pus, if necessary.

Difficulties

Sometimes the nasogastric tube cannot be passed into the stomach. In such cases a guide wire may be passed from above endoscopically or the introducer may be passed upwards through the gastrostomy, using the index finger to guide it into the lumen of the oesophagus.

Discharge

Seven to ten days after operation.

HIATUS HERNIA (extra major)

Aims

- Closure of the hiatus after reducing the hernia.
- Maintaining the oesophagogastric junction beneath the diaphragm and establishing a length of intra-abdominal oesophagus
- Fashioning an acute angle between the oesophagus and the gastric fundus.

Procedures

Nissen fundoplication
In this procedure the hernia is reduced at laparotomy and a wide-bore tube passed into the stomach. The limbs of the right crus are then approximated behind the oesophagus by sutures (one or two usually suffice). The gastric fundus is then carefully mobilized by dividing the gastrosplenic omentum and is wrapped around the lower oesophagus to form a cuff of stomach behind, in front, and on each side. The stomach is held in place by non-absorbable sutures.

Belsey Mark IV operation
This is carried out through a left sixth-interspace thoracotomy. The entire oesophagus in its lower part is freed up to the level of the aortic arch. The cardia is mobilized and pulled up through the hiatus. The acute angle of entry of the oesophagus into the stomach is then re-established by a series of mattress sutures passing from the oesophagus to the fundus and back up through the diaphragm. At the end of the procedure the right crus is approximated behind the oesophagus.

Other procedures can be performed such as the Collis operation in which the right crus is sutured in front of the oesophagus and the fundus is sutured to the undersurface of the diaphragm to re-establish the acute angle of entry or gastropexy in which the anterior surface of the stomach is sutured to the linea alba (Boerema anterior gastropexy) or the lesser curve is fixed to the median arcuate ligament (Hill posterior gastropexy). If increased oesophageal length is required, a gastroplasty (Collis) can be performed. In this a tube is fashioned from the lesser curvature to lengthen the gullet and the gastric fundus is sutured to the arcuate ligament. (See also Angelchik prosthesis, p. 148.)

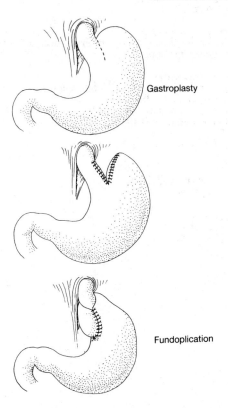

Gastroplasty

Fundoplication

Operative procedures for hiatus hernia.

GASTRECTOMY (extra major)

Indications

Partial gastrectomy
Carcinoma of distal stomach, benign gastric and duodenal ulcers, benign tumours.

Total gastrectomy
Carcinoma of proximal stomach, multifocal carcinomas, Zollinger–Ellison syndrome.

Intestinal continuity is re-established by gastroduodenal anastomosis (Billroth I) or gastrojejunal anastomosis (Billroth II or Polya).

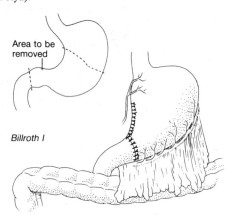

Billroth I

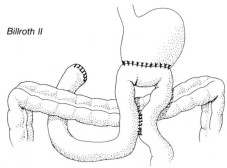

Billroth II

Polya   As Billroth II but with retrocolic anastomosis

Gastrectomy: anastomosis.

Preoperative preparation

Check haemoglobin, electrolyte, and nutritional status. Correct if necessary by replacement therapy or parenteral nutrition. Treat shock if present. Wash out the stomach if it contains food or debris. Assess cardiorespiratory status. Pre- and postoperative physiotherapy is of value. Check liver and renal function. Use prophylactic antibiotics particularly in emergencies, in patients with carcinoma, and in those who have received prolonged H_2 receptor antagonists. Consider CT or laparoscopic staging.

Incision

Upper midline or paramedian. Oblique with thoracic extension if oesophagogastrectomy is indicated.

Procedure

Identify the pathology. Assess the extent of spread of a carcinoma. Are there metastases locally or in the liver? If so, consider palliative or no surgery.

Mobilize the stomach along its curves as required. If there is a carcinoma excise the omentum and lymph nodes. At the pyloric end of the lesser curve identify, ligate, and divide the right gastric artery. On the greater curve identify, ligate, and divide the right gastro-epiploic artery. Divide the short gastric arteries and the left gastro-epiploic arteries at the cardiac end of the greater curve.

Mobilize the duodenum by dividing the peritoneum along its lateral border. Divide between clamps and oversew it. Now use the stomach as its own retractor by lifting it upwards by its distal clamp. Identify and ligate the left gastric artery at the proximal end of the lesser curve.

Divide the stomach at its midpoint between clamps, partially close the lesser curve, and perform an antecolic gastrojejunal anastomosis in two layers using an absorbable suture.

Closure

In layers. Nylon or Prolene to skin.

Special postoperative care

Insert a nasogastric tube after the operation. Aspirate it hourly for the first 12 hours to observe for haemorrhage. Begin oral fluids on the third postoperative day. Observe for evidence of gastric bloating or anastomotic leakage.

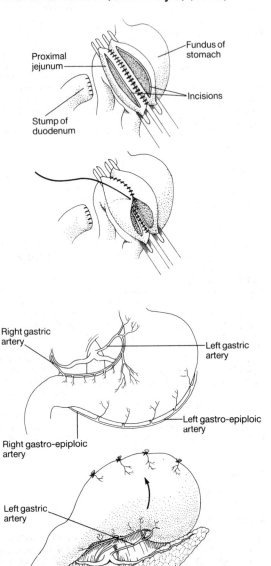

Fundus of stomach

Proximal jejunum

Stump of duodenum

Incisions

Right gastric artery

Left gastric artery

Right gastro-epiploic artery

Left gastro-epiploic artery

Left gastric artery

Gastrectomy: procedure.

Complications

Early
- Haemorrhage
- Anastomotic leakage (up to 3 days postoperatively)
- Gastric bloating

Late
- Recurrent disease
- Metabolic complications
- Postgastrectomy syndromes

Discharge

Seven to ten days after operation.

CHOLECYSTECTOMY (major, extra major)

Aim

This is an elective operation (usually) to remove the gall
bladder and its contents and to retain the anatomy of the
biliary system.

Indications

Cholelithiasis, carcinoma, cholangiohepatitis, empyema or
perforation of the gall bladder, traumatic rupture, bile duct
cancers.

Diagnosis

This is suspected by clinical signs and symptoms and confirmed by ultrasonography or cholecystography.

Special anatomy

There is great variability in the anatomy of the gall bladder
and bile ducts. You should not attempt this operation until
you are fully conversant with these.

Incisions

Several approaches may be used.
- Right paramedian incision
- Kocher's (subcostal) incision (in obese patients)
- Transverse
- Midline

The rectus muscle is reflected in a paramedian incision or
divided with diathermy in a Kocher's or transverse incision.
The peritoneum is opened between artery forceps. A self-
retaining retractor is inserted.

Procedure

A full laparotomy is performed. There is an incidence of colorectal carcinoma of about 5 per cent. If this is found, it
should be dealt with first. If a Kocher's incision has been
made, it may be necessary to close it and make a fresh incision
to obtain access.

The gall bladder is identified and the small bowel packed
downwards to expose the biliary tree. The assistant's left hand
maintains exposure. The liver is retracted with a Deaver
retractor held in the assistant's right hand.

Sponge-holding forceps are applied to the gall bladder near
its junction with the cystic duct and gentle traction applied by
the operator. The peritoneum overlying the neck of the gall
bladder is then carefully incised and the junction of the cystic

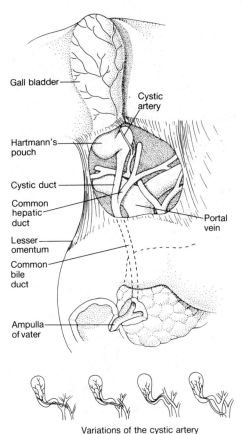

Variations of the cystic artery

Gall bladder and bile ducts.

duct with the common bile duct (CBD) carefully exposed by sweeping away the peritoneum with gauze. The cystic artery is exposed close to the cystic duct by the same method and its destination to the gall bladder is confirmed. It is then ligated at two sites and divided between the ligatures. Now the gall bladder is attached to the CBD by the cystic duct only. At this stage carry out on-table cholangiography either by passing a

CHOLECYSTECTOMY (major, extra major) (*cont.*)

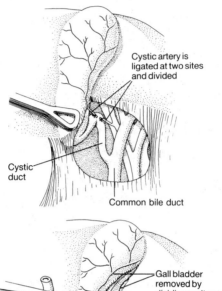

Cholecystectomy.

cholangiogram catheter into the CBD via the cystic duct or by the direct puncture technique. Take two films (or use image intensification) after injection of 2–4 ml and 6–8 ml of contrast. If this excludes stones and shows good flow into the duodenum, ligate the cystic duct almost flush with the CBD with Vicryl, ensuring that there is no narrowing.

The gall bladder can now be removed by dividing its peritoneal attachments to the liver.

Closure

Secure haemostasis in the gall bladder bed either by diathermy or by oversewing the peritoneum with catgut. Bring a suction drain (Redivac) through a separate stab wound from the gall bladder bed. Close the wound in layers with Dexon or Vicryl to the peritoneum and non-absorbable suture to the rectus sheath. Insert interrupted or continuous sutures to the skin. Stitch the drain in position. Check that the swab count is correct.

Specific postoperative care

As with all upper abdominal surgery, physiotherapy should be prescribed for at-risk patients to prevent pulmonary atelectasis. Revacuum the drain daily and measure the drainage. As it reduces, the drain may be removed between 3 and 5 days after operation. Remove the sutures between 7 and 10 days (7 days is the ideal).

Complications

Pulmonary atelectasis, subphrenic abscess, retained stones, damage to the common bile duct

Discharge

Seven to ten days after operation.

EXPLORATION OF THE COMMON BILE DUCT (major)

This is usually performed during a cholecystectomy or as a secondary procedure for retained stones. A single dose of prophylactic antibiotics is usually given, unless there is cholangitis when antibiotic treatment is indicated. Prophylactic antibiotics are routinely given.

Indications

- Stones or block seen on operative cholangiography performed as a routine during cholecystectomy
- Stones palpated in CBD
- CBD thick-walled or dilated
- Obstructive jaundice
- Retained stones

The exploration may be supraduodenal (most common), retroduodenal, or transduodenal.

Procedure

Divide the hepaticocolic ligament if not already done at cholecystectomy. Insert two stay sutures into the wall of the supraduodenal duct parallel to each other. Place a swab in the hepato-renal pouch to collect bile leakage and stones. Open the duct with a knife for about 1 cm. Note and aspirate the bile. If it is a thick sludge, consider transduodenal sphincterotomy or a choledochoduodenostomy in older patients to prevent further problems. Fortunately, most stones can be flushed out of the CBD with sterile saline injected through a soft rubber catheter inserted into the opening in the duct. Difficult stones can be removed by passing a modified Fogarty catheter past the stones, inflating the balloon, and gently withdrawing the catheter. Prevent proximal migration of stones above the choledochostomy with gentle digital pressure or a bulldog clamp. Explore the proximal duct in similar manner.

Insert the Desjardin's forceps upwards and downwards and feel for stones. Wash out the ducts with saline passed through a catheter. If stones are still felt, pass the Desjardin's forceps and try to remove them. If they cannot be removed, use the choledochoscope to visualize and remove them either complete or after crushing. The use of the choledochoscope requires considerable experience. Flush the ducts proximally and distally several times to remove clot and debris.

Prepare as small a T-tube as possible (Maingot 14) by fashioning its short limb into a gutter. Bring the long limb through a stab wound on the abdominal wall and insert the short limb into the choledochostomy. Ensure that bile flows freely up the long limb. Close the choledochostomy above the T-tube with 3/0 Vicryl.

Impacted stones

If a stone is impacted at the lower end of the duct, mobilize and open the duodenum along its convex border to expose the ampulla. Pass a Bakes' dilator, or preferably a soft rubber catheter from above. If the stone passes through, all is well. If not, slit the ampullary orifice gently until the stone passes through followed by the probe. Close the duodenostomy transversely in two layers of 00 catgut. An alternative is endoscopic sphincterotomy in selected patients. Do not use the Bakes' to dilate a stricture.

Stricture

If there is a stricture distally, perform a duodenotomy and pass a probe or a fine Bakes' dilator to mark the sphincteric orifice. Cut down on it for 1 cm or so with a knife or diathermy and divide the sphincter. Stop bleeding. Suture the duodenal mucosa to that of the CBD on each side using 4/0 Vicryl. Close the duodenotomy and insert the T-tube in the CBD. This procedure is a sphincteroplasty. Choledochoduodenostomy is an alternative to sphincteroplasty. Longitudinal incisions are made in the supraduodenal portion of the CBD and the duodenal bulb. The two are anastomosed with interrupted Vicryl, inserting all the sutures first and tying them at the end of the procedure bringing the two openings together to form a diamond-shaped anastomosis. Ascending cholangitis is a rare complication of the procedure.

231

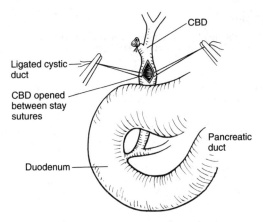

Supraduodenal choledochostomy.

TRANSDUODENAL
SPHINCTEROPLASTY (extra major)

This procedure is associated with postoperative pahcreatitis which has a high morbidity and mortality. Endoscopic papillotomy is a reasonable alternative.

Indications

• Gallstones impacted at the lower end of the CBD with or without stricture which cannot be removed by supraduodenal choledochotomy.

Procedure

If supraduodenal choledochotomy fails to retrieve stones, place two 3/0 Vicryl sutures on the duodenum opposite the ampulla. Make a 3 cm longitudinal duodenotomy using diathermy. The ampulla can then be identified by passing a soft Harris catheter through the supraduodenal choledochotomy when it will bulge into the duodenum. Make a 1 cm vertical incision using diathermy on the medial side of the duodenum over the stone and the ampulla. This is made easier by placing stay sutures on each side of the proposed incision using 3/0 Vicryl. Achieve haemostasis and suture the CBD mucosa to the duodenal mucosa with 4/0 Vicryl. Lengthen the incision upwards in stages and complete the 2 cm sphincteroplasty with interrupted 4/0 Vicryl between the CBD and the duodenal mucosa. A sphincterotomy alone risks scarring with further stenosis. Leave a T-tube in place through the supraduodenal choledochotomy. Any retained stones should now be able to pass through the widened ampulla.

Closure

Close the duodenum transversely to avoid stricture formation. Use two layers of continuous 3/0 Vicryl.

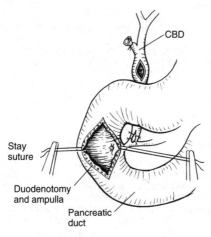

CBD

Stay
suture

Duodenotomy
and ampulla

Pancreatic
duct

233

Transduodenal sphincteroplasty.

CHOLECYSTOSTOMY (major)

Indications

- Cholecystitis or empyema associated with cholangitis or jaundice.
- As a safe alternative in the medically unwell or elderly. Interval cholecystectomy may be carried out if the patient improves clinically.

Incision

Upper midline

Procedure

If the gall bladder is tense, empty it using a suction trocar. This will remove the infected bile without spillage. Then enlarge the stab wound and remove stones through the cholecystostomy using straight Desjardin's forceps. Do not remove the gall bladder unless it is quite clearly gangrenous. When the gall bladder is empty, place a double purse-string suture of 2/0 or 3/0 Vicryl around the cholecystostomy and insert a Foley catheter which has been introduced to the abdominal cavity through a separate stab wound. Inflate the balloon and tie the purse-string suture over the balloon. A cholangiogram can be performed at 7–10 days down the catheter and may indicate the need for ERCP and removal of common duct stones through a sphincterotomy before an interval cholecystectomy is carried out. If the patient is very frail, a cholecystostomy may be all that is required provided that the gall bladder and CBD are free of stones. The Foley catheter can then be removed at about 10–14 days. The tract which has formed by this time will simply close provided that there is no distal obstruction.

BILIARY BYPASS PROCEDURES

Choledochoduodenostomy (extra major)

This is a suitable alternative in older patients in whom the bottom end of a CBD cannot be cleared.

Procedure

A vertical duodenotomy is made opposite the supraduodenal choledochotomy made for the CBD exploration. Both these incisions should be about 2 cm long and made between stay sutures which can be used to maintain both the duodenum and the CBD wide open, thereby facilitating the placement of sutures. Use 3/0 Vicryl and a round-bodied needle and start the anastomosis at the midpoint of each opening. Taking one side at a time, place 2–3 mm bites 2–3 mm apart, tying the sutures on the mucosal aspect. The duodenum is slowly rolled upwards towards the stoma. When you are at the half-way point, begin to place the bites so that the knots are tied on the outside. Eventually a 1–2 cm wide stoma is made. One or two extra seromuscular sutures keep the duodenum in place over the stoma. The anastomosis does not need stenting with a T-tube nor does it need peritoneal drainage.

The major complication of this procedure is ascending cholangitis.

Choledochojejunostomy (extra major)

Indications
- Palliative decompression of the biliary tree, usually in patients with pancreatic cancer. When the gall bladder is not distended or absent or there is obstruction of the lower end of the cystic duct.
- Strictures of the CBD.

Procedure

Prepare a Roux loop of jejunum. Identify the supraduodenal CBD and gently free it from the portal vein posteriorly. Pass a ligature around it and tie it as low as possible. Now divide the duct above the stricture. Biliary leakage can be prevented with a soft vascular clamp.

Bring up the Roux loop and anastomose its open end to the cross-clamped CBD with one or two layers of continuous or interrupted 3/0 Vicryl on a round-bodied needle. Tacking sutures between the seromuscular layer of the Roux loop will draw the bowel up over the suture line to reduce tension.

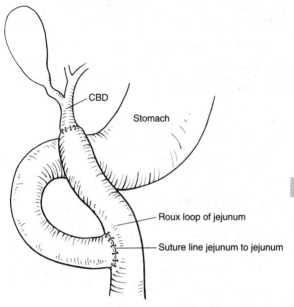

CBD

Stomach

Roux loop of jejunum

Suture line jejunum to jejunum

Choledochojejunostomy with a Roux loop of jejunum.

Cholecyst-enterostomy (major)

Indications
- Palliative relief of jaundice in patients with malignant and unresectable obstructive lesions of the lower CBD in the presence of a distended gall bladder.
- Benign bile duct stricture (occasionally)

Procedure
Identify the duodenojejunal junction by lifting the transverse colon and omentum upwards. Bring the first part of the jejunum up to the gall bladder. If the gall bladder is distended, use a trochar and cannula to aspirate it. Apply soft occlusion clamps to the gall bladder and jejunal loop. Insert seromuscular sutures to the gall bladder and small bowel. Make a 2–3 cm opening in each and insert an all-coats layer of continuous 3/0 Vicryl to create the anastomosis. Then complete the seromuscular suture. Usually no drainage is required. To ensure

BILIARY BYPASS PROCEDURES (*cont.*)

free flow of jejunal contents an enteroanastomosis is fashioned, and in patients with malignant disease a gastroenterostomy is added to prevent vomiting (triple bypass).

Complications after biliary surgery

Most patients can go home within 7 days after uncomplicated open cholecystectomy and within 1–3 days after laparoscopic cholecystectomy. However, complications can occur.

General
- Wound infection (should be less than 5 per cent)
- Chest infections, atelectasis: both can be prevented by physiotherapy and early mobilization
- Venous thromboembolism

Specific
- Biliary leak: this should settle spontaneously provided that there are no distal stones on cholangiography.
- Subhepatic, subphrenic abscess: these can be diagnosed and monitored by ultrasound and drained percutaneously.
- Jaundice: may be due to CBD damage at the time of surgery or scarring subsequent to devascularization of the common ducts.
- Retained stones: may be seen on T-tube cholangiography on the seventh or eighth post-surgery day. They can be dealt with by flushing methods, dissolution endoscopic surgery, or open surgery (in some cases).

238

Triple=bypass procedure for inoperable carcinoma of the head of the pancreas: (1) cholecystojejunostomy; (2) entero-anastomosis; (3) gastro-enterostomy.

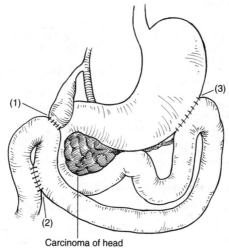

(1)

(3)

(2)

Carcinoma of head
of pancreas

239

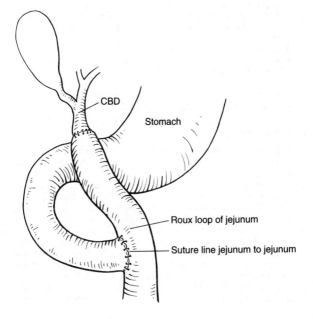

CBD

Stomach

Roux loop of jejunum

Suture line jejunum to jejunum

SMALL BOWEL RESECTION AND ANASTOMOSIS

Indications

- Congenital atresias, stenosis, and intussusception.
- Diverticula commonly causing perforation or bleeding. Rarely, causing nutritional problems (because of blind-loop syndrome).
- Trauma: blunt or penetrating which causes damage to bowel or mesentery.
- Infective conditions: Crohn's disease, salmonella, or tuberculous disease leading to stricture obstruction, perforation, or bleeding.
- Neoplastic diseases (rare).
- Vascular complications following strangulated hernia, volvulus, or mesenteric embolus.
- Fistulae due to unsuccessful or inadequate surgery.

Ideals for successful anastomosis

Anastomoses in the small bowel are sound provided that the bowel is viable and free from disease. This is different from large bowel resection which often needs exteriorization, particularly when unprepared or in the presence of perforation or obstruction.

- Exposure must be adequate.
- The bowel should be as empty as possible.
- There should be good and even approximation of the two ends.
- There should be no tension.
- There should be no peritoneal soiling.
- Defects in the mesentery must be closed to prevent internal herniation.
- There should be no complicating factors (e.g. poor blood supply to cut ends, anaemia, malnutrition, radiotherapy).

Procedure

Select the section of bowel to be resected and gently lift it out of the wound. Hold the bowel to the light so that the vascular pattern can be seen and choose the line for resection. If the resection is for benign disease the vessels can be divided and ligated close to the bowel. If it is for malignant disease, a generous V-shaped portion of mesentery should be resected with the affected segment. Divide the near-side layer of mesentery with scissors in a V-shape and gently ligate and divide the vessels between artery forceps. Do this up to the bowel wall. Apply light crushing clamps (Kocher or Stevenson) from the antimesenteric border and angle them to include more of the antimesenteric border than the mesenteric border. Apply a second pair of crushing clamps parallel to these at the same angle, and again at the same angle apply soft occlusion clamps about 8 cm away from the double clamps after first emptying the bowel by milking the contents in either direction. Now divide between the crushing clamps and remove the resection specimen. Resection can be carried out without clamps, in selected patients.

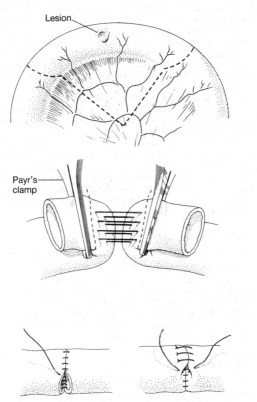

Anastomosis in two continuous layers

Intestinal resection and anastomosis.

241

SMALL BOWEL RESECTION AND ANASTOMOSIS (cont.)

End-to-end anastomosis

Ask your assistant to hold the crushing clamps to bring the two ends of the bowel together. Now gently turn the clamps back on themselves and join the adjacent walls of the small bowel with a seromuscular Lembert suture. When this has been completed, cut across the bowel beneath the crushing clamps and remove them. Now join the bowel together with an all-coats over-and-over suture using 2/0 chromic catgut or Vicryl. The stitches should be less than 0.5 cm apart and pick up about 0.5 cm of bowel wall. Continue this layer round the corner and on to the anterior wall and tie it at the other corner. Remove the non-crushing clamps and complete the seromuscular Lembert stitch on the other wall; tie it when completed. Now place interrupted sutures in the mesenteric defect to close it, taking care not to pick up mesenteric vessels. The use of a double-ended suture makes end-to-end anastomosis even easier.

NB To turn the corner pass the needle from the mucosa outwards on one corner to the serosa inwards on the other followed by the mucosa outwards on the same side to the serosa inwards on the other, thus forming a series of loops on the mucosal surface (the Connell suture, which is not haemostatic at the edges). Once the corner is passed, continue with the over-and-over suture.

Disparity of the lumen

When the lumina of the bowel are of different sizes the anastomosis can be effected by longitudinal division of the antimesenteric border of the bowel with the smaller lumen. Anastomosis is then carried out as above. This procedure is commonly indicated in cases of obstruction where the bowel distal to the obstructive lesion is collapsed.

Linear and side-to-side stapling instruments can also be used for anastomosis (see Chapter 7).

Other procedures

There is some clinical and experimental evidence that small bowel inverting anastomoses are safer, although many stapling techniques evert with safety.

End-to-side or side-to-side anastomoses should follow similar principles. They are alternatives when stenosis is possible, particularly when there is disparity between bowel ends.

Side-to-side anastomosis can be made easier using twin-bladed clamps (Lane's), but they are cumbersome and the trauma that they cause may outweigh their function of preventing spillage from the bowel.

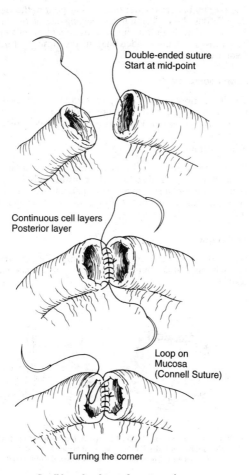

Double-ended suture
Start at mid-point

Continuous cell layers
Posterior layer

Loop on
Mucosa
(Connell Suture)

Turning the corner

Small bowel end-to-end anastomosis.

ILEOSTOMY

The terminal ileum is exteriorized as a spout in the right iliac fossa. Effluent is collected in a collecting bag (ileostomy bag). The procedure is an option in the treatment of inflammatory bowel disease, familial adenomatous polyposis, and proximal colonic obstruction.

Loop ileostomy

This is exteriorization of a loop of terminal ileum, usually as a temporary procedure to decompress obstruction or protect a distal anastomosis (e.g. following restorative proctocolectomy).

Preparation

Counsel the patient. As for colostomies, the ileostomy should be sited in the right iliac fossa clear of the umbilicus and anterior superior iliac spine. The patient should wear an ileostomy bag for 24 hours before siting to determine the best spot.

Technique

Divide the terminal ileum between clamps. Remove the distal part with the colon if this is a total colectomy. If not, close the distal end.

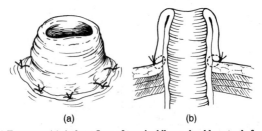

(a)   (b)

(a) Ileostomy (a) At least 5 cm of terminal ileum should protrude from the abdominal wall. (b) The mucosa is everted with Babcocks tissue forceps and sutured to the skin of the abdominal wall.

Pick up the skin marked for the ileostomy with tissue forceps and excise a circular area. Divide the underlying aponeurosis and muscle. Do not divide the peritoneum if the ileostomy is to be extraperitoneal. Divide the peritoneum if the ileostomy is going to traverse the peritoneal cavity.

For an extraperitoneal ileostomy make a tunnel under the peritoneum from the caecal reflexion to the anterior abdominal wall (preferred method).

For transperitoneal ileostomy draw the ileum through the opening on the anterior abdominal wall so that it protrudes for several centimetres. Insert a few interrupted stitches between the aponeurosis and the ileum to anchor it. Close the lateral peritoneal space to prevent herniation and then close the main abdominal wound. Now trim the bowel ends if required and gently evert the edges with Babcock's forceps to draw them down to skin level, thus forming a spout which should be at least 5 cm from the skin to permit close application of the ileostomy bag with discharge of effluent well away from the skin. Stitch the mucosa to the skin with interrupted catgut sutures.

Complications

Prolapse, retraction, necrosis, recurrence of disease (usually Crohn's disease).

EXCISION OF MECKEL'S DIVERTICULUM

In infancy embryological remnants may present as an abscess with perforation, obstruction, or fistula. In adults indications for surgery are as follows.

- Inflammation leading to perforation and peritonitis. If the appendix is normal always search for an inflamed Meckel's diverticulum.
- Bleeding: heterotopic 'peptic' epithelium may be the cause.
- Intussusception.

Incision

McBurney or Lanz (a lower midline laparotomy when the diagnosis is uncertain).

Procedure

Isolate the segment of ileum containing Meckel's diverticulum and apply light non-crushing paediatric Doyen clamps after milking the contents of the ileum away from the area. Protect the wound and peritoneum with abdominal packs. The diverticulum can be excised after applying light crushing clamps longitudinally and cutting the specimen away using a scalpel against the clamps. The enterostomy is closed transversely in two continuous layers to avoid stenosis.

If the diverticulum is large and encroaching upon the intestinal lumen or presenting as an impacted intussusception, a limited small bowel resection is required. There is rarely any need to excise mesentery in this resection.

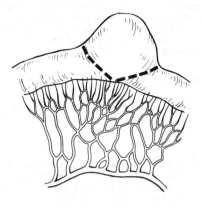

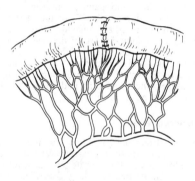

Excision of Meckel's diverticulum.

SPLENECTOMY (major)

The spleen plays a vital role in normal immunological function. It may be removed electively in cases of hypersplenism and massive splenomegaly. It may also be removed as an emergency after trauma. Every effort should be made to preserve the normal spleen.

Elective procedure

Incision
Midline incision extending to umbilicus or beyond. This may be extended transversely or into the chest for very large spleens.

Procedure
Identify the splenic artery arising from the coeliac axis and running along the superior border of the pancreas. Tie it first in continuity. This is done by opening the lesser sac of the peritoneum and isolating the artery before passing a ligature around it.

Now place the left hand, palm downwards, over the top of the spleen and draw it medially. Divide the peritoneum lateral to the spleen proximally and distally. Draw the spleen forwards, lifting the splenic flexure of the colon and the tail of the pancreas. Identify the splenic pedicle, tie the vein and the artery separately, and divide them. Now divide the other attachments of the spleen: the phrenicosplenic ligament and the lienorenal ligaments. Identify and divide the short gastric arteries and remove the spleen.

Emergency procedure

The assistant retracts the left side of the abdominal wall and the left hand of the operator is passed over the spleen which is then drawn forwards; and the peritoneum lateral to and above it is divided. The splenic pedicle is then identified, and the artery and the vein are ligated and divided in turn. The procedure is then continued as for an elective splenectomy.

Closure

The wound is closed in layers with a suction drain brought out through a separate stab wound and Nylon or Prolene to skin.

Complications

- Haemorrhage
- Acute pancreatitis from damage to the tail of the pancreas
- Subphrenic abscess
- Overwhelming post-splenectomy infection (OPSI)

Salvaging the spleen

OPSI is a major complication and may cause death in around 5 per cent of splenectomized patients. Some patients (25 per cent) may be managed conservatively if they are stable with no other intra-abdominal injury and if the extent of splenic damage is minimal on CT scan, radionuclide scanning, or laparoscopy.

At laparotomy splenic artery ligation is valuable for preservation, particularly for multiple tears of the hilar region. Partial splenectomy may also be effected by ligation of individual branches of the splenic artery. Other methods include ligation of the short gastric arteries to control bleeding, the insertion of mattress sutures, staples, or the application of collagen-impregnated packs.

If the spleen has to be removed, autotransplantation of sliced spleen into the omentum may provide protection. Otherwise long-term antibiotics or vaccination are necessary.

249

References

Buyukunal, C., Danismend, D., and Yeker, D. (1987). Spleen saving procedures in paediatric splenic trauma. *British Journal of Surgery*, **74**, 350–2.

APPENDICECTOMY (major)

The clinical presentation varies according to the anatomical position. Classically, tenderness is maximal over McBurney's point.

Preoperative preparation

Give the patient one suppository of metronidazole per rectum when the diagnosis is made. If there is peritonitis, preoperative IV antibiotics will be required. Nasogastric intubation, antibiotics, and IV fluids may be indicated if there is severe peritonitis.

Incision

Lanz or right gridiron centred on McBurney's point. The muscles are split in the line of their fibres. The incision may be extended upwards and laterally or downwards and medially to gain access to a retrocaecal or a pelvic appendix respectively (muscle cutting if necessary).

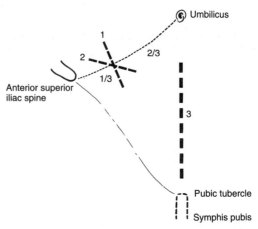

Incisions for appendicectomy: *1*, McBurney; *2*, Lanz; *3*, Midline.

Procedure

Identify the peritoneum and open it between artery forceps. Extend the opening to gain access. Insert the index finger. Identify the caecum by grasping a taenium and deliver it. The appendix is at its base. Alternatively, the appendix may be delivered directly and Babcock's forceps applied to its tip.

Secure the appendiceal artery with forceps. Clamp, divide, and ligate it. The appendix mesentery can then be divided. Clamp the base of the appendix with two artery forceps and divide it between them. Place the appendix and the instruments in a dirty dish, taking care during and after division not to soil the wound or peritoneum. Ligate the appendix stump with Vicryl and bury it with a purse-string suture.

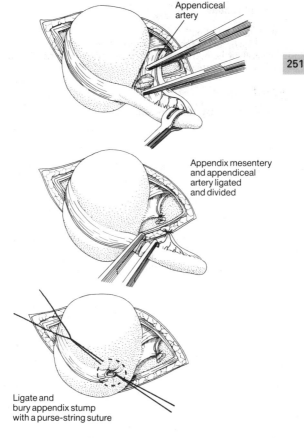

Appendiceal artery

Appendix mesentery and appendiceal artery ligated and divided

Ligate and bury appendix stump with a purse-string suture

Appendicectomy.

251

APPENDICECTOMY (major) (*cont.*)

Closure

Close the peritoneum with continuous Vicryl. Then close the muscle layers with loosely inserted Vicryl sutures. Insert interrupted Nylon or subcuticular Prolene to skin.

Special postoperative care

Encourage early oral fluids. If there has been peritonitis proceed cautiously, introducing fluids orally only when bowel activity returns.

Complications

- Wound infection
- Pelvic or abdominal abscess formation
- Paralytic ileus: treat with IV fluids and nasogastric suction
- Incisional herniation (rare)

Discharge

Three to five days after operation.

LARGE BOWEL RESECTION AND ANASTOMOSIS

Indications

- Diverticula complicated by perforation, bleeding, or obstruction.
- Penetrating or blunt trauma: resection or exteriorization is more likely than in the small bowel, particularly in the presence of mesenteric damage.
- Infective conditions causing bleeding or perforation.
- Inflammatory conditions including Crohn's disease or ulcerative colitis, including failure of medical treatment.
- Neoplastic diseases: adenoma carcinoma, premalignant conditions such as familial adenomatous polyposis, or refractory ulcerative colitis. Benign neoplasms rarely require resection.
- Vascular complications (e.g. infarction, strangulation in a hernia or volvulus), ischaemic colitis.
- Rare congenital disorders or intussusceptions.

Anastomoses are less sound in the large bowel and exteriorization–resection is safer if viability appears compromised. Resection is better than bypass as a palliative procedure for colonic cancers.

Ideals for successful large bowel anastomosis

- Adequate mechanical bowel preparation and antibiotic prophylaxis.
- Adequate blood supply, particularly in the splenic flexure and low anterior resection.
- Early pedicle ligation which may determine the resection line and prevent tumour dissemination.
- Avoid anastomosis in the presence of perforation, obstruction, inflammation, ischaemia, systemic sepsis, or shock.
- Avoid 'gathering-in' of mesentery.
- Take care in mesenteric defect closure.
- Avoid wide disparity of bowel lumina.

Preoperative preparations

All patients undergoing colonic or rectal surgery should be counselled and warned that in some cases a stoma (either temporary or permanent) may be necessary. The site should be clearly marked preoperatively and the patient should have the opportunity of wearing a bag over it.

Effective antimicrobial and antiembolic prophylaxis is mandatory. In addition, some sort of mechanical cleansing is required. Patients with stenosing malignancies or inflammatory disease may develop obstruction, with increased morbidity and mortality, and so limited mechanical cleansing is used in stenosing lesions.

A low roughage diet for 4–5 days before surgery should ensure an adequate protein and calorific fluid intake. Enemas

24 hours before surgery clear the colon distal to the disease but may be ineffective for proximal loading. Oral mannitol is preferred as a laxative to magnesium sulphate or Picolax. Bowel preparation using 5–10 litres of normal saline rapidly infused through the nasogastric tube is highly effective but is very distressing for patients. There is a particular need to monitor older patients in case of dehydration following laxative preparation (measure plasma osmolality).

Procedure

In benign or premalignant disease resection can stay close to the bowel, whereas in malignant disease clearance is mandatory. A high mesenteric tie should be undertaken for cancer operations as it allows accurate staging (Dukes C1–C2) even if it does not improve prognosis. If the diagnosis between diverticulitis or cancer is obscure, cancer clearance principles should be obeyed.

Identify the major vessels on which the resection is going to be based and transilluminate the mesentery if possible to help in the identification of vessels. After the pedicle has been ligated before resection, ensure that the bowel ends are viable and can be anastomosed without tension.

Protect the wound and peritoneum from soiling. Ligate the mesenteric vessels based on the chosen pedicle. Empty the bowel contents into the specimen and apply clamps as for small bowel resection. If bowel preparation has been adequate and effective, clamps may not be required. Following resection, the bowel ends should bleed freely.

Isolate the prepared bowel ends using antiseptic packs. Lay the ends together for end-to-end anastomosis. It is conventional to use a two-layer technique starting with the back seromuscular layer using interrupted sutures (Lembert). Prevent gathering of the mesentery by rotating one bowel end by 90°. Sutures should be placed 2–3 mm from the bowel edge and 2–3 mm apart. It is easier to insert all the sutures of this first layer before tying them, particularly in procedures like anterior resection. The bowel can then be parachuted down until the ends meet. Leave the two outside sutures long as markers with artery forceps attached. The inside haemostatic all-layer sutures are then placed continuously. Use a double-ended suture and start halfway along the closed back layer using a Connell loop on the mucosa at the corners if necessary. When this layer is complete, the clamps can be removed and the front interrupted Lembert suture layer completed. This will ensure inversion, but it is difficult in low pelvic anastomosis when a single layer is preferable. Vicryl or a non-absorbable 2/0 or 3/0 silk can be used for the seromuscular layer and an absorbable 2/0 or 3/0 chromic catgut or Vicryl (preferable) for the inner haemostatic layer.

If a single-layer anastomosis is used, the sutures are placed 2–3 mm from the edge and 2–3 mm apart and can be combined with a mattress inversion suture on the back wall. The knots are tied on the luminal side in the back layer and on the outside in the front layer. Close mesenteric defects with care to prevent devascularization of the anastomosis. If you have doubts do not take risks but refashion the anastomosis ensuring viable bowel ends. Use disposable continuous low suction drains if required, placing the tip with its multiple perforations at the site of resection.

Complications

Morbidity and mortality vary depending on the pathology and the type of procedure (elective versus emergency).

Local and general complications can occur as in other major abdominal surgery. However, he most significant disaster is anastomotic leakage as a result of poor surgical technique (tension at the anastomotic site, resection of distended bowel, heavy faecal loading) or ischaemia of the bowel itself.

Suspect leakage if there is continuing abdominal pain and distension in a toxic patient with a raised temperature and pulse rate. There may be guarding and rebound or even discharge of faeces through the wound.

In many patients leakage is local, leading to abscess and fistula formation. Most respond to conservative therapy of nil orally and IV feeding/antibiotics until spontaneous closure occurs.

In others complete anastomotic breakdown will lead to faecal peritonitis with great risk to the patient's life. Swift intervention with broad-spectrum antibiotics, early laparotomy, exteriorization of the anastomotic ends, and peritoneal lavage is vital to prevent further deterioration.

257

RIGHT HEMICOLECTOMY (extra-major)

This procedure is most frequently performed for malignant disease affecting the caecum, the ascending colon, and the hepatic flexure.

Incision

Midline or transverse

Procedure

Insert a self-retaining retractor and carry out a laparotomy. Is the tumour resectable? Does the liver contain metastases? If so are they localized to one lobe only? Consider subsequent hepatic lobectomy. If there are multiple metastases, is resection of the primary lesion worthwhile?

Use large packs to pack the small bowel to the medial side of the abdomen away from the right hemicolon. Incise the lateral peritoneal attachment of the right colon and mobilize it from the posterior abdominal wall. Identify and preserve the spermatic or ovarian vessels, the ureter, and the second part of the duodenum. Mobilize the hepatic flexure by dividing the greater omentum from the right extremity of the transverse colon. If the omentum is involved with tumour, it should also be removed. Avoid handling the carcinoma itself to prevent dissemination of the cancer cells.

When the right hemicolon is mobilized note the ileocolic and right colic vessels. Ligate and divide them near their origins to preserve the small bowel blood supply. The branches of the middle colic vessel can now be identified and preserved as required. Next divide the mesocolon from the distal ileum (to be used for the anastomosis) to the mid-transverse colon. Ensure that there is at least 5–10 cm clearance on either side of the tumour and divide the transverse colon and the terminal ileum between clamps. The transverse colon can now be closed using loose over-and-over Vicryl sutures with the clamp as a retractor. Remove the clamp and pull the suture line tight. Bury the first suture line by inserting a second line of Vicryl sutures, picking up serosa only.

Gastrointestinal continuity

This is established by an ileotransverse end-to-end or end-to-side anastomosis (less conventional) in two layers of absorbable or non-absorbable sutures. Control of leakage of the GI contents is maintained by using non-crushing intestinal clamps. Bring a suction drain out through a separate stab wound in the abdominal wall and lay it near the anastomosis.

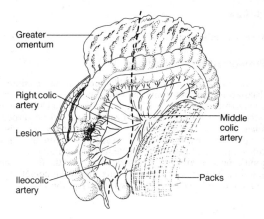

End-to-End anastomosis

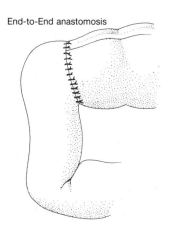

Right hemicolectomy.

RIGHT HEMICOLECTOMY (extra-major)
(*cont.*)

Closure

Mass with interrupted Nylon to skin.

Postoperative complications

As for other major abdominal surgery, the most important disaster is leakage from the anastomosis. This may occur owing to poor surgical technique or as a result of intestinal ischaemia or poor general perfusion. It should be suspected when there is abdominal pain and distension with a rise in temperature accompanied by guarding or rebound. Early reoperation is the best management. Those patients with peritonitis need drainage, peritoneal lavage with an antiseptic solution, and broad-spectrum antibiotics. (See complications of large bowel resection and anastomosis, p. 186.)

TRANSVERSE COLECTOMY (extra-major)

This operation is indicated for resection of malignant disease of the transverse colon and more rarely for benign disease. In malignancy the omentum, the transverse colon, and the mesentery are included in a wedge resection based on the middle colic artery.

Incision

Upper midline.

Procedure

Detach the stomach from the colon and its omentum by serial division of the gastrocolic omental connections, dividing them between Frazer Kelly forceps and ligating with Vicryl. Avoid damage to the gastroepiploic arcade. Identify the middle colic artery at its origin and, with minimal handling of the tumour, divide the artery early in the procedure between two Roberts clamps on the proximal side and one on the distal side. Ligate the vessel with 2/0 Vicryl. Divide the mesenteric peritoneum with McIndoe scissors and the vascular arcade between Frazer Kelly forceps with 2/0 Vicryl ties. Fashion a V-shape in the mesocolon to give clearance of at least 5–10 cm on each side of the tumour. This can be extended to the right or left, depending on the site of the tumour, but should include the omentum. The hepatic or splenic flexure may need to be mobilized to allow a tension-free anastomosis. An end-to-end anastomosis is then performed in one or two layers.

Closure

Close the abdomen with mass sutures (PDS or Nylon) and the skin with Nylon or Prolene. Drainage is not usually necessary.

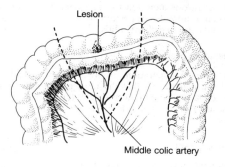

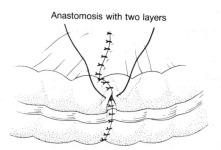

Transverse colectomy.

LEFT HEMICOLECTOMY (extra-major)

This procedure is indicated for malignant disease of the left hemicolon. It may also be performed in benign disease such as severe and extensive diverticulitis.

Preoperative preparation

Standard bowel preparation. Ensure preoperative catheterization of the patient and that the table can be tilted into the Trendelenburg position if necessary. If the lesion is low in the sigmoid colon or rectum, place the patient in the lithotomy position.

Special consent

All patients undergoing large bowel surgery should be advised whether or not a stoma will be necessary and counselling should be provided.

Incision

Lower midline extended proximally if required.

Procedure

Mobilize the left hemicolon by dividing the peritoneum lateral to it and extending the mobilization around the splenic flexure. This is often best done by first mobilizing the transverse and descending colons, drawing them downwards into the wound and dividing the phrenicocolic ligament.

The extent of resection depends on the size and site of the tumour and the possible involvement of regional lymph nodes. If the procedure is a radical left hemicolectomy, anastomosis is established between the transverse colon (which must then be mobilized) and the rectosigmoid colon. Less extensive resections (segmental resections) involve resection of the affected portion of colon with its mesentery and affected lymph nodes with end-to-end anastomosis of the descending colon to the rectosigmoid junction. Such lesser procedures are carried out for small tumours or in the elderly and frail patient. The inferior mesenteric artery can be left intact, with the vessels being ligated and divided close to the bowel wall.

Radical left hemicolectomy involves ligation of the inferior mesenteric pedicle, the sigmoid vessels, and the middle colic vessels at their left extremity.

Closure

The wound is closed in layers. A suction drain is brought out through a separate stab wound and Nylon or Prolene sutures are applied to the skin.

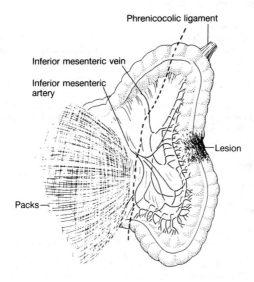

Phrenicocolic ligament

Inferior mesenteric vein

Inferior mesenteric artery

Lesion

Packs

265

Anastomosis of bowel and mesentery

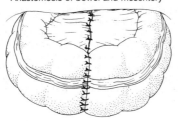

Left hemicolectomy.

SIGMOID COLECTOMY

Indications

- Carcinoma
- Benign polyp(s)
- Diverticular disease associated with stricture, fistula formation, or pericolic inflammation.

Specific preoperative preparations

Ensure that the stoma nurse marks the best site for a left iliac colostomy in case of technical difficulties when Hartmann's procedure may have to be carried out. Warn the patient of this during counselling and obtaining consent.

Incision

Lower midline. Extend it proximally if necessary.

Procedure

To mobilize the sigmoid divide its lateral peritoneal attachments. Identify and preserve the left ureter which may be more at risk in patients with diverticular disease because of pericolic inflammation. Mobilize the colon as far as required for safe clearance. In benign disease the mesocolon can be divided close to the wall of the bowel, ligating and dividing the sigmoid branches of the inferior mesenteric artery. However, adequate resection proximally and distally with high ligation of the vessels is necessary in patients with cancer. The sigmoid loop is then removed between crushing clamps and end-to-end anastomosis is carried out in a single interrupted layer of Vicryl. Alternatively, a seromuscular and all-coats layers can be inserted, with the inner layer being continuous with Connell sutures at the corners.

Access to the mobilized sigmoid usually permits a tension-free anastomosis. A proximal colostomy and drainage need to be considered in each case. If there is doubt about the anastomosis, do both.

Closure

Mass with Nylon or Prolene to skin.

TOTAL COLECTOMY

Indications

- Complicated ulcerative colitis, e.g. fulminant, toxic mega-colon, perforation, or haemorrhage; long-standing disease.
- Complicated Crohn's disease.
- Premalignant disease such as familial adenomatous polyposis.

Preoperative preparation

Antimicrobial and venous thromboembolic prophylaxis are given. In very severe disease bowel preparation may not be possible, and antibiotics may need to be continued as therapy. Try to correct anaemia or poor nutrition and dehydration as far as possible. Mark the stoma site on the abdominal wall for the ileostomy.

Position of patient

Supine unless a panproctocolectomy is considered when the Lloyd Davies position should be adopted for the rectal excision as in abdominoperineal excision of the rectum.

Incision

Full-length midline.

Procedure

Total colectomy is undertaken as a combination of right and left hemicolectomy with anterior resection bringing out the ileum as a right iliac fossa ileostomy. Unless there is malignant change, high ties of the mesenteric vessels are not necessary. The rectal stump may be oversewn or excised. In emergency procedures it may not be possible to consider mucosal protectomy or ileal pouch surgery as a one-stage procedure because of the state of the patient, but an ileorectal anastomosis or a J or W pouch can be planned for elective operations.

269

COLOSTOMY (major)

Colostomies have to be fashioned for a variety of reasons. They may be temporary or permanent. The stoma itself may be the loop, end, or double-barrelled type.

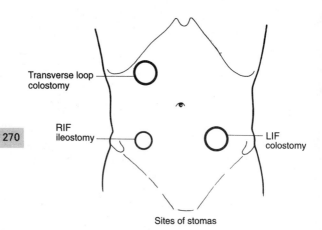

Sites of stomas

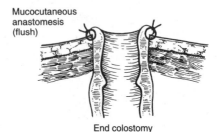

End colostomy

Colostomy types.

Loop colostomy

These are usually placed in the right upper quadrant and are fashioned from the right transverse colon to the right of the middle colic artery pp. 273–4. They are bulky, difficult to manage, and lead to complications such as prolapse or hernia. Fortunately, they are usually temporary and are fashioned:

- to protect a distal anastomosis
- to defunction bowel when resection and anastomosis distally is not possible
- to defunction bowel before radiotherapy or chemotherapy
- as the first stage of a three-stage procedure for distal obstruction
- to defunction bowel when there is distal perforation, sepsis, fistula, or incontinence due to tumour.

Loop colostomies should be avoided if possible because management is difficult. Hartmann's procedure or on-table lavage with primary anastomosis and caecostomy is preferable to a three-stage operation for obstruction of the distal colon. Inexperienced surgeons should seek help with this.

Incision
Vertical, 4 cm lateral to the midline through the right rectus muscle. Extend if necessary when there is gross obstruction and distension.

Procedure for colostomy closure
With the patient anaesthetized insert silk stay sutures at positions 3, 6, 9, and 12 in the skin close to the stoma. Attach artery forceps to each and applying traction in turn incise the skin close to the stoma, taking care not to cut the sutures. When the skin and subcutaneous tissue has been completely incised, mobilize the bowel by a combination of blunt and sharp dissection from the muscle layers. As the bowel becomes free, apply occlusion clamps on each side of the loop. Now excise the skin circle around the stoma and tidy the ends for anastomosis. Close the loop transversely with interrupted all-layers 2/0 or 3/0 Vicryl on a round-bodied needle. If required, invert it with seromuscular sutures and return the bowel to the peritoneal cavity. Add a drain if you feel it is necessary.

Closure
The abdominal wall defect can be closed with mass Nylon with Prolene or Nylon to skin.

End colostomy

This is part of an APER for cancer, but can be used in Hartmann's procedure either as palliative treatment for cancer or in an emergency case where the rectum or sigmoid cannot be anastomosed because of obstruction, perforation, or doubtful viability. In Hartmann's procedure the rectal stump is oversewn with sutures or closed with a linear stapling device.

In elective surgery mark the best site for the stoma preoperatively ensuring that you have informed consent.

Procedure

After sigmoid colectomy or abdominoperineal excision of rectum the proximal clamped colonic end is drawn to the surface through the defect in the abdominal wall fashioned for the stoma. This is prepared by applying Littlewood's forceps to the proposed site, tenting the skin, and making a 2–3 cm full-thickness circular defect using the scalpel. Underlying fat is excised and a cruciate incision made into the anterior rectus sheath. The muscle is then split and the peritoneum opened. If the colostomy is to be permanent, the clamped colon can be drawn extraperitoneally to the site of the stoma to prevent internal herniation or prolapse. Alternatively, close the lateral space using interrupted Vicryl ensuring that there is no tension and that the bowel is viable. Do not remove the clamp until the main abdominal wound is closed and protected by a dressing.

Hold the colonic end with two Babcock's tissue forceps before dividing the bowel next to the clamp with a scalpel. If there is obstruction, anticipate spillage and protect the stoma wound. Suture the mucocutaneous junction using 2/0 Vicryl on a cutting needle. Usually 12–16 interrupted sutures will suffice. Ensure that full-thickness 4–5 mm bites are taken. Persistent bleeding requires diathermy. Clean the skin and dry it well around the stoma (compound benzoin tincture or Friar's Balsam on the surrounding skin is useful). Fashion an appropriate colostomy bag with a hole which is large enough to fit around the stoma without compromise. Place the bag laterally, as the patient will be nursed supine for the first few hours, and ensure that the clip on the bag is in place.

Closure of Hartmann's end colostomy

This can be safely undertaken 6–8 weeks postoperatively, but it can be difficult. Check the length of the rectal stump with rigid sigmoidoscopy. Give appropriate antimicrobial and venous thromboembolic prophylaxis as well as rectal washouts. Position the patient as for anterior resection and mobilize the colostomy with a combination of sharp and blunt dissection. Clamp the colon proximal to the stoma and open the abdomen through a lower midline incision. Identify and mobilize the oversewn rectal stump. This can be done by passing a sigmoidoscope from below. Carry out an end-to-end tension-free anastomosis as in a low anterior resection with a stapling device or by hand.

Close the abdominal and colostomy wounds with mass Nylon and subcuticular Prolene or Nylon. A right iliac fossa suction drain to the anastomotic site is conventional.

Double-barrelled colostomy, Paul Miculicz colostomy, and mucous fistula

Whenever possible the distal colon should be brought out as a mucous fistula because this makes closing the colostomy much easier. Following emergency sigmoid resection (for diverticular disease or obstructing volvulus with ischaemia) a left iliac fossa colostomy can be brought out with enough distal bowel length to form a separate mucous fistula which can be sited in the lower end of the abdominal wound. If the mucous fistula is brought out adjacent to the end colostomy, subsequent closure is easier. The two ends of bowel can be double-barrelled together for 3–4 cm using a Vicryl 2/0 suture along their antimesenteric borders. Mobilization and closure of the stoma 6–8 weeks later can be carried out by anastomosing half the circumference of the bowel using one or two layers of 2/0 Vicryl (preferably intraperitoneally).

273

Paul Miculicz double-barrelled colostomy was originally devised for obstruction. A glass tube and draining soft rubber tube are tied into the proximal stoma to decompress the bowel. The mucous fistula is double-barrelled with the proximal stoma for a longer length to allow the application of an enterotome. The enterotome is placed over the spur between the two stomas 1–2 weeks postoperatively and gradually tightened until the crushed tissue sloughs, allowing its removal. The double-barrelling in this procedure needs to be long to prevent interposition of the small bowel or other viscus and its subsequent damage by the enterotome.

Transverse colostomy

This can be carried out as a decompressive colostomy for intestinal obstruction or as a protective colostomy for a more distal anastomosis, but it should be avoided if possible as management is difficult.

Incision
Vertical, 4 cm lateral to the midline through the right rectus muscle.

Procedure
Open the peritoneum, identify the transverse colon, encircle it with the fingers, and draw a segment of colon through the wound as far to the right as possible. Hold the segment of colon to the light so that the mesocolic vessels can be seen and choose as avascular a site as possible. Make a hole through

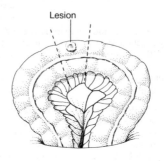

274

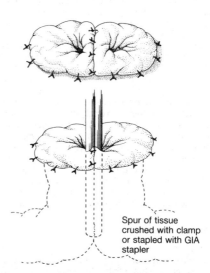

Procedures for dealing with colonic obstructive lesions (exteriorization resection method—Paul Mikulicz

this close to the bowel wall with large artery forceps. Pass a glass rod or plastic colostomy bridge (Hollister) through this window. Draw the colon out of the wound and gently suture the serosal surfaces of the afferent and efferent limbs together for a distance of about 3–4 cm. Allow the colon, except for the glass rod or bridge, to fall back into the abdomen. Close the wound in layers above and below the colostomy loop. Apply a dressing.

Opening the colostomy

If the bowel is obstructed, open the colostomy at the time of surgery and apply a colostomy bag. If there is no obstruction you can wait for 24–48 hours before opening the colostomy on the ward with diathermy by making a small cross-shaped incision at its most prominent surface. Many patients do not like this procedure, and so colostomies are probably best opened in theatre.

Caecostomy—on-table lavage

Caecostomy is rarely used for decompression or defunctioning a distal anastomosis because it is not as effective as a loop colostomy, but it is useful for on-table lavage. In emergency, colonic surgery a single-stage resection and anastomosis procedure can safely be undertaken.

Procedure

Determine whether resection and primary anastomosis is feasible in cases of colonic obstruction due to perforation, haemorrhage, or poor viability.

Following laparotomy, prepare the appendix as for appendicectomy with two encircling 2/0 Vicryl purse-string sutures. Keep the needles on and leave the suture ends long. If the appendix has been removed at an earlier operation, mobilize the caecal pole so that the catheter can easily reach the caecum from the abdominal wall. Make a stab incision in the right iliac fossa near McBurney's point and pull through a 28F Foley catheter. Surround the area with antiseptic-soaked protective abdominal packs and have the purse strings ready to tighten. Make the caecostomy, insert the catheter, tie the purse strings, and inflate the catheter balloon. In obstruction, liquid faeces and gas will come out under pressure and the caecum may be at risk of rupture. Lead the bowel contents by siphonage into a closed container via the catheter and tubing. If obstruction is minimal, spiggot the catheter. Approximate the caecum to the abdominal wall stab incision by traction on the catheter and secure it to the abdominal wall with the long ends of Vicryl (with extra sutures to exclude the chance of leakage). The balloon of the catheter can be placed into the ileum later to divert the liquid contents completely.

Proximal to an obstructing lesion or at the proximal end of the proposed specimen place two or three 2/0 Vicryl purse-string sutures on the antimesenteric border of the colon. Make a colotomy wide enough to accommodate the lumen of a long anaesthetic scavenger tube and insert this in a proximal direction using the purse-string sutures to prevent spillage. In obstruction or when spillage is anticipated, protect the area with antiseptic-soaked abdominal packs. Make a mesenteric

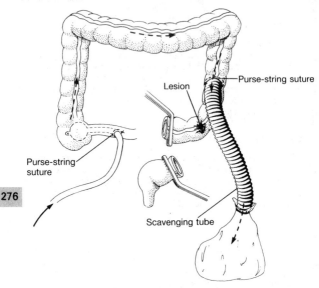

On-table lavage and colectomy.

window and pass through a linen tape which can be tied
tightly over the tubing (once in place) to prevent spillage.
Before making the colotomy the bowel contents can be
milked into the proposed specimen and the colotomy protected between non-crushing intestinal clamps.

Lavage the colon through the caecostomy tube until the
effluent from the scavenger tubing, led into a closed recep-
tacle on the theatre floor, is clear. This may need 10–12 litres
of warmed normal saline. An antiseptic (Savlon, chlorhexi-
dene, or betadine) can be added to the irrigating fluid which
may need to be milked around the colon. Hold-ups can occur
at the colonic flexures (see diagram).

Once the colon is empty it may appear normal or more
viable. Mobilization of the area bearing the lesion is then
easier and more complete. Remove the scavenger tube with
the specimen and undertake a primary anastomosis.

Leave the caecostomy on free drainage into a urinary bag.
Spigot it and deflate the balloon when the patient has passed
flatus or faeces (usually at 7–10 days). If no complications
develop, spigot the catheter for 2–3 days and remove it (at

10–12 days postoperatively). There may be a faecal fistula but this will close quickly. Usually there is a minor purulent discharge for 1–2 days which can be managed with simple absorptive dressings.

ANTERIOR RESECTION (complex)

Introduction

This procedure is undertaken for malignant disease of the rectum with end-to-end anastomosis by hand or with an end-to-end stapling device (see large bowel anastomosis). A very low colo-anal anastomosis is only possible in relatively slim women with a favourable tumour grade. In obese men, adequate cancer clearance must not be compromised by injudicious attempts to avoid abdominoperineal excision. Failure to clear the pelvis and mesorectum risks a suture line recurrence of over 10 per cent.

Preoperative preparations

A urinary catheter should be inserted after the induction of anaesthesia to ensure that fluid balance is maintained, particularly in older patients. Ask the stoma therapist to mark the best sites for a right transverse loop or left iliac fossa end colostomy if unforeseen complications occur.

Position of patient

Position the patient supine with the legs in the Lloyd Davies position and head-down tilt. There must be access to the perineum for abdominoperineal excision, to allow the introduction of an end-to-end stapler, or carry out a pull-through technique. The catheter (and scrotum in males) should be taped to a leg out of the way.

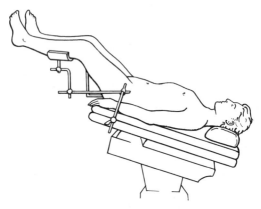

Lloyd Davies, lithotomy—Trendelberg.

Incision

Lower midline which may need extension upwards if the splenic flexure has to be mobilized for a tension-free anastomosis.

Procedure

Undertake a careful laparotomy. Assess the tumour and the extent of its spread without undue manipulation. Look for synchronous colonic tumours and palpate the liver for metastases. It is usually easier to pack the small bowel superiorly with the patient in head-down tilt. This manoeuvre maintains the pelvis empty of small bowel. Insert a self-retaining retractor to allow your assistant to retract the anterior pelvic contents. In women, a bulky uterus can be temporarily sutured anteriorly to permit access.

Mobilize the congenital adhesions (the 'white line') on the lateral abdominal wall from the sigmoid. Incise the peritoneum on the right side of the sigmoid loop and, by dissection on both sides of the sigmoid mesentery, identify the inferior mesenteric pedicle at its junction with the aorta. Ligate and divide it at this level (the high tie). Divide the inferior mesenteric vein at the same level. The high tie will devascularize the lower left colon and, if there is any tension, the need for splenic mobilization (and a larger operation) is almost certain. Therefore in some cases (very obese, the elderly, or patients undergoing palliation) the left colic branch can be spared. The peritoneal incisions made on the right and left of the sigmoid colon are carried down to meet anteriorly in the deepest part of the pouch of Douglas. As the sigmoid is mobilized, anticipate and identify the gonadal vessels and the left ureter.

Open the presacral plane posteriorly, avoiding damage to the sacral plexus. If possible, identify and divide the mesorectum and excise it with the specimen. The anterior plane is opened next. Dissection in Devonvillier's fascia is facilitated by instructing your assistant to use a deep St Mark's style pelvic retractor. The bladder, seminal vesicles, and prostate in males, and the uterus and vagina in females, can be separated by a combination of sharp and blunt dissection. Avoid the anterior venous plexus, and diathermy or tie bleeding vessels. In low anterior resection the lateral ligaments can be divided (with diathermy or ties to the middle rectal vessels), allowing access to the lower third of rectum. A 2 cm clearance below a rectal neoplasm is ideal.

Apply a non-crushing angled clamp below the rectal lesion at the proposed site of division and wash the rectum out per anum (aqueous chlorhexidine or povidone-iodine) with an antiseptic to clear faecal debris or intraluminal viable cancer cells. Place crushing and non-crushing clamps at the proposed division site in the sigmoid or descending colon. Divide the bowel and clean the proximal bowel end with a Savlon-soaked swab. Check that there will be no tension at the proposed anastomosis. Place three stay sutures in the seromuscular distal rectum to prevent its retraction and divide it above a non-crushing Hayes Lowe clamp. Long Babcock's forceps can also be used, but may traumatize the bowel.

Single-layer anastomosis

This is carried out using horizontal mattress sutures. The posterior wall is completed first and the knots are tied on the inside. When the posterior wall is completed, the anterior wall anastomosis is carried out using interrupted mattress sutures.

If doubt remains about anastomotic integrity consider a right transverse loop defunctioning colostomy.

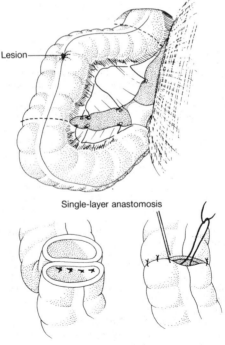

Lesion

Single-layer anastomosis

Anterior resection.

Completion of the anastomosis with the stapling gun

Most surgeons use a stapling gun (end-to-end anastomosis EEA) passed from below by an assistant. The bowel ends are closed over the open instrument with purse-string sutures. The gun is then fired. A circular knife within the instrument removes two 'doughnuts' of bowel which should be inspected for completeness after the gun has been gently removed.

Closure

A suction drain is brought out through a separate stab wound, and if required the gap between the mesocolon and parietal peritoneum is closed to prevent herniation. The abdominal wall is closed with continuous mass nylon and subcuticular prolene or interrupted nylon to skin.

PROCEDURES FOR DEALING WITH COLONIC OBSTRUCTIVE LESIONS

There are several procedures other than than abdomino-perineal resection which can be used to deal with cancers of the colon, pericolic infection, intussusception, or volvulus.

Hartmann's procedure

This is ideal in the frail elderly patient. The affected colon is excised with full protocol through a left lower paramedian incision. The proximal colon is brought through the abdominal wall as a colostomy. The distal rectal stump is either over-sewn or covered with peritoneum. The pelvic cavity may be drained through the anus.

Exteriorization resection method (Paul Mikulicz procedure)

This can be used for gangrenous small bowel, colonic cancers with obstruction and proximal distension, volvulus, or localized diverticular infection. The affected segment of bowel is exteriorized at laparotomy and the abdominal wound is closed. The bowel is then resected between Kocher clamps after anchoring the two loops to skin. This procedure reduces the risk of contamination of the peritoneal cavity and allows decompression of the bowel. The spur of tissue between the double-barrelled colostomy can be crushed with an entero-tome and the colostomy closed 10 days after the procedure, although it is more common to wait for 6–12 weeks and then close it formally.

Palliative decompressive colostomy

This should be done only if senior help is not available. If primary resection is not possible at the time of surgery, a transverse colostomy should be fashioned in the right upper quadrant. This permits decompression of the bowel and the formal resection can be carried out later. The colostomy is closed at a third operation (the three-stage procedure). Equally, if disease is advanced and the patient is obstructed, a palliative transverse or left iliac colostomy will relieve obstruction. (NB The blood supply to the left colon is poor, making later closure risky.)

Local procedures

Polyps and small tumours can be resected transanally using a resectoscope similar to that used for transurethral resection of the prostate. The instrument makes use of a cutting diathermy loop, Frankenfeldt snares for polypoidal lesions, and electro-coagulation.

On-table bowel lavage

Following removal of an obstructive lesion, the proximal bowel should be washed out before fashioning the anastomosis. A large Foley catheter is passed into the caecum from the distal ileum and held in place with a purse-string suture. The proximal bowel is mobilized to bring it out of the wound, and a length of anaesthetic scavenging tube is inserted into it and secured with Nylon tapes tied onto the corrugations. Packs are then applied to the abdominal cavity and wound to collect spillage. The distal end of the tubing is now tied into the neck of a double-plastic bag and led over the table. Physiological saline or Hartmann's solution at body temperature are then instilled, and faeces are broken down through the bowel wall with finger pressure. Wash-outs are continued until the fluid appears clear on entry to the bag. Suction of the colon into the tube is prevented by a large-bore needle introduced through the colonic wall to act as a vent.

283

ABDOMINOPERINEAL EXCISION OF THE RECTUM (complex)

This procedure is indicated for rectal carcinomas too close to the anal margin to permit adequate clearance by anterior resection. Other malignancies include those of the anal canal. Inflammatory bowel disease, such as severe Crohn's disease with multiple fistulae, can be treated by anorectal excision, and occasionally the procedure needs to be part of panprocto-colectomy for total severe ulcerative colitis.

Preoperative preparation

As for anterior resection. Ask the stoma therapist to mark the site for a left iliac fossa end colostomy.

Position of patient

Modified lithotomy with the legs flexed to about 45° and the sacrum raised on a sandbag to allow exposure for the perineal operator. The table should have a slight head-down tilt and the anal skin should be sutured using two 1 or 0 silk encircling sutures to make the orifice watertight. Tape the catheter and scrotum (in males) to the leg out of the operative field.

Incision

Lower midline.

Procedure

Undertake a laparotomy as in anterior resection. There is no need to carry out a high tie in inflammatory disease or pallia-tive operations. Mobilize the sigmoid colon as in sigmoid colectomy and the rectum as in anterior resection. Anticipate and identify the left gonadal vessels and ureter. At this stage it will be apparent whether the operation is feasible and the perineal dissection can begin.

The perineal dissection is undertaken by a separate surgeon, a scrub nurse, and instruments (synchronous combined abdo-minoperineal excision of rectum). Begin by applying Little-wood's forceps to the perianal suture and make an elliptical incision around it, taking care not to cut it. Deepen the in-cision and insert a self-retaining retractor. Now deepen the incision posteriorly, securing bleeding vessels by diathermy or ligation, through the perirectal fatty tissues to reach the coccyx and Waldeyer's fascial plane. The tip of the coccyx can be divided and taken with the specimen. Laterally the levator ani is divided from posterior to anterior. At this stage make con-tact with the abdominal operator above and work together to divide the superficial transverse muscles anteriorly. When the rectum is freed a glove can be placed over the sutured anus to prevent contamination and the specimen removed through the perineum. In women the posterior vaginal wall can also be excised if the tumour is bulky anteriorly. In inflammatory disease, particularly ulcerative colitis, the perineal dissection can be made intersphincterally. At the abdominal end the bowel is divided between a De Martell or Zachary Cope instrument followed by the fashioning of a left iliac fossa end colostomy. The pelvic peritoneum can then be closed or a mesh inserted to keep the small bowel out of the pelvis in case postoperative radiotherapy is required.

Closure

The abdomen is closed *en masse* with Nylon or PDS and prolene or nylon to skin. The perineum is closed approximating the ischiorectal fat, oversewing the edges of the vagina in women and suturing the perineal skin with 2/0 subcuticular Prolene or Vicryl. A suction drain is brought out through a separate stab wound.

Specific complications

See complications after large bowel resection and anastomosis (pp. 256)
- Necrosis of the colostomy. Its viability must be regularly checked. If it does not move within 72 hours a suppository may be inserted.
- Necrosis of the perineal wound may occur. This requires daily irrigation and dressing with antiseptic packs until healing occurs.

HAEMORRHOIDS

In patients with haemorrhoids include in the differential diagnosis Crohn's disease (for which haemorrhoidectomy is not indicated) and also perianal cancers such as basiloid and squamous tumours, or even melanomas. These diagnoses can usually be excluded by sigmoidoscopy, colonoscopy, or barium studies.

Indications

- Prolapse with or without minor incontinence
- Discharge with or without pruritis ani
- Excoriation, bleeding, or pain associated with strangulation or thrombosis
- Reassess pregnant women with piles 6–8 weeks after delivery

Operative haemorrhoidectomy or excision with cryosurgery, laser, or diathermy should only be reserved for thrombosed, strangulated, or tertiary prolapsed haemorrhoids.

Injection therapy (minor)

This is reserved for uncomplicated bleeding. On the first occasion draw up between 10 and 20 ml of 5 per cent phenol in almond oil in a glass syringe with a shouldered Gabriel needle. With the patient in the left lateral position, carry out sigmoidoscopy to exclude other disease and then pass the proctoscope and identify the left lateral, right anterior, and posterior internal haemorrhoids. Inject 3–5 ml of phenol submucosally into each haemorrhoid. This technique can often control bleeding and may also be useful for small anterior mucosal prolapses. Review the patient at 6 weeks and repeat the procedure if necessary.

Banding of haemorrhoids (minor)

This can be undertaken in the out-patient clinic or at examination under anaesthetic. In out-patients the patient lies in the left lateral position. If a general anaesthetic is used, the patient lies in lithotomy. Carry out sigmoidoscopy, identify the haemorrhoids one at a time, and band up to two of them, usually the two largest, by inserting the haemorrhoid gun through the proctoscope, grasping the redundant mucosa of the internal haemorrhoids in alligator forceps, and firing the rubber band over the mucosa. Before firing ensure that the application of the alligator causes no pain and that you are above the anorectal ring. Approximately 0.5 cm diameter of haemorrhoidal mucosa will be banded. Assure the patient that more bleeding than usual may be experienced for the next 1–2 days and that within 4–7 days there may also be a risk of secondary haemorrhage when the rubber band falls off, exposing an ulcer. Patients should be reviewed at 6 weeks and the procedure repeated taking a third haemorrhoid if necessary.

Examination under anaesthetic and Lord's anal dilatation

This is carried out for anal fissure or primary haemorrhoids when there is a degree of sphincter spasm. Avoid stretching the sphincter. Under general anaesthetic with the patient in the left lateral or lithotomy positions insert one finger at a time until four fingers can easily be rotated within the anal canal and lower rectum. Resist pulling the fingers apart as the risk of bleeding and incontinence is increased.

Haemorrhoidectomy (intermediate)

This can be combined with a caudal block or injection of local anaesthetic and adrenaline into the haemorrhoidal mucosa.

Position of patient

Lithotomy. Carry out a sigmoidoscopy, an examination under anaesthetic, and Lord's anal dilatation.

Procedure

Prepare the skin with aqueous cetrimide or chlorhexidine and towel-up. Identify the three haemorrhoids in the left lateral, right posterior, and anterior position. Sit down facing the anus, apply tissue forceps to the internal and external component of each haemorrhoid and pull it gently downwards. Make an incision with curved scissors at the base of each haemorrhoid and identify the external sphincter. Push the skin laterally with a swab and dissect the submucosa upwards to leave a 1 cm pedicle which can then be transfixed using 2/0 Vicryl. Make sure that there is a bridge of mucosa left between each excised area. Achieve haemostasis with diathermy, but if oozing persists with adrenaline apply Sterispon or a similar haemostatic agent. When there is a large external component, the skin should be closed externally.

As a variant diathermy or laser can be used to excise the haemorrhoids.

Complications
- Incontinence
- Faecal impaction
- Acute pain
- Retention of urine
- Haemorrhage, reactionary or secondary
- Stenosis
- Chronic pain associated with fissure

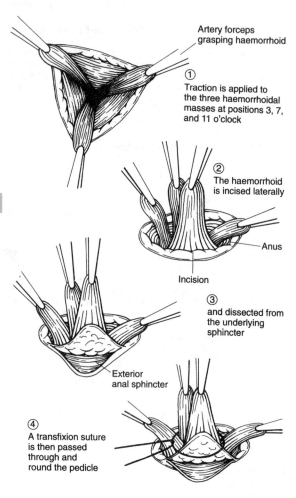

Artery forceps
grasping haemorrhoid

① Traction is applied to
the three haemorrhoidal
masses at positions 3, 7,
and 11 o'clock

② The haemorrhoid
is incised laterally

Anus

Incision

③ and dissected from
the underlying
sphincter

Exterior
anal sphincter

④ A transfixion suture
is then passed
through and
round the pedicle

288

Haemorrhoidectomy.

Thrombosed external pile (syn. external plexus haematoma) (minor)

This presents with severe pain and perianal swelling. The pain may be relieved by spontaneous bursting, but otherwise injection around the swelling with local anaesthetic and simple incision is all that is required to treat the condition. There is often an external skin tag which may need subsequent removal.

Fibroepithelial polyps (external skin tags and sentinel piles related to anal fissure) (minor)

These can usually be removed under local anaesthetic with transfixion of the stalk of a polyp for example. Skin may be closed with sutures.

ANAL WARTS

If these do not respond to podophylline consider operation. Under general anaesthetic the perianal skin bearing the polyps is injected with 1 per cent local anaesthetic and adrenaline 1:200 000. This has the effect of raising up the warts and they can then be easily removed at their small bases using scissors. Little skin is lost using this technique and the wounds heal well.

ANORECTAL POLYPS

Small anorectal polyps can be removed with biopsy forceps, but if they are larger a general anaesthetic is required. Pedunculated polyps can be resected using a diathermy snare through an operating sigmoidoscopy or resectoscope. Sessile or villous polyps can be removed perianally with the operating proctoscope. They should be raised from the muscular layers by submucosally injecting local anaesthetic and adrenaline 1:200 000. The polyp can then be excised from the underlying sphincter with scissors. Histological assessment is easier if the area removed can be pinned out on a cork board. Diathermy loops such as the Frankfelt snare can be used for pedunculated polyps greater than 1 cm. The wire can also be used to achieve haemostasis at the base of the polyp after removal.

RECTAL CANCER

Inoperable rectal cancers can be debulked with the resecto-scope and diathermy. Lasers can also be used.

FISSURE IN ANO

Consider other pathologies such as inflammatory bowel disease or malignancy. In women fissures tend to occur anteriorly and are usually related to childbirth. In men they are more common posteriorly. Medical treatment with lignocaine gel or an anal dilator is rarely successful.

Examination under anaesthetic and Lord's dilatation (simple)

Position of patient
Left lateral or lithotomy. If there is a large sentinel pile it is more easily excised in lithotomy. Lord's dilatation is achieved by inserting four fingers, one at a time, and rotating them through 360° within the anal canal. Do not overstretch the sphincter or you will risk incontinence. This is usually successful for acute fissures.

Lateral sphincterotomy (intermediate)

Indications
- Failure of examination under anaesthetic and Lord's dilatation
- Chronic fissure in ano

Position of patient
Lithotomy.

Procedure
Infiltrate local anaesthetic with 1:200 000 adrenaline. The operation may be open or closed. In the open procedure a circumferential lateral incision is made outside the external ring, and the white external sphincter fibres are divided up to the dentate line. The wound is then closed.

A long-bladed knife is used in the closed operation. The non-dominant index finger is inserted in the anal canal. The knife can then be placed lateral to the external anal canal and the external sphincter divided against the index without opening the mucosa, which increases the risk of fistula. With sphincterotomy there may be long-term problems such as incontinence. Wide excision of fissure in ano is no longer practised.

PERIANAL ABSCESS

Differential diagnosis

Cancer and Crohn's disease. Exclude by examination under anaesthetic. Most perianal abscesses result from an anal gland infection bursting through the external sphincter and they may develop into ischiorectal abscesses.

Position of patient

Lithotomy.

Procedure

Prepare the skin with aqueous antiseptic. Towel up and make a cruciate incision over the abscess. Remove the corners of the incision to permit drainage. Take a bacteriology swab, curette the abscess wall, and send a piece for histology. Pack the cavity with either alginates or Silastic foam dressings. These allow both haemostasis and painless dressing changes. Alternatively, close the wound primarily with antibiotic cover.

FISTULA IN ANO

Exclude underlying pathology like inflammatory bowel disease, tuberculosis, or neoplasia by examination under anaesthetic, sigmoidoscopy, and biopsy. Carry out the procedure even if the fistula in ano appears to be idiopathic.

Position of patient

Lithotomy.

Procedure

Low fistula (intermediate)

Low fistulas are subcutaneous, submucous, and intersphincteric, and lie below the anorectal ring. High fistulas should not be treated by this technique.

Prepare the operative site with an aqueous antiseptic and towel up. If the fistula in ano is low insert a grooved director through the external opening into the anal canal. Most obey Goodsall's rule: an anterior fistula is straight, whereas a posterior fistula is usually horseshoe-shaped. Cut down onto the grooved director and lay open the fistula. Curette and send the granulation tissue for biopsy. Apply an alginate dressing on the open fistula to provide haemostasis and easy change of dressings.

High fistula (major)

These are fistulas in which the internal opening is above the anorectal ring (high transphincteric and supralevator types). They are an operative minefield because if they are badly treated incontinence can result. Healing depends on good drainage which is best achieved in specialized centres.

With the patient in Sim's or lithotomy position carry out sigmoidoscopy to exclude inflammatory bowel disease or carcinoma. Take tissue for biopsy. Attempt to locate the internal opening using binocular loop magnification. This is usually in the region of the anal crypts (dentate line), and finger pressure over the fistula may allow some pus to escape to identify it. A probe may then be passed from the external to the internal opening taking great care not to create a false passage. If this is not possible, the track should be excised in stages by dividing the tissue over the probe and curetting it as far as possible under vision. Do no more than this and wait to see if healing occurs.

If there is an obvious internal opening, a seton suture may prevent abscess formation and increase the patient's comfort. A seton suture is a ligature of braided silk, Nylon, or even

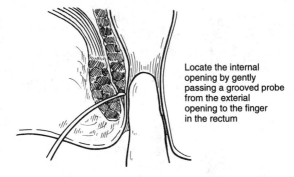

Locate the internal opening by gently passing a grooved probe from the exterial opening to the finger in the rectum

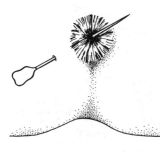

Bring the probe out through the anal fistula

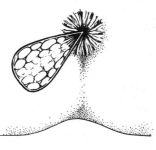

Excise and lay open the fistulous track

Excision of a low fistula.

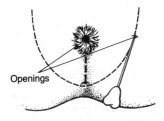

Management of a
low posterior (horseshoe)
fistula

Insert the grooved probe
into an external opening

Provided it passes easily
the overlapping skin can
be excised

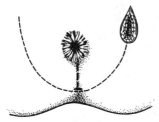

and the track laid
open

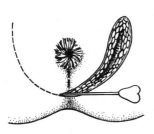

Progressively, work
around the horseshoe
exising and laying
open the track

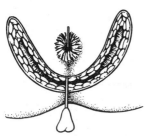

Finally, locate the
internal opening
and excise the track

Low fistula with multiple openings.

rubber, and the technique has been used since the time of Hippocrates. It is passed up the fistula into the internal opening in the rectum and tied loosely after being brought through the anus and left for 4–8 weeks. Discharge usually increases initially but then reduces. After 8 weeks the ensuing fibrosis may permit easier fistulotomy.

INGROWING TOENAIL

This procedure can be performed under local or general anaesthesia. If there is cellulitis, give the patient perioperative broad-spectrum antibiotics.

Procedure

Simple nail avulsion
This is indicated for the relief of suppuration, but regrowth and recurrence of the problem is common.

Wedge excision
The lateral or medial nail and nailbed are removed with granulation tissue and a wedge of the nailfold. The tissue is excised down to the periosteum of the lateral or medial side of the phalanx distal to the joint.

Zadik's procedure (complete excision of the nailbed)

The nail is avulsed, and incisions are then made on each side of the skin covering the matrix of the nail. Thus a flap is fashioned and drawn back, and the germinal matrix so exposed is completely excised ensuring adequate lateral and medial dissection. The skin flaps are loosely sutured with interrupted Nylon sutures.

Complications

- Recurrence. Common after simple avulsion. Uncommon if adequate lateral and medial dissection of the germinal matrix is carried out. Nail spikes are difficult to manage.
- Wound infection. This responds to antiseptic dressings rather than antibiotics unless there is cellulitis.
- Osteomyelitis and septic arthritis can also occur occasionally and need treatment with antibiotics.

INGUINAL HERNIA

Indications

- Elective: all symptomatic hernias need operation, particularly if indirect
- Emergency: irreducible or strangulated hernias.

Preoperative preparation

Check for cardiorespiratory disease and renal function. IV fluids, antibiotic prophylaxis, and nasogastric suction are required in emergency situations associated with intestinal obstruction.

Incision

Curved inguinal incision in skin crease approximately 2 cm above the medial two-thirds of the inguinal ligament. Incise fat and fascia, ligating the two or three veins which cross the line of the incision.

Procedure

Identify the external ring. Divide the external oblique aponeurosis along the line of its fibres over the inguinal canal. Apply artery forceps to the edges. Turn back the edges and identify the internal oblique and conjoint tendon above the cord and the inguinal ligament below. Steps now include identification and clarification of the sac after picking up the cord at its medial end, splitting its investing fibres in the line of the cord, and dissection of the sac to its origin. Excise the sac after transfixion of its base in indirect hernias, except when a sliding hernia is suspected. Repair the transversalis fascia margins of the internal ring and repair the posterior wall of the inguinal canal with non-absorbable sutures.

In direct hernias push the sac inwards and repair the posterior wall. If the sac is very large, it may be necessary to divide the sac near its origin and leave the distal portion open. In sliding hernias reduce the sac and viscus into the abdomen and repair the posterior wall.

Repair

Use non-absorbable sutures in darn fashion. Bassini, Halsted, and Shouldice are common methods of repair. In cases of recurrence the testis may be removed in elderly men to achieve repair.

The mesh repair (Leichstenstein) is now a popular procedure. The mesh is used to reinforce the posterior wall of the inguinal canal. It is less painful and has a low recurrence rate.

Bassini repair

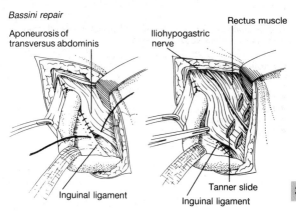

Aponeurosis of transversus abdominis

Inguinal ligament

Rectus muscle

Iliohypogastric nerve

Tanner slide

Inguinal ligament

307

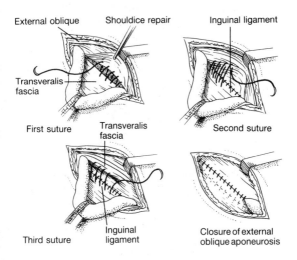

External oblique

Shouldice repair

Transveralis fascia

First suture

Transveralis fascia

Third suture

Inguinal ligament

Inguinal ligament

Second suture

Closure of external oblique aponeurosis

Inguinal hernia.

INGUINAL HERNIA (cont.)

Closure

Approximate the external oblique and close the wound in layers
with clips or adhesive strips to skin.

Complications

- Urinary retention
- Haematoma
- Infection
- Exacerbation of prostatic symptoms
- Recurrence

REPAIR OF FEMORAL HERNIA

There are several approaches to the repair of femoral hernia which are all safe, but the operator must witness all of them and decide which procedure suits his needs most.

McEvedy approach

Incision
Oblique vertical or transverse over the femoral canal with the lower part of the incision over the sac.

Procedure
First isolate the sac by a preperitoneal approach through the external oblique aponeurosis and conjoint tendon. Open the transversalis fascia and dissect between it and the peritoneum to the neck of the sac. The inferior epigastric vessels may now have to be divided in this plane. Reduce the sac by manipulating it from above and below. Then isolate it, open it, ensure that it is empty, and transfix, ligate and divide it. Carry out the repair of the hernia by uniting the inguinal and pectineal ligaments for a distance of 0.5–1 cm laterally without constricting the femoral vein. Use monofilament nylon or braided Ethibond or Ethiflex. Retract the vein laterally with an index finger, insert the stitch into the inguinal ligament, have your assistant detract the ligament upwards, and take a large bite of the pectineal ligament. A single stitch may be all that is required. If not, insert a further stitch.

High approach

Incision
Inguinal incision about 1 cm above the medial two-thirds of the inguinal ligament.

Procedure
Identify the external oblique aponeurosis. Split it as for the approach to an inguinal hernia repair and then displace the cord or round ligament upwards. Incise the transversalis fascia in line with the incision to identify the neck of the sac and the external iliac vein. Gently isolate the sac, open it, and empty it. Then transfix, ligate, and divide it. Effect the repair by placing non-absorbable sutures between the pectineal ligament and the inguinal ligament. Do not constrict the femoral vein.

Low approach (not recommended for strangulation)

Incision
Incision 6–12 cm long in the line of the groin crease centred between the anterior superior iliac spine and the symphysis pubis. Deepen the incision to identify the hernial sac. Ligate veins as necessary. Clean the sac, open it, empty its contents, transfix, ligate, and divide it, and carry out the repair as above.

Closure
The skin wounds are closed in layers with interrupted Nylon to skin.

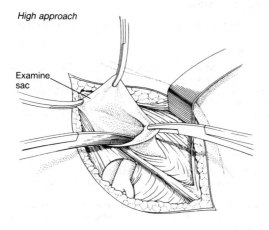

High approach

Examine sac

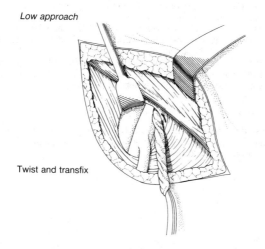

Low approach

Twist and transfix

Repair of a femoral hernia.

REPAIR OF INCISIONAL HERNIA

Aim

To close the abdominal wall defect and prevent recurrence by side-to-side suture of healthy aponeurosis, overlap of the defect edges, or interposition of a prosthetic patch or mesh.

Position of patient

Since most hernias are midline, the patient is usually supine.

Procedure

Excise the old scar and deepen the incision around the margins of the hernia until healthy aponeurosis is identified. Then dissect towards the free edges of the defect. Return the sac, intact if possible, to the peritoneal cavity and suture its margins together. 'Clean' the edges of the defect so that they are free all round.

Options

1. If the defect edges come together easily, suture them with continuous (mass type closure) or interrupted Nylon sutures.
2. Create a two-layer closure by incising along the edges of the muscular defect. Suture the opposing sides together in two layers.
3. Overlap the edges of the defect in two layers of sutures. Do this only if no tension is created.
4. The 'keel' repair involves inversion of the sac with suture of its margins followed by several layers of sutures to invert the edges of the defect.
5. If the defect is very large, use a mesh (Marlex) or a patch (Teflon) to close the defect. Suture the prosthesis all the way round the palpable margins of the defect.

Closure

Close the skin with interrupted Nylon sutures. Bring a suction drain through a separate stab wound. When using a prosthesis give prophylactic antibiotics.

THYROIDECTOMY

Indications

Absolute
- Suspicion of malignant change
- Compression of the trachea by a benign lesion

Relative
- Treatment of thyrotoxicosis
- Unsightly goitre

Choice of operation

- *Thyroid nodule*: thyroid lobectomy
- *Thyroid cancer*: total thyroidectomy
- *Nodular colloid goitre* (with hyperthyroidism): subtotal thyroidectomy

Preoperative preparation

Investigations may include indirect laryngoscopy, thyroid function tests, serum calcium, ECG, thyroid antibodies, fine-needle aspiration, and ultrasound to exclude malignancy. Patients with thyrotoxicosis need preoperative preparation with carbimazole, iodine, or possibly beta blockade. Informed consent must be obtained beforehand, and in particular it should include advice on possible change in voice and possible hyperthyroidism or damage to the recurrent nerve.

Position of patient

Supine with neck extended at 20°–25° and the table foot down. Place the head on a padded ring with a pillow or pad beneath the shoulders. Place packs on either side of the neck. Use a double towel as a head set. Stand on the side opposite the lobe to be removed.

Incision

Look for skin creases. Mark the incision beforehand with ink or a 2/0 thread pressed on the skin. Make a transverse incision near to midway between the thyroid cartilage and manubrial notch, in a crease if possible. The incision should reach the sternomastoid on each side.

Procedure

Use a no. 15 blade. Deepen the incision through fat, platysma, and cervical fascia to expose the strap muscles. Reflect skin flaps proximally and distally. Begin with the knife and then use gauze dissection. Stop bleeding. Insert a Joll retractor.

Divide the strap muscles in the midline. The deep-layer

muscles (sternothyroids) may be stretched or adherent to the gland. When they are split the gland is exposed.

Thyroid lobectomy
Palpate both lobes to assess the extent of disease. Ligate the middle thyroid veins. Now draw down the upper pole. Identify the superior thyroid vessels. Ligate them with care using 2/0 Vicryl. Draw the upper pole down with a Kocher forceps and divide the vessels below the ligature with a scalpel. The upper pole can now be peeled downwards under gentle traction.

315

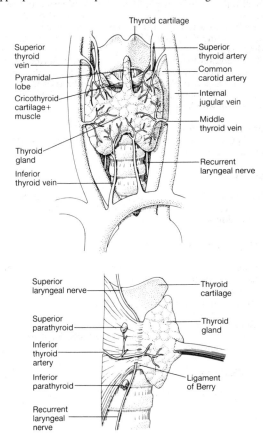

Thyroid gland.

THYROIDECTOMY (*cont.*)

Apply gentle traction on the forceps to rotate the pole to the opposite side. Wipe away the fascia on its undersurface to identify the superior parathyroid. Divide any vessels between thus thyroid and parathyroid, thus keeping them safe.

Now pay attention to the recurrent laryngeal nerve and the inferior thyroid artery. Move the assistant's retractor to exert a pull laterally. Apply a small swab to the gland and exert a medial pull with the left hand to expose the fascia overlying the inferior thyroid artery, the recurrent laryngeal nerve, and the inferior parathyroid. Gently divide the fascia longitudinally to identify the nerve close to the ligament of Berry. Do not disturb the inferior parathyroid. Simply locate it. Ligate the artery in continuity and then the inferior thyroid veins. The lobe is now free and can be removed by dividing the isthmus, dissecting the gland off the trachea, and oversewing the isthmus with Vicryl.

In a subtotal lobectomy the gland is not dissected off the trachea. Instead, several small haemostats are applied along the lateral aspect of the gland anterior to the recurrent nerve and the tissue anterior to the forceps is excised. The remnant is oversewn with Vicryl if possible.

Total thyroidectomy

Total lobectomies are performed on each side with or without radical neck dissection.

Closure

Close in layers. Bring suction drains (one on each side) through separate stab wounds. Close the platysma with Vicryl and the skin with clips.

Postoperative care

1. Check the vocal cords postoperatively. The anaesthetist usually does this (but the appearance of the cords may be misleading).
2. Ensure an adequate airway. If haematoma develops open all the layers of the wound.
3. Remove drains on day 2. Check serum calcium daily.
4. Home on day 3–5. Surgical out-patients department and thyroid function tests after 6 weeks.

Complications

These can be early, intermediate, or late.

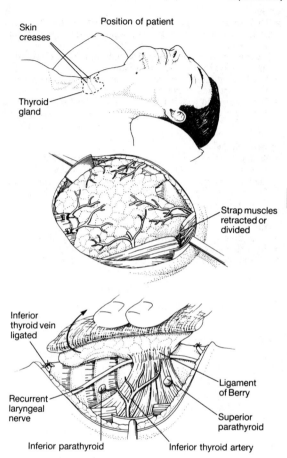

Position of patient

Skin creases

Thyroid gland

Strap muscles retracted or divided

317

Inferior thyroid vein ligated

Recurrent laryngeal nerve

Inferior parathyroid

Ligament of Berry

Superior parathyroid

Inferior thyroid artery

Thyroidectomy.

THYROIDECTOMY (*cont.*)

Early
- Thyrotoxic storm is rare after thyroidectomy for thyrotoxicosis but needs treatment with antithyroid drugs and beta blockade.
- Bleeding may be reactionary within hours of the operation and requires urgent decompression.
- Tracheal collapse is usually recognized by the anaesthetist and requires re-intubation.
- Paralysis of the recurrent nerves or superior laryngeal nerve damage usually presents as a voice change if not recognized early.

Intermediate
- Wound infection and hypocalcaemic tetany which usually occurs within a week of surgery. Always check the serum calcium preoperatively before the patient goes home. Tetany is treated by intravenous infusion of calcium and then oral administration of vitamin D.

Late
- Hypothyroidism—confirmed by measuring thyroxine levels.
- Hypertrophy of the scar.
- Keloid is rare except in the dark-skinned races.

PARATHYROIDECTOMY

Indications

Parathyroid adenomas, carcinoma, secondary- or tertiary-hyperparathyroidism (all four glands).

Preoperative preparations

Frozen section facilities should be available. The laboratory should be informed.

Position of patient

Supine with the head on a neck ring, the neck extended, and a 20°–25° downward tilt.

Incision and access

The same approach as for subtotal thyroidectomy is used (p. 00).

Procedure

Mobilize the thyroid gland and retract its upper and lower lobes forward. Also asssess its areolar bed. The normal parathyroid glands are difficult to identify but lie posterior to each of the four poles of the thyroid. Each gland is yellowish and is flattened with a small vascular pedicle.

If there is an adenoma carefully remove it. If the patient has secondary- or tertiary-hyperparathyroidism, remove all four glands.

Apply tissue or dissecting forceps to the gland and dissect it free by a combination of sharp and blunt dissection. Diathermize bleeding vessels. If you are in doubt about the nature of the tissue send biopsies for frozen section. Sometimes an adenoma can be found in the mediastinal region or in relation to the superior or inferior thyroid arteries.

Closure

Layers. Clips to skin. Suction drainage.

Postoperative care

- Observe for signs of hypocalcaemia and haematoma.
- Remove the drain at 2–3 days.
- Repeat serum calcium daily to observe the trend.
- Most patients can have their sutures removed on day 4 or 5 and go home.
- Arrange surgical out-patients department appointment in 6–8 weeks.

Complications

- Haemorrhage.
- Nerve injury
  - Unilateral recurrent laryngeal nerve injury: hoarseness
  - Bilateral recurrent laryngeal nerve injury: stridor
  - Superior laryngeal nerve: change in 'timbre' of voice
  - Cervical sympathetic chain: Horner's syndrome.

ADRENALECTOMY

Indications

- Cushing's disease
- Aldosteronoma (Conn's syndrome)
- Phaeochromocytoma.
- Advanced breast cancer (now rare)

Preoperative care

- Locate tumours by CT scan or arteriography.
- Check serum potassium (Conn's syndrome).
- Prevent alkalosis due to hypokalaemia which leads to tetany.
- Check and correct serum sodium which contributes to hypertension.
- Estimate serum catecholamine levels.
- Rogitine (phentolamine) test for phaeochromocytoma. Blood pressure falls for a short time in response to drug.
- Use beta-blocking agents to control blood pressure for several days before surgery to allow adequate expansion of plasma volume. Discontinue for 24 hours presurgery.

Anaesthetic

General anaesthetic. In cases of phaeochromocytoma tranquillizers are given as premedication because opiates stimulate catecholamine release. IV lignocaine, propranolol, and phenotolamine are at hand to correct dysrhythmias or blood pressure changes.

Approaches

- *Anterior*: both glands.
- *Lateral*: obese patients, tumour localized to one side.

Position of patient

- *Anterior*: patient supine, foot down 30°, lateral tilt.
- *Lateral*: patient in full lateral position, table broken to 30° over ribs 10 and 11.

Strap the patient to the table for both approaches.

Incisions

- *Anterior*: long left paramedian. Extend laterally through the transpyloric plane if access is difficult.
- *Lateral*: over rib 11 from lateral border of sacrospinalis to abdominal wall.

Procedure

Anterior approach
Left adrenal   Pack small intestine downwards. Retract costal margin upwards. Place left hand over spleen and divide the posterior parietal peritoneum from the splenic flexure to the oesophageal hiatus. Apply several pairs of forceps to retract the peritoneum downwards. Identify the kidney with the adrenal gland above it. Identify and divide between ligatures the adrenal vein which drains into the left renal vein. Mobilize and remove the gland by blunt dissection. Cauterize bleeders.

Right adrenal   Retract liver upwards and hepatic flexure downwards. Note the vena cava and kidney. Divide the posterior parietal peritoneum along the upper pole of the kidney to the vena cava. Identify the gland. Divide the two or three adrenal veins which drain into the vena cava between ligatures. Remove the gland by blunt dissection. Secure haemostasis.

323

Lateral approach
Deepen the incision in the rib bed. Beware of the pleura. Use a self-retaining retractor. Identify kidney and upper pole. Divide its fascia. Remove the gland carefully as in the anterior approach.

Closure

Layers. Suction drain. Nylon to skin.

7 Laparoscopy and laparotomy in general surgery

Introduction   326
Laparoscopic cholecystectomy   328
Laparoscopic appendicectomy   334
Exploratory laparotomy   338
Second-look abdominal surgery   340

325

INTRODUCTION

Laparoscopy is a relatively new technique in general surgery. It involves a completely different approach to surgery within the abdominal cavity and allows the whole surgical team to see clearly with the use of a camera and television. Good assessment of the abdominal contents can also be made by laparoscopy. Indeed, in the past few years laparoscopic cholecystectomy and other laparoscopic procedures have become standard practice. New instrumentation is allowing manipulation to become easier, with the placement of ties, clips, and anastomosis using stapling devices. Drains can also be inserted through the laparoscope and a whole new range of operations, including oesophagectomy, vagotomy, Nissen fundoplications, colectomy, and hernia repair, are now being undertaken by laparoscopic means.

Although laparoscopic cholecystectomy is now an accepted first option for surgical treatment, laparoscopic appendicectomy was much slower in gaining widespread acceptance. However, it should be remembered that open appendicectomy should not be lost from the training programme.

LAPAROSCOPIC CHOLECYSTECTOMY (extra-major)

The indications are as for open surgery and the procedure can be performed electively or as an emergency.

Preoperative preparations

Normal liver function tests, normal calibre common bile duct (assessed with ultrasound), preoperative insertion of a nasogastric tube to decompress the stomach, and catheterization of the bladder before inducing a pneumoperitoneum with a Verres needle. None of these precautionary procedures is strictly necessary. The facility to undertake intraoperative cholangiography should be available.

Anaesthetic

Unless otherwise stated, these procedures are performed under general anaesthesia with the patient supine.

Incision

Four ports are usually used for the operation. Two 10 mm ports are used, one located a third of the way from the xiphisternum to the umbilicus and the other subumbilically. The latter is inserted first after induction of a pneumoperitoneum using a Verres needle. Two 5 mm ports are placed in the right flank, usually in the anterior and mid-axillary lines. If the ports are too close together, the instruments and telescope obstruct each, making access more difficult. Carbon dioxide is insufflated; usually approximately 3–4 litres is required for an adequate pneumoperitoneum. Ensure after the Verres needle has been inserted that the flow of gas is not impeded and that the pressure is not unduly high. Fortunately, most modern insufflation machines have settings for this to avoid the danger. After induction of the pneumoperitoneum it is safer to use a disposable 10 mm trocar with a safety guard.

When there has been previous upper abdominal surgery open insertion of a 10 mm port is safer. Gynaecologists rarely bother, but general surgeons tend to undertake the Palmer test where a 20 ml syringe containing saline is placed on the Verres needle prior to connection to carbon dioxide insufflation. If normal saline is seen to run into the peritoneum easily, then it is safe to proceed further. Reducers down 10 mm ports are needed in order to insert the instruments. This is usually the case with the upper mid-line port.

The telescope is inserted through the umbilical port and a laparotomy should be undertaken. Fogging of the lens system can be prevented by warming the telescope in warm water. Diathermy or laser can be used for the cutting procedures.

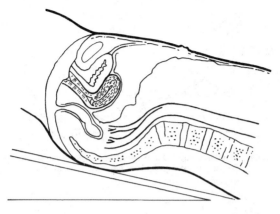

With the patient in the head-down position the small bowel shifts
cephalad, permitting easier and safer insertion of the needle.

329

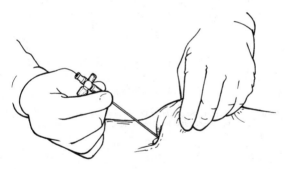

With the patient in the Trendelenburg position, grasp the abdominal
wall. Insert the Veress needle towards the pelvis.

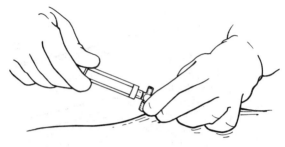

Before insufflation check that the needle is safely placed; blood or faeces in the syringe indicate improper placement.

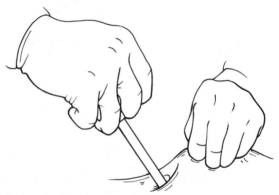

As the trocar is inserted direct its tip towards the pelvis; gently rotate the tip to ensure that the tissue is incised rather than torn.

Procedure

Identify the gall bladder and gently divide the adhesions that may exist between it and the omentum. This is usually achieved using non-toothed forceps. Grasp the fundus of the gall bladder with a toothed instrument through the most lateral 5 mm port and push the fundus superiorly. This usually exposes the rest of the gall bladder, allowing further dissection of omentum from it as well as tenting up the cystic duct. Most of this dissection is undertaken through the superior 10 mm port. As the gall bladder becomes further exposed, the second 5 mm port can be used for another toothed forceps to lift up the cystic duct. At all times keep close to the gall bladder wall. In at least one-third of patients the cystic artery may not be seen.

Grasping
forceps

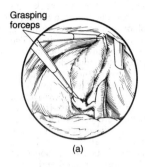

(a)

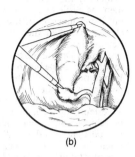

(b)

(a) The gall bladder is pushed upwards over the edge of the liver to expose the cystic duct and artery.
(b) The cystic artery and duct in turn have staples applied to them

331

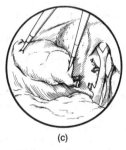

(c)

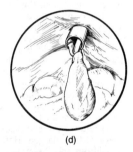

(d)

(c) The gall bladder is dissected from the liver bed.

(d) The dissected gall bladder is then drawn into the portal on the anterior abdominal wall. It can usually be removed by gentle traction. If there are large stones the port incision may need to be enlarged.

Steps in laparoscopic cholecystectomy.

LAPAROSCOPIC CHOLECYSTECTOMY
(extra-major) (cont.)

Identify the body of the gall bladder, then the neck, and then the cystic duct. The common bile duct is often not seen, but if the junction of the gall bladder with its cystic duct is clearly identified then it is safe to mobilize the duct. The Petelin dissector is useful for opening the plane behind the cystic duct. Once it has been identified, place three clips adjacent to the neck of the gall bladder. Use scissors through the upper 10 mm port to divide the cystic duct, leaving two clips on the non-specimen side. The cystic artery may then be seen and it can be divided between the clips in the same way. If it is inadvertently opened, do not apply diathermy. Haemostasis can be achieved by placing a pledget down the upper 10 mm midline port and bleeding will be minimized after a few minutes. Then the arterial end can either be clipped or a loop knot can be placed around it. Loop knots are pre-tied and easily tightened down the trocar.

If an operative cholangiogram has to be performed, first place a clip on the cystic duct distally leaving as much cystic duct visible as possible. Make a small hole into the cystic duct lumen and pass an umbilical catheter or a similar cannula into the cystic duct via one of the lateral ports. There are several devices which hold this in place, allowing cholangiography to be carried out without leakage. The gall bladder can then be removed from the liver bed with a combination of diathermy or laser and irrigation. Usually it is the peritoneum which needs to be divided and this can be done with hooked diathermy or spoon. The gall bladder is then removed through one of the large ports. This is made easier by putting the specimen into a plastic bag to prevent the loss of stones when it is being removed. A final check for bleeding in the gall bladder-bed can then be made before the final adhesion is removed from the liver.

To remove the gall bladder the upper 10 mm port incision needs to be enlarged. Before this is undertaken, bile can be sucked out and the stones can either be crushed or removed with Desjardin forceps. Few units have a lithotripter suitable and available for this procedure.

If there is any concern about bleeding or a bile leak, a drain can be placed into the gall-bladder bed through one of the right flank ports. It is usually unnecessary to close the deep layers unless the incisions have been extended, in which case they can be closed with 2/0 Vicryl or 2/0 PDS. Subcutaneous Vicryl or Steristrips can be used to close skin.

LAPAROSCOPIC APPENDICETOMY (major)

Laparoscopic appendicectomy should be avoided in pregnancy or in the resolving phase of acute appendicitis when a mass or abscess is a possibility. More experienced surgeons may not regard these as contraindications.

Incision

Two 10 mm ports need to be inserted, one subumbilically for the telescope and one in the lower right iliac fossa for manipulation and to remove the appendix. A high 5 mm port in the mid-clavicular line at umbilical level or a low port on the left iliac fossa should also be inserted.

Procedure

The vessels to the appendix need to be exposed and clipped or ligated. Two pre-tied loops may be placed on the appendix before its amputation and removal through the 10 mm right iliac fossa port, which may need to be enlarged.

Slip knots with catgut for the appendix base are preferable to clips which do not fit a large appendix and are in danger of coming off. Indications for drains and closure are the same as for laparoscopic cholecystectomy.

Complications

If technical difficulties due to extensive adhesions, unsuspected abdominal pathology, abnormal anatomy, acute inflammation, or excessive bleeding develop during either of these procedures, the procedure must be converted to an open operation immediately.

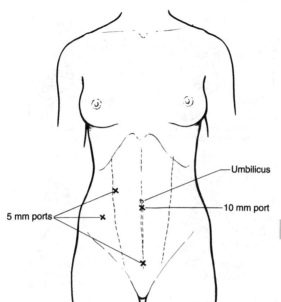

5 mm ports

Umbilicus

10 mm port

Laparoscopic appendicectomy.

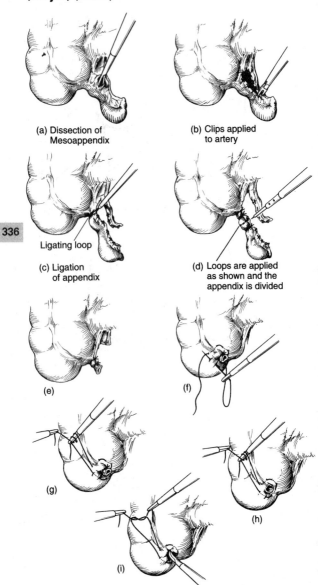

(a) Dissection of
    Mesoappendix

(b) Clips applied
    to artery

(c) Ligation
    of appendix

Ligating loop

(d) Loops are applied
    as shown and the
    appendix is divided

(e)

(f)

(g)

(h)

(i)

336

(a–e) Steps in laparoscopic appendectomy; (f–g) inserting the purse-string suture.

EXPLORATORY LAPAROTOMY (major)

This operation is indicated in elective patients when investigations have failed to confirm the diagnosis or when the operability of a condition is in doubt. In emergency cases laparotomy may be indicated to determine the diagnosis and subsequent treatment in the patient with an acute abdomen. All abdominal procedures should be combined with a laparotomy.

Preoperative assessment

Appropriate haematology and biochemistry results should be at hand. Resuscitation should be as complete as possible in emergency cases. Cefuroxime 1500 mg IV and metronidazole 500 mg IV should be given on induction if septic peritonitis is suspected. Be prepared to start intravenous antibiotics by ensuring that an IV line has been established.

Incision

Mid-line skirting the umbilicus.

Procedure

Open the peritoneum (paramedian). Is there free fluid or pus? Take a bacteriology swab if there is. Now examine the abdominal contents systematically. Begin by examining the lobes of the liver. Are there metastases? Next examine the gall bladder (are there stones?) and spleen. Examine the oesophageal hiatus, stomach, and pylorus. Is there a perforated duodenal ulcer? Are the bile ducts normal?

Palpate the right kidney and head of pancreas. Then lift the greater omentum out of the wound and pass the right hand down behind it to examine first the body and tail of pancreas, then the left kidney, then all the transverse colon, both the ascending colon and caecum, and then the descending, sigmoid, and pelvic colon as far as possible. Is there diverticular disease or a carcinoma? Now inspect the root of the mesentery with its vessels and, proceeding from the duodenojejunal flexure, examine all the small bowel to the appendix. Is there inflammation (Crohn's disease?), a Meckel's diverticulum, or appendicitis? (If obvious pathology is found early (e.g. appendicitis), it is best dealt with first and then followed by a laparotomy.)

Finally, examine the pelvic organs and hernial orifices. Note whether there is dilatation of the ureters (hydronephrosis). Does the uterus contain fibroids? Are the tubes and ovaries inflamed (salpingitis)? Is there tubal bleeding (ruptured ectopic pregnancy)? Note should also be made of the retroperitoneal structures. Is there an aortic aneurysm? (This is usually extremely obvious!) Are there abnormalities of the iliac vessels? Is there a retroperitoneal mass? Once the diagnosis has been confirmed, carry out the definitive procedure indicated in the circumstances.

Closure

Mass closure with interrupted or subcuticular Nylon to skin. Suture any drain in position, bringing them out through a separate stab wound.

Special postoperative care

Maintain the IV infusion until bowel sounds return. Then start oral fluids. Monitor temperature, respiration, and urine output. Continue antibiotics if indicated.

Complications

See Chapter 1 (postoperative care (pp. 42) and late postoperative complications (pp. 52)).

339

Discharge

Seven to ten days after operation in uncomplicated cases.

SECOND-LOOK ABDOMINAL SURGERY
(major complex)

Laparotomy can also be used in second-look abdominal surgery.

Indications

- Suspicion of a leaking anastomosis.
- Suspicion of a venous mesenteric thrombosis.
- To reassess cancer. This may be up to six months after colorectal surgery. Markers like carcinoembryonic antigen (CEA) are not of consistent help, and second-look surgery after cancer is still controversial.
- Suspicion of persistent sepsis.
- Suspicion of necrosectomy in pancreatitis.

The technique of laparostomy with the insertion of an abdominal zipper has been used for acute conditions in other countries, but has not gained popularity in the United Kingdom to date.

8 Stapling in surgery

Introduction   344
Stapling technique in anterior resection   346
Stapling technique in oesophagojejunostomy
    (Roux loop) after transabdominal total
    gastrectomy   348
Stapling technique for transection of
    bleeding oesophageal varices   350
Stapling technique for transection of
    duodenum   352
Stapling technique for gastroenterostomy   354
Stapling technique for bowel resection and
    functional end-to-end anastomosis   356

INTRODUCTION

The first linear stapler used successfully in surgery was described by Professor Humer Hultl in Hungary in 1908. This large instrument weighed 5 kg and took 2 hours to load. In 1921 von Petz described a much lighter instrument which was easier to use. These early instruments inserted a double row of staples giving a B-closure which achieved haemostasis without necrosis of the suture line. Modern instruments are now disposable and some have a multiple-fire facility allowing them to be used several times without the need to re-open a basic unit. Some of these instruments have different staple heights which can be adapted for use in different thicknesses of tissue.

End-to-end staplers

These instruments insert a double row of staples in circular fashion and are used for visceral end-to-end anastomosis. The gun is fired to insert the staples against an anvil and there is a knife which cuts the tissue within the lumen of the bowel at the same time as it staples (see section on stapling technique in anterior resection). Some of the instruments are curved with a detachable or rotatory anvil which allows much greater adaptability, particularly when transecting oesophageal varices or carrying out transabdomino-oesophagojejunal anastomosis or a low anterior resection. The action of end-to-end staplers is to invert the bowel edges. There are varied diameters between 21 and 133 mm to accommodate the bowel lumen being anastomosed.

Linear staplers

These insert two parallel staple lines. The lengths vary from 30 to 90 mm, with the shorter ones being used for closing a small bowel enterotomy, for example, the intermediate ones for closing the duodenal stump after a partial gastrectomy, and the longer ones for creating a new lesser curve after distal gastrectomy.

Side-to-side staplers

Here four parallel staple lines are inserted with a cutting blade between. The lengths vary from 50 to 90 mm permitting side-to-side anastomosis. This is particularly useful if speed is important or in less accessible operations. These instruments can also be used for laparoscopic work, allowing bowel anastomosis down 10 mm ports.

Accessories are available, for example the tissue-measuring and purse-string-inserting devices. Some operations are made easier or carried out more quickly with staples, and this justifies their cost in many cases.

STAPLING TECHNIQUE IN ANTERIOR RESECTION (complex major)

Preparation, anaesthetic, and incision are as for hand-sewn anterior resection. The table should be in Lloyd Davies position to allow per anum access.

Procedure

As for anterior resection. Be certain that the proximal colon reaches the pelvis easily and mobilize the splenic flexure if not. Place a purse-string suture in the proximal colonic resection line using a disposable purse-string device, a modified Furness clamp, or by hand. Use 2/0 Prolene on a round-bodied needle. Start extra-luminally and then continuously over and over taking full thickness bites, in and out, to invert the bowel edge. The two ends will be on the outside of the bowel. The ideal siting is on the anterior aspect so that tightening of the purse-string suture later is facilitated. The distal purse-string is placed on the rectal stump and is best performed by hand. Metal sizers used to assess which size of stapler to use can be traumatic, and simple measurement with a ruler is safer. However, when a sizer is introduced through the anus it can lift a very low anterior rectal stump into the pelvis, making the insertion of the purse-string easier. Again, try to place the two suture ends anteriorly.

If the end-to-end stapler being used can be set for tissue thickness, take the mean of the tissue thicknesses. Choose the

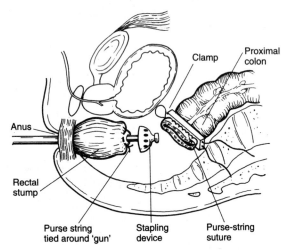

Stapling technique in anterior resection.

largest stapler that can safely be introduced into the two bowel lumina. A curved instrument usually makes this easier. If the pelvis is narrow, use an instrument with a head which can be revolved (roticulator). Introduce the stapling device per anum with its safety catch on. Open the instrument to separate the firing end from the distal anvil. Tie the purse-string sutures over the separated ends. A perineal operator can move the instrument from below to make this easier. Close the instrument and ensure that no extraneous tissues enter it by keeping a hand around the proposed anastomosis. When closed remove the safety catch and fire the instrument. Open the anvil two to three turns and rotate the stapler through 360°, which should be easy. Remove the stapler through the anastomosis carefully as if undoing a button from a buttonhole, but keeping your left hand around the anastomosis.

When the stapler is removed detach the anvil and remove the two colon ends. Both should be complete 'doughnuts', confirming a complete anastomosis which is secure. If these are not complete, it may be necessary to redo the anastomosis or repair the defect. Some surgeons test the anastomotic integrity by filling the pelvis with saline containing a weak antiseptic and looking for air leaks with air insufflation below. If the omentum is free encourage it to lie in the pelvis.

347

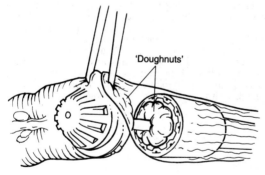

Buttonholing out of end-to-end stapler after firing (note 'doughnuts').

STAPLING TECHNIQUE IN OESOPHAGOJEJUNOSTOMY (ROUX LOOP) AFTER TRANSABDOMINAL TOTAL GASTRECTOMY (major)

This is a major procedure. Preparation, anaesthetic, position, and incision are the same as in abdominal total gastrectomy.

Procedure

Fashion a Roux loop of jejunum, either retrocolic or antecolic. This can be done quickly using a multifire side-to-side stapler. Leave the end of the proximal jejunum open, ensuring that it can reach the oesophagus below the hiatus. Prevent proximal retraction of the oesophagus by applying a soft clamp above stay sutures which have been inserted into the mucosa. Place a 2/0 Prolene purse-string suture as for a stapled anterior resection ensuring that the ends are outside the lumen. Include full thickness, particularly the strong mucosa.

Insert an appropriately sized end-to-end stapler with the anvil removed through the open end of the jejunal loop. Ensure that the safety catch is on, that the stapler is the largest you can safely use, and that you have checked staple heights and tissue thickness. Push the spindle spike through the jejunum 4–5 cm within the bowel end on the antimesenteric side. No purse-string is necessary. A curved stapler with a detachable roticulating head makes this easier. Tie the purse-string in the oesophageal resection line over the anvil and join the stapler. Close the stapler and fire it after removing the safety catch. Open the stapler two to three turns and rotate it through 360°. Then remove it, holding the anastomosis with your left hand and using the buttonhole technique. Feel the anastomosis through the open jejunum and ensure that it is intact and that the efferent long loop is open. Close the open jejunum with a linear stapler or by hand using two layers of Vicryl.

Stapling technique in oseophagojejunostomy (Roux loop) after
transabdominal total gastrectomy (major)

349

STAPLING TECHNIQUE FOR TRANSECTION OF BLEEDING OESOPHAGEAL VARICES (major)

When varices continue to bleed despite medical therapy resuscitation and insertion of Sengstaken tubes, transection should be considered. Gastric varices and other sources of GI bleeding must be excluded. Preparation, anaesthetic, position on the table, and incision are the same as for other variceal procedures.

Procedure

Divide the phreno-oesophageal ligament and dissect free the lower oesophagus. Place an atraumatic sling around it, taking care not to damage the vagal nerves.

Make a small gastrostomy high in the anterior surface of the stomach to accommodate the largest end-to-end stapler that has been judged to fit in the oesophagus with adjustments calculated for staple height and tissue thickness. Insert the complete stapler into the oesophagus with the safety catch on. Open the stapler three or four turns so that there is a gap between the anvil and the firing end. Tie a 2/0 silk or other easily tied braided suture into the gap, thereby inverting the whole circumference of the oesophagus into the gun. Close and then fire the gun with a protective hand around the site of anastomosis. Open the gun two or three turns and rotate it through 360° before removing it with the buttonhole technique. Check the doughnuts and the anastomosis which should be 2–3 cm above the oesophagogastric junction.

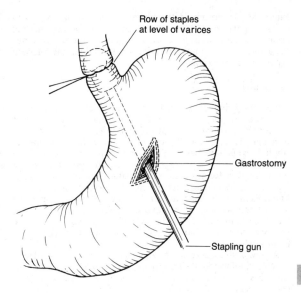

End-to-end transfixion ligation of oesophageal varices.

STAPLING TECHNIQUE FOR TRANSECTION OF DUODENUM (major)

Linear staple closure of the bowel is safe, haemostatic, and quick to perform. Closure of the duodenum by this method applies equally well to closure of other bowel segments. Preparation, anaesthetic, position on the table, and incision are as for gastrectomy.

Procedure

After mobilizing the stomach during total or Polya gastrectomy, prepare the duodenum for transection. Place a linear stapler (30 or 60 mm long) just distal to the proposed transection line. Ensure that the catch is on and that the correct staple heights have been taken into account. Place a crushing clamp (Parker-Kerr or Payrs) adjacent and proximal to the linear stapler. Remove the safety catch and fire the stapler. Divide the duodenum between the stapler and clamp using a knife. Remove the specimen or displace it medially. Open the jaws of the stapler and remove it. Check the staple line for bleeding. If there is a bleeding vessel, underrun it. Drainage to cover the risk of blow out is no more necessary than after hand-sewn closure.

A new lesser curve to the stomach during distal gastrectomy can be fashioned similarly using the longer 90 mm linear stapler. Continuity can be re-established with a gastroenterostomy using a side-to-side stapler (Polya) or an end-to-end stapler to the duodenum (Billroth 1).

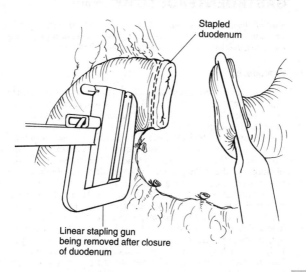

Stapled
duodenum

Linear stapling gun
being removed after closure
of duodenum

353

Stapled closure of duodenum.

STAPLING TECHNIQUE FOR
GASTROENTEROSTOMY (major)

Stapled gastroenterostomy using a side-to-side technique is
easy and rapid to perform in distal gastric resection or palliative proximal bypass for unresectable antral cancer.

Procedure

After resecting the distal stomach or realizing that the antral
cancer cannot be resected, bring up a loop of duodenum ante-
or retrocolically so that it reaches the stomach without tension.
In palliative surgery exclude the distal stomach (the 90 mm
linear stapler is ideal for this). Position the jejunal loop with
the afferent loop to the lesser curve so that the proposed
stoma lies in the most dependent part of the stomach. Plan the
position of the stomach and jejunal loop for stapling and
ensure that vessels in the gastric arcade and jejunal mesentery
are not embarrassed. Hold the proposed suture lines adjacent
with four Babcocks' forceps. Make two enterotomies opposite
each other in the duodenum and stomach with diathermy.
These should admit the jaws of a side-to-side stapler and be
approximately 1 cm across. Insert the open jaws of the stapler
fully into each viscus and approximate the proximal end first.
Ensure that the vessels and other structures are not incorpo-
rated and fire the stapler. Open the stapler and remove it. The
anastomosis can be inspected for completeness and bleeding
through the now single enterotomy. Close the enterotomy
with two layers of continuous 2/0 Vicryl or with a linear
stapler. It is not necessary to reinforce the staple line, but a
Vicryl suture placed seromuscularly at each end of the anastomosis may take the strain off it.

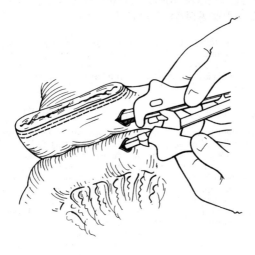

355

Gastroenterostomy using side-to-side stapler.

STAPLING TECHNIQUE FOR BOWEL RESECTION AND FUNCTIONAL END-TO-END ANASTOMOSIS (major)

After bowel resection, e.g. right hemicolectomy, an end-to-end anastomosis can be fashioned quickly using the side-to-side stapler. Preparation, anaesthetic, position on the table, and incision are the same as for conventional hand-sewn anastomosis.

Procedure

After right hemicolectomy line up the distal ileum and transverse colon with their open lumina adjacent using Babcock's tissue forceps. Be sure that the mesentery of each viscus is as far away from the proposed anastomosis as possible. Ideally the staple line should run along the antemesenteric border. Insert the open jaws of the stapler down each bowel limb, close, and fire. Open and remove the stapler and inspect the long side-to-side join. Close the open ends of the ileum and colon with two layers of continuous 2/0 Vicryl or by using a linear stapler. A similar palliative gastoenterostomy bypass can be fashioned quickly for an unresectable cancer by lining up two loops of bowel as in gastroenterostomy.

Stapling can be justified when operative procedures can be undertaken more quickly and easily. Other more complex operations are further facilitated by stapling, which is the method of choice for many surgeons. Such operations include small bowel pelvic pouches and Koch reservoir ileostomy, vertical banded gastroplasty (for obesity), and reverse gastric tubes. Oesophageal replacement using stomach, colon, or small bowel is also quicker using stapling techniques

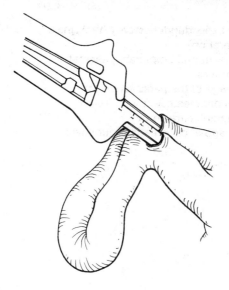

357

Functional end-to-end anastomosis.

9 Pancreatic surgery

Pancreaticoduodenectomy (Whipple's
    operation)   360
Enucleation of ampullary pancreatic
    tumours   364
Drainage of the pancreatic duct   366
Distal pancreatectomy   368
Total pancreatectomy   370
Drainage of pancreatic pseudocyst   372

PANCREATICODUODENECTOMY (WHIPPLE'S OPERATION) (complex)

Ensure that the patient is on an X-ray table so that inter-operative X-rays can be taken.

Incision

Upper mid-line or gable (two subcostal incisions meeting in the mid-line). Access can be improved with a self-retaining ring retractor or a sternal retractor.

Procedure

Carry out a laparotomy to assess the extent of disease and operability. Evaluate the lesser sac via the greater omentum. Examine the root of the mesocolon and the porta hepatis, if need be with frozen section.

If the carcinoma appears to be operable, Kocherize the duodenum fully and identify the common bile duct, the hepatic artery, the right gastric artery, and the gastroduodenal artery. Mobilize the neck of the pancreas whilst raising the duo-denum and identify the superior mesenteric vein along the inferior border of the neck of the pancreas. This leads to the portal vein. Assess operability by lifting the pancreas off the portal vein. There are usually no veins passing directly posteriorly from the neck of the pancreas to the structures beneath, and the superior and inferior borders of the neck of the pancreas can be opened, gently dissecting with the index fingers of each hand. If the portal vein is clearly involved, the tumour is not resectable. Many vessels pass from the right side of the portal vein to the head of the pancreas and unci-nate process. Avoid damaging these until operability is con-firmed. The pancreas can be dissected free anteriorly if there is no involvement, and a ligature can be passed around its neck anterior to the portal vein. The neck can then be divided using diathermy when a dilated pancreatic duct can often be seen. If the ligature has already been passed behind the neck of the pancreas, haemostasis can easily be achieved by gently tightening this.

Ligate the gastroduodenal artery, avoiding damage to the hepatic artery. Mobilize the supraduodenal common bile duct and gall bladder. Remove the gall bladder and divide the common bile duct. A soft vascular clamp will prevent leakage of bile from above. A distal gastrectomy *en bloc* with the pancreatic specimen can then be achieved using the linear stapler (see section on gastrectomy and stapling). This leaves the stapled gastric remnant and a stapled jejunum distal to the resection specimen.

Divide the ligament of Treitz and mobilize the duodeno-jejunal flexure. Transect the upper jejunum and advance this through the mesocolon. The specimen can now be freed

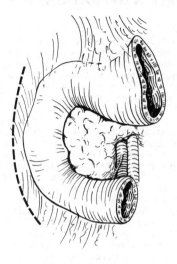

Kocherization of duodenum.

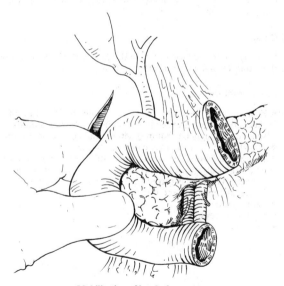

Mobilization of head of pancreas.

PANCREATICODUODENECTOMY (WHIPPLE'S OPERATION) (complex) (*cont.*)

together with the distal stomach, the duodenum, the first part of the jejunum, and the lower common bile duct.

The anastomosis can now be fashioned. Start with the pancreaticojejunal side-to-end anastomosis. The conventional method of doing this is to 'ink-pot' the jejunum (invert the antimesenteric border of the jejunum over the cut end of the pancreas) in two layers over the whole of the remaining pancreatic neck. 3/0 Vicryl can be used for this and strengthened with an external suture such as silk. When there is a large obstructed pancreatic duct, direct ductal suture to the jejunal mucosa end-to-side can be carried out by removing some seromuscular tissue from the jejunum to allow direct mucosal apposition. A 4/0 or 5/0 Vicryl suture is used. With direct duct to jejunal sutures splint the anastomosis with a catheter from the pancreatic duct into the jejunum, particularly if the pancreatic duct is small. The common bile duct is anastomosed using interrupted 3/0 Vicryl end-to-side to that portion of jejunum distal to the pancreaticojejunostomy. Ensure that there is no tension and splint the anastomosis with a T-tube. Finally, fashion a gastroenterosotomy. This should be retrocolic and can be stapled. The anastomosis will be of the Polya type incorporating a Hofmeister valve (see section on gastrectomy operations).

Closure

Leave two large suction drains in the pancreatic bed and bring them out through separate stab wounds.

Complications

- Postoperative bleeding. Suspect if the patient becomes shocked or there is excessive blood in the drainage bottles. A second look may be required within hours of the operation.
- Anastomotic leakage may cause peritonitis.
- Pancreatic fistula formation. This can present as peritonitis or a high-output fistula through the drain site or the main wounds. The fluid is turbid with a high amylase content.
- Pancreatic necrosis and infection.
- Wound infection.
- Hypergylcaemia.
- Diabetes.

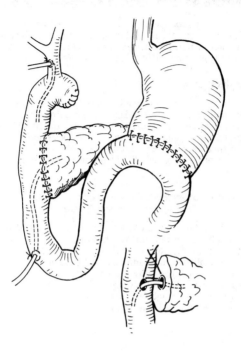

363

Pancreaticoduodenectomy (Whipple's operation) showing three anastomoses.

ENUCLEATION OF AMPULLARY PANCREATIC TUMOURS (extra-major)

This procedure can be carried out for localized carcinoma, particularly in the elderly and frail. The operative mortality is much lower than that for pancreaticoduodenectomy and survival is generally good provided that the cancer is localized.

Procedure

After the duodenum has been Kocherized carry out a duodenotomy and excise the ampullary tumour submucosally using diathermy to ensure a clear margin. Carry out a sphincteroplasty at the lower end of the common bile duct. If the pancreatic duct is small, it will need stenting. Close the duodenotomy in two layers of 3/0 Vicryl, usually in a transverse manner to prevent stenosis.

Enucleation of endocrine tumours (insulinoma, gastrinoma, Zollinger–Ellison syndrome)

When these tumours have been localized by CT scanning, angiography, or intraoperative ultrasound, they can be enucleated. However, this procedure is not indicated if the tumour is malignant or multiple. If there are metastases in the presence of Zollinger–Ellison syndrome, a truncal vagotomy and pyloroplasty is also required. The pancreas is exposed through the gastrocolic omentum, thereby gaining access to the lesser sac and the whole of the gland.

DRAINAGE OF THE PANCREATIC DUCT (major)

Indications

- Chronic pancreatitis
- Obstructing carcinoma
- Internal drainage of a fistula
- Stenosis following trauma

Preoperative preparation

The size of the duct can usually be ascertained from CT scan, ultrasound or pancreatography, and ERCP.

Incision

Upper mid-line.

Procedure

Open the lesser sac through the gastrocolic omentum. Locate the duct digitally or identify it by needling. Place some stay sutures in the pancreatic capsule and then open the duct with scissors, knife, or diathermy longitudinally along its dilated segment. Divide any strictures within the dilated duct. Prepare a Roux loop of the upper jejunum and bring its distal limb through the colonic mesentery. Use an avascular mesenteric defect to the left of the middle colic artery.

With 3/0 Vicryl make a continuous seromuscular anastomosis between the duct and a jejunostomy in side-to-side fashion. Open the jejunum to match the duct size. Splint the anastomosis with a T-tube brought out via the jejunum or the posterior gastric wall.

It is possible to excise the pancreatic tail to expose a dilated duct and to place a Roux loop of jejunum over the pancreas (as in Whipple's operation), but complications such as leakage are more likely.

367

DISTAL PANCREATECTOMY
(extra-major)

Procedure

After carrying out laparotomy remove the spleen. This will then allow mobilization of the tail of the pancreas along its superior and inferior borders. Divide the short gastric veins and then expose the splenic vein and follow it to its junction with the superior mesenteric and inferior mesenteric vein. Divide it at this junction. Avoid damaging the middle colic vein during the procedure.

Expose the splenic artery and ligate it along the superior border of the pancreas adjacent to the proposed resection line. Transect the neck of the pancreas over the portal vein in the same fashion in Whipple's operation. Again, a ligature or alternatively a Doyen clamp can allow temporary haemostasis. As the clamp or ligature is gradually released, ligation or diathermy to any vessel is facilitated.

Pancreatography should then be undertaken. If there is free flow into the duodenum, the pancreas may be ligated at its neck or more distally. If there is any suggestion of obstruction, a Roux jejunal loop should be brought over the open pancreatic duct. Drainage is conventional.

TOTAL PANCREATECTOMY (complex)

This procedure may be undertaken as a combination of Whipple's operation with distal pancreatectomy. It is usually easier to work from left to right, starting with the tail. The indication is usually for complete pancreatitis. Diabetes and problems with the exocrine pancreas are inevitable.

DRAINAGE OF PANCREATIC PSEUDOCYST (major)

Indications

Symptomatic or recurrent cysts confirmed by ultrasound and unsuitable for percutaneous external drainage.

Incision

Upper mid-line.

Procedure

Carry out a laparotomy and confirm that the swelling is cystic by passing a wide-bore needle into it through an avascular portion of the greater omentum. Make an anterior gastrostomy between stay sutures. Make a similar 5 cm posterior gastrostomy into the cyst wall which should be mature. Aspirate the contents and anastomose the cyst wall to the posterior gastrostomy with continuous 3/0 Vicryl. Interrupted sutures do not prevent haemorrhage. Close the anterior gastrostomy with continuous 3/0 Vicryl.

An alternative is to use a Roux loop brought to the most dependent part of the cyst, usually through the transverse mesocolon. Carry out the anastomosis in a single layer of continuous 3/0 Vicryl.

10 Surgery of the breast

Incision and drainage of breast abscess   376
Microdochectomy   378
Hadfield–Adair operation   380
Fine-needle aspiration of the breast   384
Trucut biopsy of breast   386
Open-breast biopsy   388
Breast biopsy of inpalpable lesions   390
Wide-excision lumpectomy of breast   392
Simple mastectomy   394
Axillary node dissection   398
Reconstruction of the breast   400

INCISION AND DRAINAGE OF BREAST ABSCESS (intermediate)

Most large breast abscesses will occur in late pregnancy, in the early postnatal period, or during lactation. Periareolar breast abscesses are usually related to duct ectasia and can occur in the absence of pregnancy. Beware of simple incision and drainage of these abscesses as this may cause a mammillary fistula and a more formal Hadfield–Adair procedure may be required (see p. 380). These abscesses often respond to conservative measures. An infected tubercle of Montgomery can be treated as any kind of infected epidermoid cyst.

Incision

Periareolar or cosmetic-dependent. Make sure that the incision is long enough.

Procedure

Incise into the abscess. Take a swab for culture. Break all loculi down with your finger and remove part of the cyst wall for histology. Curette the cavity to remove the abscess wall. If the incision is dependent, it is not usually necessary to insert the tube drain, but in a large abscess in the upper part of the breast a dependent tube drain is useful for 1–2 days. Packing the cavity is unnecessary.

Closure

Primary closure can be used if the abscess is incised and drained under antibiotic cover. Both incision and drainage and primary closure are usually followed by rapid healing.

MICRODOCHECTOMY (intermediate)

Indications

This should be undertaken for bleeding from a single duct which may be related to a benign papilloma or, less commonly, an intraductal cancer.

Position of patient

Supine with the arm at 90°.

Incision

Radial.

Procedure

Identify the single duct using a probe or a ductogram at mammography. Usually the duct is dilated towards the areolar side of a papilloma and easily allows the probe to be passed. Cut down from the nipple along the line of the probe beneath. There is no need to excise skin. Take a margin of at least 0.5 cm of breast tissue around the probe, thereby removing the probe with a specimen. Be sure that haemostasis is perfect and try to avoid using a drain.

Closure

Avoid the use of subcutaneous or fat sutures. Use a subcuticular 2/0 or 3/0 Prolene or Vicryl suture.

HADFIELD–ADAIR OPERATION
(intermediate)

Indications

- Complicated duct ectasia (particularly when there is a mamillary fistula)
- Subareolar biopsy of a breast lump
- Nipple inversion relating to duct ectasia

Position of patient

Supine with the arm by the side or at 90° on an arm rest.

Incision

Subareolar. Take care to prevent undercutting the skin by asking your assistant to stretch it. Avoid going more than half way around the circumference of the areolar as this may endanger its viability.

Procedure

Disconnect the nipple from the underlying terminal ducts and breast tissue, taking care not to buttonhole it or make the skin too thin. Your assistant can make this easier by lifting the areola up with skin hooks like a trap-door or you can use a scalpel. In duct ectasia large ducts may be seen and they will exude purulent secretion. Small true abscesses may also be encountered. If you think that the material is infected send a swab for microbiological analysis. Ensure that all central ducts are divided and achieve perfect haemostasis. Once the ducts are divided, excise a truncated pyramid of tissue with a base 3–4 cm across underneath the nipple reaching back into the breast tissue. Send this for histology. If the nipple is inverted, evert it and maintain in that position by using a Vicryl 2/0 purse-string. If you have any doubts about haemostasis insert a small suction drain.

Closure

Use a 3/0 Prolene or Vicryl subcutaneous suture. Cover the nipple with a transparent polyurethane adhesive dressing and place a pressure dressing using cotton wool and strapping over the skin dressing.

Complications

Fistula, scarring, and persistent infection. These should occur in less than 10 per cent of cases.

Axilla

Periareolar incision
below the nipple

Raised nipple
flap

Division of all central
ducts and excision of
truncated pyramid of
tissue beneath

381

Purse-string suture on
the undersurface of the flap
to evert the nipple

Hadfield–Adair operation.

HADFIELD–ADAIR OPERATION
(intermediate) (*cont.*)

Mamillary fistula

This results because of ignorance of its cause. In a non-lactating or perimenopausal breast a central abscess related to the areola is almost always connected to an underlying duct ectasia. The previous history is typical. Such an abscess usually responds to conservative management with appropriate antibiotics. If the material inside the abscess is fluid, it can be aspirated. Simple incision as for breast abscesses is inappropriate because a mamillary fistula will result. If conservative measures fail, a Hadfield–Adair procedure should be considered.

FINE-NEEDLE ASPIRATION OF THE BREAST (less than minor)

Aims

Cytocological diagnosis of any soft tissue swelling.

Indications

- Cystic swellings including haematomas and infective lesions.
- Malignant lesions. The risk of implantation of malignant tissue along the needle tract is overstated and rarely occurs. The information obtained usually far outweighs the risk.

Contraindications

- Vascular abnormalities
- Haemangiomas
- Aneurysms

Preoperative preparation

Explain what you are going to do to the patient. Written consent is not required, but the patient should be informed that minor complications relating to bleeding may occur.

Anaesthetic

Local anaesthetic. This is often unnecessary in breast tissue.

Procedure

Use a sterile disposable 20 ml syringe with a 19G (green) venepuncture needle. Clean the microbiological slides and the slide holder (to convey smears to the cytocological laboratory). The syringe can be held in a Cameco gun which gives suction by pulling on a trigger when the tip of the needle attached to the syringe is accurately placed into the breast lesion. Alternatively, it can be held in the dominant hand and suction applied manually when the needle reaches the lesion. Try both methods to find which one suits you best. When the needle is in position make four or five passes through the suspicious area with full suction (the barrel of the syringe drawn back to the 20 ml mark). Keep the needle under suction as it is removed. Place a swab or cotton-wool ball on the aspiration site and ask the patient to apply pressure with the flat of her hand for about 5 minutes to prevent bruising. Place a small adhesive dressing on the site. This can be removed 12 hours later.

Inject the contents of the syringe on to clean glass slides (the side which bears the ground glass for writing the patient's name in pencil). Five or six slides may be needed. Remove the needle and inject any remaining material in the syringe on to a slide. The contents of the hub of the needle should also be harvested. Then smear the material on each slide evenly using a sweep of another clean slide. If there is excessive contamination by clot try to remove this before smearing. Air dry the slides and place them in their holder. Label each slide and holder with the patient's name, number, and date. Match it with the clinical data on the request form and give the cytologist as much information as possible. Place the needle and syringe in the disposable sharps box. More cells can be recovered from the syringe and needle by aspirating saline and centrifuging the fluid.

Scrapings can be taken from a lesion suspected to be due to Paget's disease of the nipple by stroking a scalpel blade over the infected areolar skin. Air dry the scrapings on a slide and send them for cytology.

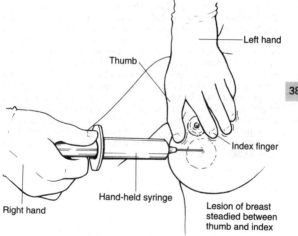

Fine-needle aspiration of the breast. As an alternative to the hand-held syringe a Cameco gun can be used.

TRUCUT BIOPSY OF BREAST

Aims

The histological diagnosis of many soft tissue swellings.

Indications

As for fine-needle aspiration excluding vascular abnormalities, haemangiomas, aneurysms, and possibly cystic swellings.

If fine-needle aspiration can be performed it should take precedence over Trucut biopsy. Remember that a lesion may be missed in the breast with Trucut and occasionally a second attempt may be required.

Procedure

Raise a bleb of local anaesthetic in the skin and infiltrate the underlying tissue. When it has taken effect make a small stab incision through the bleb using a size 11 blade. This permits easy passage of the Trucut needle.

Check that the Trucut needle is working and familiarize yourself with the technique and the way that the inner-needle works. There is no need to use gown or gloves, but a careful no-touch technique is indicated with hand-washing before the procedure.

Hold the lesion in the breast between the finger and thumb of the non-dominant hand. If an assistant is available he may steady the breast and reassure the patient. Insert the closed needle through the small stab incision and advance the outside sheath well within or just beyond the lesion. Now advance the inner needle of the Trucut device, keeping the outer sheath still. Remove the Trucut biopsy needle from the breast and examine the material within the inner sheath. If the procedure has been successful, a long core of tissue will be obtained. This should be placed in formalin and sent for histology. If the lesion has been missed or the specimen is inadequate, take another core of tissue in a slightly different direction. Apply a small plaster over the stab incision. Suturing is not usually necessary.

OPEN-BREAST BIOPSY (intermediate)

Indications

- When fine-needle aspiration or Trucut biopsy have failed to exclude malignancy
- When the patient elects to have the lesion removed for diagnostic or cosmetic reasons

Preoperative preparations

Examine the patient to check the side and the site of the breast lump. Ask her to indicate the lump to you.

Position of patient

Supine with the arm by the side or on a side-board.

Incision

Periareolar whenever possible. However, when the lump is mobile, such as a fibroadenoma, and is at some distance from the nipple a cosmetic or inframammary incision may be used. Try to place the incision in a Langer's line in the bikini line.

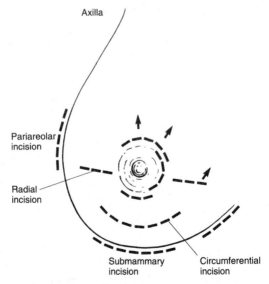

Incisions for open-breast biopsy of the right breast.

388

Procedure

Incise the fat underlying the skin and reflect it to identify breast tissue proper. Take a representative sample if there is only dysplasia. Try to achieve complete haemostasis using diathermy. This dispenses with the need for a drain. When dysplasia is a likely diagnosis remove as much abnormal-feeling tissue as possible for the patient's sake, otherwise she may feel that the operation has not been completed.

When the lump is a fibroadenoma it can easily be enucleated with a rim of normal breast tissue around it. However, when the procedure is being undertaken to exclude cancer a skin ellipse over the lesion should also be removed. The incision line should be placed in such a position that any subsequent wide-excision lumpectomy or mastectomy can easily be carried out to include this first scar. If the lump is suspicious, aim to clear at least a 1 cm margin around it. After the skin has been incised, grasp the lump with Allis forceps. Excise the breast tissue using scalpel, scissors, or diathermy. Try all these methods in different operations to determine which you feel is best.

Closure

Be careful not to produce dimpling if sutures are inserted underneath the skin as this tends not to disappear with time. If haemostasis is not perfect, a small suction drain may be brought out through a separate stab wound. Close the skin with 2/0 or 3/0 Prolene or 2/0 or 3/0 Vicryl for subcuticular closure. Cover the suture line with a transparent dressing. Place some cotton wool over the dressing and mould the breast using an adhesive strapping to give some pressure. Sutures can be removed after 7–8 days and drains within 24 hours.

BREAST BIOPSY OF INPALPABLE LESIONS (intermediate)

The patient will arrive in theatre with a mammographically placed needle of either the Hawkins 2 or Reedy type, or with some dye placed in the suspect area.

Position of patient

Supine with the arm at 90°.

Incision

Elliptical around the needle entry point.

Procedure

Follow the needle down to its hook. Quality assurance insists on small biopsies with screening mammography. Once the hook has been removed with skin, breast tissue, and the suspect lesion, ensure that haemostasis is achieved and close the skin in the usual way. There is usually no need for drainage. Confirm with an X-ray of the specimen that the entire suspect lesion has been excised. This should be done before waking the patient. If there is any doubt, a further specimen of breast tissue should be removed.

WIDE-EXCISION LUMPECTOMY OF BREAST

Indications

Breast cancers less than 2 cm in size particularly in the upper outer quadrant. A good cosmetic result is usually achieved and adjuvant radiotherapy may be given afterwards. The axillary nodes can be taken *en bloc* with an upper outer quadrant lump or can be removed with a separate axillary incision.

Position of patient

Supine with the arm on the affected side at 90°.

Incision

Elliptical over the lesion to include the previous biopsy site, fine-needle aspirate, or Trucut biopsy site. Ensure a minimum 2 cm margin around the lump. Whenever possible, use a cosmetic incision along Langer's lines.

Procedure

In addition to a 2 cm margin of skin be sure that you also have a 2 cm margin around the lump. Achieve haemostasis with diathermy as in open-breast biopsy. Extend the dissection into the axilla to assess the nodal status.

Closure

Subcutaneous or fat sutures may deform the breast and should be avoided. Close the skin with subcuticular 2/0 or 3/0 Prolene or Vicryl. If haemostasis is not perfect, insert an 8–10 mm disposable suction drain and apply a transparent film dressing and a pressure dressing over the wound as in open-breast biopsy.

SIMPLE MASTECTOMY (major)

Indications

- Carcinoma of the breast
- Severe mammary dysplasia (in patients with a strong history of cancer)
- Fibrocystic disease (when there is chronic infection and unremitting pain the patient often requests mastectomy)

Position of patient

Supine with the patient's arm at right angles to the trunk on a board.

Incision

Elliptical to include the nipple and the tumour position. Usually this will be oblique or transverse with a tumour in the upper outer quadrant, and the incision should be marked out with a marker pen. Beware of taking too much skin which may predispose to flap necrosis owing to tension during closure. Remember the need to assess the axilla when placing the incision and try to include the site of any previous open-breast biopsy, fine-needle aspiration, or Trucut biopsy within the skin ellipse.

Procedure

Aim for at least a 2 cm clearance of both the skin overlying the tumour and the tissue around the tumour itself. Once the incision is made, apply tissue forceps (e.g. Littlewoods forceps) to the flaps but do not put them directly onto the skin. Rather, apply them to the subcutaneous tissue. Identify the plane between the skin and the breast and avoid making thin flaps or buttonholing the skin using scalpel, scissors, or diathermy. Diathermy carries the risk of burning the skin. Using a scalpel held obliquely or scissors are the best methods. Achieve haemostasis as you proceed. Continue the dissection between the skin and the breast superiorly, inferiorly, and medially until the muscle fascia can be seen. The breast can then be removed from the underlying fascia from medial to lateral side. Two-thirds of the breast is on the pectoralis major and one-third on the serratus anterior. Unless the tumour is invading muscle, which is rare, avoid damaging the muscle itself as it tends to bleed. The tissue plane can be found much more easily if the assistant lifts the tissue forceps placed on the skin edge straight up. Apply tension by pulling the breast away from the skin flap with your non-dominant hand. The plane between the muscle fascia is then easily identified. Diathermize any perforating muscular vessels as you meet them and allow the specimen to fall naturally as the dissection in the fascial plane between the breast and the muscles is continued. Avoid going too far laterally or posteriorly with the dissec-

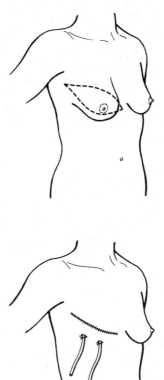

Simple mastectomy.

tion, remembering that the long thoracic nerve and the nerve to the serratus anterior are at risk. A total mastectomy must include the axillary tail of the breast and associated axillary nodes.

Begin the axillary dissection by following the inferior margin of the pectoralis major in the axillary cone. Once you enter the axilla open the brachiopectoral fascia and dissect with a gauze swab on the finger. Combine with scissor dissection to remove the truncated pyramid of axillary tail and nodes, achieving haemostasis as you go. Look out for the apical veins which drain into the axillary vein and tie them. As an alternative, the dissection can begin at the axillary vein at the apex of the axilla. Look for and avoid the lateral thoracic vessels and the nerve to the serratus anterior. The intercostobrachial nerve can be sacrificed. Continue the gauze dissection until the axillary vein is seen which gives a level I axillary dissection and includes all the anterior pectoral node group which should allow good staging. The venous tributaries can be difficult to identify in a fat breast. Avoid diathermy which may cause more damage.

Closure

After haemostasis insert two disposable suction drains (14 mm). Bring them out inferior to the lower skin flap. Place one drain in the axilla and one in the pectoral area. These should remain for 48 hours. Close the skin with subcuticular 2/0 or 3/0 Prolene or Vicryl taking care to avoid 'dog ears' at each end of the incision. An appropriate skin ellipse should prevent this. Steristrips can be applied to the wound if there is any gaping. Then cover the wound with a transparent polyurethane dressing. Apply cotton wool and a pressure dressing for about 12 hours.

Complications

- Flap necrosis.
- Haematoma, wound infection, seroma. These may need drainage by a needle and syringe inserted through the wound edges. This procedure may have to be repeated on several occasions.
- Arm and shoulder stiffness. This should respond to physiotherapy.
- Nerve paresis or section.
- Swollen arm. This is commonest after operations which incorporate lymphadenectomy, and radiotherapy. It is unusual with level I axillary dissection.

AXILLARY NODE DISSECTION (major)

This is most easily undertaken by opening the brachiopectoral fascia and subcutaneous tissue in the axilla. If there is an attached breast specimen, this allows retraction. Dissection can then be undertaken with scissors or a gauze on a finger, which could be regarded as being safer and easier (see section on mastectomy for details of level I dissection).

Axillary dissection may be more radical. Examples include the Patey mastectomy and radical mastectomy.

Patey mastectomy

This operation involves division or excision of pectoralis minor with the mastectomy specimen and allows dissection to level II. The pectoralis major is retracted upwards. The specimen does not need marking for the pathologist's orientation as in simple mastectomy where there may be very little in the way of an axillary tail.

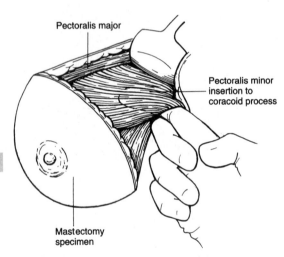

Pectoralis major

Pectoralis minor insertion to coracoid process

Mastectomy specimen

Patey mastectomy.

Position of patient
When towelling the patient after skin preparation place the drapes to allow abduction of the arm during operation which gives best access to the axilla.

Procedure

Following the axillary dissection described for simple mastectomy divide and remove the pectoralis minor from the coracoid process and then turn the muscle downwards. This allows exposure of the apex of the axilla. Divide the insertion of the pectoralis minor on the ribs using diathermy. The medial pectoral nerve is sacrificed with this procedure, but the lateral pectoral nerve and pectoral artery from the acromiothoracic artery should be preserved. The axillary dissection then continues beyond the axillary vein at the level I dissection. The venous tributaries can easily be seen and divided.

Radical mastectomy

In this operation, which is rare in the United Kingdom, the pectoralis major is removed with the pectoralis minor.

Procedure

Divide the pectoralis major tendon on the humerus and turn it down with the pectoralis minor. In this operation the lateral pectoral nerves to the pectoralis minor/major are taken with the medial pectoral nerve and the vessels from the acromiothoracic trunk. Identify the axillary venous tributaries and divide them as they enter the axillary vein. Do not damage them, as the haemostasis using diathermy on this site is difficult. Dissect the axillary contents from latissimus dorsi, subscapularis, and serratus anterior, thereby stripping the whole of the axillary vein. In this operation the intercostobrachial nerve is divided with the lateral intercostal vessels, but the nerve to the latissimus dorsi and serratus anterior must be seen and preserved. The breast is removed together with the pectoralis major and minor. The muscular attachments can be divided by diathermy.

399

RECONSTRUCTION OF THE BREAST

Tissue expansion and implantation following simple or subcutaneous mastectomy (major)

A tissue expander can be placed under the pectoralis major. Avoid the old mastectomy scar after simple mastectomy and use a separate submammary. Develop a pouch underneath the pectoralis major using your fingers and make this large enough to accommodate the tissue expander. Bring out the port separately, laterally and inferior to the breast position. The tissue expander can then be enlarged at 50–100 ml a week using the subcutaneous port until the appropriate breast size is achieved. At a second operation the tissue expander is replaced by an appropriately sized implant. Antibiotic prophylaxis is recommended for both procedures.

Myocutaneous flap reconstruction (complex)

Latissimus dorsi or rectus muscle myocutaneous flaps can be raised to give substance and extra skin when required. An expander can be placed beneath with later replacement by an implant. The added tissue helps to match the ptosis of the remaining breast.

Nipple fashioning

This can be undertaken using a free-flap transfer of pigmented skin from the vulva or the ear.

Reduction mammoplasty (complex) and breast augmentation (major)

Reduction requires careful measurements and preservation of the nipple which needs to be resited. Augmentation is usually easy and is achieved with either implants or myocutaneous flaps.

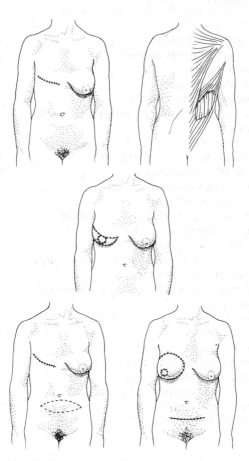

Methods of reconstruction of the breast after mastectomy.

11 Vascular surgery

Arterial anastomosis 404
Access to various arteries 408
Profundaplasty 414
Endarterectomy 416
Carotid endarterectomy 418
Excision of an aneurysmal internal carotid
  artery 422
Excision of a carotid body tumour 426
Transaxillary sympathectomy 428
Cervical sympathectomy 430
Axillo-bifemoral graft 434
Brachial embolectomy 438
Establishing an arteriovenous fistula 440
Lumbar sympathectomy 442
Aortic bifurcation graft 446
Resection of an abdominal aortic aneurysm 448
Femoral embolectomy 452
Extra-anatomical bypass femoro-femoral
  cross-over graft 456
Bypass surgery below the inguinal
  ligament 458
Femoropopliteal bypass grafting 460
Harvesting the long saphenous vein for
  bypass grafting 464
In situ saphenous vein bypass graft 466
Lower limb amputations 468
Surgery for varicose veins 472

ARTERIAL ANASTOMOSIS

Aims

The aim of anastomosis in arterial surgery is to effect a water-tight closure without tension on the vessels concerned whilst maintaining the normal lumen. This is best achieved by first excising the adventitia. It is vital that the intimal surface remains undamaged.

Materials

Vascular sutures of non-absorbable material are used. These are usually produced with a needle at each end. In general 3/0 sutures are used for large vessels such as the aorta, with 4/0 and 5/0 sutures being reserved for smaller vessels. Micro-surgical anastomosis may be performed with 8/0 to 10/0 sutures. Synthetic non-absorbable sutures such as prolene, braided polyester (Ticron) and PTFE (Gortex) are used. Taper-pointed needles permit penetration of atheromatous vessels.

Techniques

Anastomosis may be end-to-end or end-to-side. Insertion of sutures inside to outside the lower vessel of the anastomosis avoids raising intimal flaps.

End-to-end
1. Insert one of the double-ended needles from the inside to the outside of the proximal end of the artery. Insert the other from inside to outside of the distal end. Tie sutures. Now take each needle and suture round the vessel using an over-and-over stitch. Avoid tension and intimal damage. Tie the sutures at the front of the vessel.
2. Where possible to rotate the vessel insert a double-ended suture inside to outside at each corner of the vessel. Tie knots. Now complete the anterior and posterior walls with over-and-over sutures. Complete the anterior wall first, tie the knot, and then pass the opposite suture under the vessel, maintaining traction on the other to turn the vessel over. Complete the posterior wall and tie the stitch.

End-to-side
This technique is useful for femoropopliteal grafting and on-lay aortic grafting. Use a double-ended suture. Tailor the two free vessel edges (or vessel and graft) to suit each other. The anastomosis may be fashioned with the vessels at right angles to each other or at an angle. Insert one needle into the apex of the arteriotomy from inside to outside. Insert the other into the graft from inside to outside. Now tie the knot. Proceed

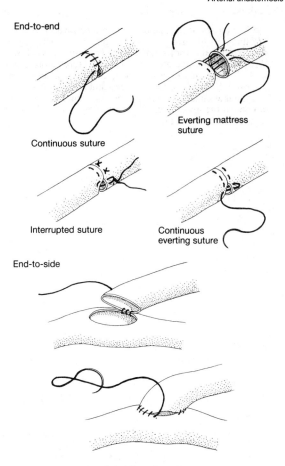

End-to-end

Continuous suture

Everting mattress suture

Interrupted suture

Continuous everting suture

End-to-side

Arterial anastomosis.

down each side of the anastomosis passing the needles from outside (graft) to the inside of the artery. Take one suture around the lowermost part of the anastomosis and tie the knot from the lower angle.

Variations

1. The first passes of the needles can both be made from outside the graft to inside the apex of the arteriotomy. Then, without tying the knot, complete the anastomosis as above. This permits the operator to place the sutures more accurately in tricky anastomoses. The graft can be gently snuggled onto the arteriotomy at the end and the knot tied.
2. Two double-ended sutures can be used, one at the apex and one at the lower end. The anastomosis is completed as in the rotation technique.

ACCESS TO VARIOUS ARTERIES

Aim

To expose arteries effectively for anastomosis or repair. This permits complete control of the arteries and their branches before performing any procedure.

Carotid bifurcation

The patient lies supine with the head turned so that the side to be operated on is uppermost.

Incision
2 cm below the mandible along the line of sternomastoid to 2–3 cm above its insertion.

Procedure
Deepen through the platysma. Incise the deep fascia along the anterior border of sternomastoid. Identify the internal jugular vein and free it from the common carotid artery and divide the fascia overlying it with scissors. Pass tape around the artery. Proceed now to expose the external carotid artery (the superior thyroid is its first branch) and the internal carotid artery by carefully dividing the fascia with scissors. Pass tapes around them. The vagus nerve is lateral to the artery. The hypoglossal and carotid sinus nerves are above the artery.

Subclavian artery

Proceed as for cervical sympathectomy (p. 430). After division of the scalenus anterior muscle (preserving the phrenic nerve), the artery is visible. Pass tapes around it and its internal mammary and thyrocervical branches.

Exposure of the abdominal aorta and iliac bifurcation

Incision
Long mid-line, paramedian, or transverse.

Procedure
Place self-retaining retractors in the wound. Lift the transverse colon out of the wound or pack it under the xiphisternum and lower thorax. Lift the small bowel out of the wound and retract it within moist warm towels or pack it into the right upper quadrant. Identify the peritoneum over the aorta and divide it over the bifurcation and upwards to the right of the inferior mesenteric artery. At the upper end displace the duodenum to the right to avoid damaging it.

To expose each common iliac lift the overlying peritoneum with forceps and carefully divide it. Diathermize bleeding points and beware of damage to the ureters (which cross the iliac bifurcation) and iliac veins (which are often adherent to the arteries).

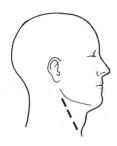

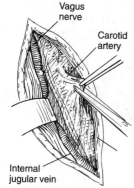

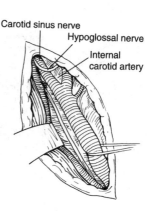

Bifurcation of the carotid artery.

409

The common femoral artery and its bifurcation

Incision
Make a 10–12 cm vertical incision two finger breadths lateral
to the pubic tubercle, one-third above and two-thirds below
the inguinal ligament. Feel for the pulsation with your fingers.

Procedure
Incise fat and fascia between the muscles of the femoral triangle.
Expose the artery using careful sharp dissection. Some minor
veins may require ligation and division. Continue sharp dissection to expose the common femoral artery, the profunda
femoris, and the superficial femoral. Pass slings around them.
The common femoral often appears to narrow at its bifurcation because a posterior muscular branch is also given off.

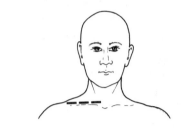

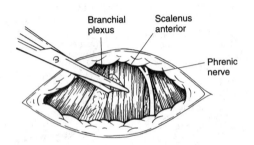

Branchial plexus

Scalenus anterior

Phrenic nerve

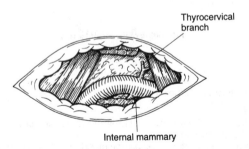

Thyrocervical branch

Internal mammary

Subclavian or vertical arteries in the neck.

410

The popliteal artery

Above the knee

Incision Vertical 10–15 cm long extending from the medial femoral condyle along the posterior border of vastus medialis.

Procedure Incise fat and deepen the incision through the fascia. Retract the sartorius downwards to expose the neurovascular bundle below the hiatus in adductor magnus. Dissect the venae comitantes and the popliteal vein from the artery whilst preserving the geniculate vessels. Expose the popliteal artery for about 5 cm. Pass slings around it.

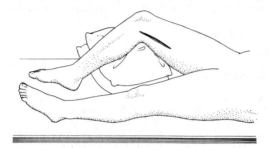

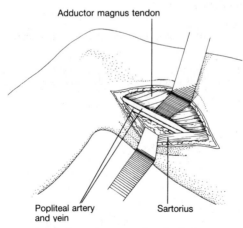

Adductor magnus tendon

411

Popliteal artery
and vein

Sartorius

Approach to and exposure of popliteal artery.

ACCESS TO VARIOUS ARTERIES (*cont.*)

Below the knee

Incision 0.5–1 cm behind the medial tibial condyle extended distally parallel to the medial tibial border for 10–12 cm. Preserve the saphenous vein.

Procedure Incise the deep fascia and retract the medial head of the gastrocnemius downwards. This exposes the fascia over the neurovascular bundle which can then be incised. The vessel can then be exposed and slings passed round it.

Tibioperoneal trunk

The tibial vein is divided through the above incision and tibioperoneal trunk dissected by incising the soleus muscle.

Peroneal artery

Incision
Vertical from the head of the fibula for 6–10 cm downwards along the fibula.

Procedure
Dissect the muscle from the fibula, incise its periosteum throughout the length of the incision, and strip it from the bone. Divide the fibula above and below. Remove the segment. The peroneal artery lies in the bed of the fibula. The fascia is incised and the vessel is isolated from its accompanying veins.

Anterior tibial artery

Incision
Vertical 15–20 cm long, lateral to anterior tibial border.

Procedure
Divide the deep fascia. Identify the plane between the tibialis anterior medially and the extensor digitorum longus laterally. The vessels lie deeply and should be carefully dissected until clearly seen. Good retraction is essential.

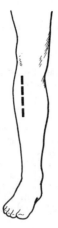

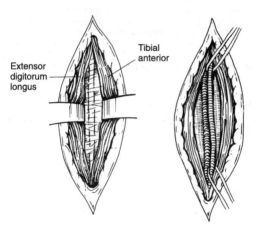

Anterior tibial artery.

413

PROFUNDAPLASTY (major)

Aim

Restoration of blood flow in the profunda femoris artery.

Indications

Atheromatous stenosis of the origin and proximal segment of the profunda femoris artery.

Exposure

Expose the common femoral, profunda femoris, and superficial femoral arteries in the groin. Pass slings around them. Dissect the profunda downwards, ligating the small vein which crosses it. After doing this, the first bifurcation will be seen followed by the main profunda vein which should also be ligated. The dissection can then proceed distally, controlling vessels as they appear until about 10 cm of the profunda is exposed. Identify and control with slings any posterior muscular branches arising directly from the common femoral artery.

Give 5000 IU herapin IV and select a suitable soft area for arteriotomy. Apply proximal and distal clamps to control bleeding. Extend the arteriotomy to the common femoral artery. Check on releasing the distal clamp that there is back-bleeding. If there is proximal atheroma, perform an endarterectomy (p. 416). Check forward bleeding. If this is satisfactory close the arteriotomy with a Dacron or vein patch using 6/0 vascular sutures. Release the proximal and distal clamps in turn.

Closure

Bring a suction drain through a separate stab wound. Close the wound in layers with interrupted Nylon or clips to skin.

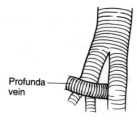

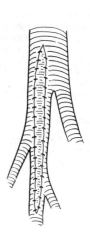

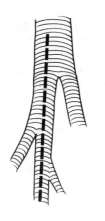

Profundaplasty.

ENDARTERECTOMY (major)

Aim

Restoration of blood flow within an artery by removing atheromatous occluding or stenosing material.

Indications

Short blocks or stenoses when the artery is otherwise normal above and below.

Procedure

Expose the diseased artery and make a longitudinal incision over the affected area. Separate the atheroma from the vessel wall using a Watson–Cheyne dissector or the tips of closed Spencer–Wells forceps. Be gentle! Start at each edge and work towards the middle until the affected area is mobilized. Lift it out and excise it above and below with scissors. Place a few (four to six) sutures through the lower edges to prevent dissection once flow has been re-established.

Closure

Close the arteriotomy with interrupted Prolene. Use a vein patch in smaller arteries if you feel that it will lead to stenosis.

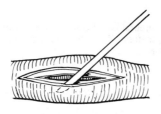

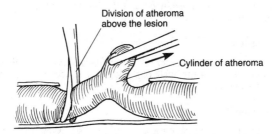

Division of atheroma
above the lesion

Cylinder of atheroma

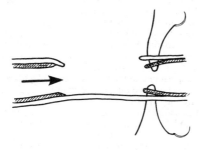

417

Endarterectomy.

CAROTID ENDARTERECTOMY (complex)

Aims

To restore the cerebral circulation by removal of atheromatous occluding material from the carotid bifurcation and, internal carotid artery.

Indications

Symptomatic carotid occlusive disease.

Position of the patient

Supine with neck extended and the head turned away from the operator.

Incision

Along the outer border of sternomastoid from two finger breadths below the angle of the jaw to just above the muscle insertion.

Procedure

The carotid bifurcation is exposed (p. 408). Avoid extensive manipulation of the area at the bifurcation to reduce the risk of embolus. Have all instruments (clamps and shunt if required) to hand before proceeding. There are various devices which permit the shunt to be haemostatically fitted (ring clamps, snugging devices). Pass tapes around the arteries.

Give 5000 IU heparin. Wait for 2–3 minutes and cross-clamp the internal carotid first to prevent arterial debris entering it, followed by the common carotid and external carotid. Make an incision into the common carotid and extend it proximally to the palpable and visible limit of the diseased section of the internal carotid.

Insert the shunt beyond the diseased portion of the internal carotid and back-bleed it whilst releasing the internal carotid clamp. During this process insert the proximal end of the back-bleeding shunt into the common carotid artery. Occlude the shunt and check for air bubbles by releasing the common carotid clamp before restoring to obtain a flush and haemostatic fit at both ends of the shunt.

The endarterectomy should now be carried out using a fine artery forceps or dissector. The atheroma should be removed proximally and distally clear of the external carotid lumen. In the internal carotid the endarterectomy should proceed proximally and stop at the limit of disease. If this is not possible, the part to be removed should be divided transversely and dissection prevented with three 7/0 sutures as described on (p. 416). Any remaining debris can be washed out with saline and the arteriotomy closed with a continuous Prolene suture

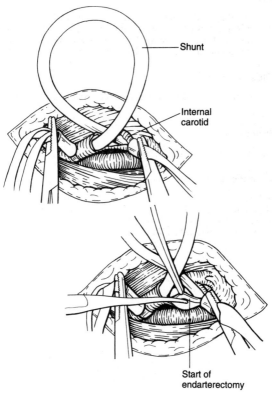

Shunt

Internal
carotid

Start of
endarterectomy

419

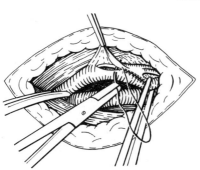

Carotid endarterectomy.

CAROTID ENDARTERECTOMY (complex) (*cont.*)

to the level of the shunt. Clamp the common and internal carotids and flush the vessels with heparinized saline. Finish suturing. Release the clamps in the following order: external carotid, common carotid, and internal carotid.

Closure

Close the wound in layers with staples or Nylon to skin. Suction drain.

Prophylaxis

Third-generation cephalosporin.

Complications

- Stroke
- Haematoma
- Haemorrhage
- Hypertension (if the bifurcation is extensively manipulated)

EXCISION OF AN ANEURYSMAL INTERNAL CAROTID ARTERY (extracranial) (complex)

Aim

To restore normal circulation and to prevent rupture, embolus, and thrombosis associated with aneurysm formation.

Indications

Established aneurysm of the extracranial internal carotid artery.

Preoperative preparations

Anaesthetic assessment of the patient. Angiographic detail of the circulation of the neck and circle of Willis. MRI or CT scan of neck.

Position of patient

Supine with the neck extended and the head turned away from the operator.

Incision

Along the anterior border of sternomastoid from two finger breadths below the angle of the jaw to just above the muscle insertion.

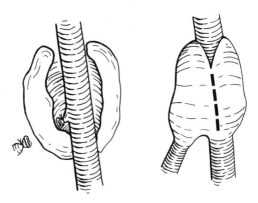

Repair of extracranial internal carotid artery aneurysm.

Excision of an aneurysmal internal carotid artery (extracranial) (complex)

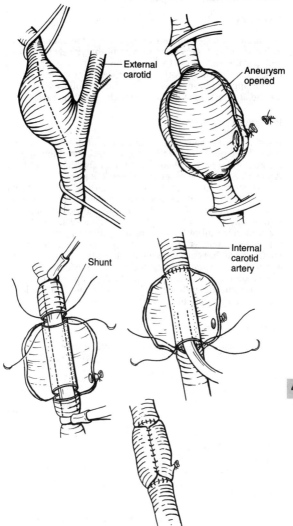

423

EXCISION OF AN ANEURYSMAL INTERNAL CAROTID ARTERY
(extracranial) (complex) (*cont.*)

Exposure

Be careful in dissection not to manipulate the aneurysm and dislodge the clot. It is safer to control the vessels proximally and distally first, pass loops around them, and ligate and divide the external carotid artery. Give 5000 IU heparin IV before applying clamps to the common carotid and internal carotid arteries. Open the aneurysm along its long axis.

Procedure

Insert a Jawaid shunt into the common carotid artery. Pass it through the preclotted synthetic graft, back-bleed the internal carotid, and pass the shunt into it after flushing with blood. Apply ring clamps or snuggers to keep it in place.

Now suture the graft end-to-end, starting at the internal carotid. The neck of the aneurysm is usually clearly visible. Start in the middle of the posterior wall and work round each side to the front wall. Complete a continuous suture line to the posterior wall of the external carotid but ligate it at each side when completed. Insert a series of interrupted sutures to the front wall but do not tie them. Clamp the common carotid and internal carotid arteries and remove the shunt. Release the external carotid clamp briefly to flush out clot or debris and wash out the graft with heparinized saline. Tie the interrupted anterior wall sutures and release the clamps.

Closure

Layers, suction drain, and Nylon or staples to skin.

EXCISION OF A CAROTID BODY TUMOUR (complex)

Carotid body tumours are rare. They are extremely vascular and their excision may sometimes involve replacing the origin of the internal carotid artery. Extensive manipulation of the tumour may lead to swings in blood pressure. Therefore dissection should proceed extremely carefully.

Preoperative preparations

Accurate localization of the tumour by CT or MRI scanning. Anaesthetist's assessment of the patient.

Position of patient

Supine with the neck extended and the head turned to the side away from the incision.

Incision

Along the anterior border of sternomastoid from 2–3 cm above its insertion to two finger breadths below the angle of the mandible.

Procedure

Expose the carotid bifurcation (p. 408). The tumour can easily be separated from the surrounding tissue. Expose the common carotid proximally, and the internal and external carotids distally. Pass tapes around them in the usual manner. Identify and preserve the hypoglossal nerve which crosses the internal and external carotids above the bifurcation.

Develop the plane between the tumour and the common carotid artery. In fact this lies between the adventitia and media of the artery. The dissection is often very vascular and small vessels require to be diathermized to maintain an adequate field of vision and prevent extensive bleeding.

As dissection proceeds proximally, the tumour should be split along its mid-line. It is often necessary to ligate the external carotid and divide it to remove it completely. If you cannot positively identify the external carotid, extend the dissection beyond the bifurcation on both vessels.

Then the tumour can usually be removed completely, without causing injury to the internal carotid artery, by continuing the dissection around the vessel on each side.

If the tumour cannot be removed safely. Heparinize the patient (5000 IU IVI) and excise the bifurcation after ligating the external carotid, clamping by passing and dividing the internal carotid. Re-establish vascular continuity with a synthetic graft. (See excision of aneurysmal internal carotid artery.)

426

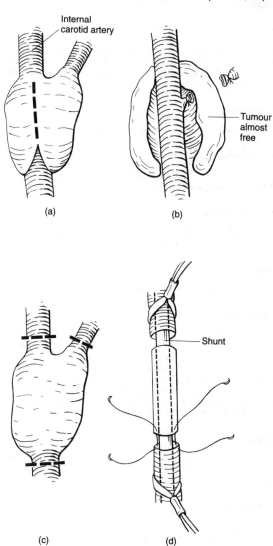

Internal
carotid artery

Tumour
almost
free

(a)

(b)

Shunt

(c)

(d)

Excision of carotid body tumour.

427

TRANSAXILLARY SYMPATHECTOMY
(major)

Aim

To achieve permanent sympathetic blockade by division of the cervical sympathetic chain, usually at the level of the fourth and fifth ganglion (the first thoracic ganglion is not easily accessible).

Indications

Raynaud's phenomenon and hyperhidrosis.

Preoperative preparation

Chest X-ray: this procedure should be avoided in patients who may have apical pleural adhesions (e.g. old tuberculosis lesions).

Position of patient

Lateral position with the arm abducted at right angles and maintained so with a sling.

Incision

Transverse/oblique in line of third rib about 15–20 cm long.

Procedure

Deepen through fat of axilla. Identify and retract the long thoracic nerve and local muscles to expose the periosteum of the third rib. This is then incised for the full length of the incision and a section of the rib is removed. Incise pleura and open the chest with a rib-spreading retractor. Displace the lung downwards to expose the sympathetic chain which lies under the mediastinal pleura. Expose the chain and excise the fourth and possibly the fifth ganglion.

428

Closure

Haemostasis. Chest drain. Allow the lung to reinflate. Approximate the ribs. Close periosteum and muscle with continuous Nylon. Subcuticular Nylon or Vicryl to skin.

Postoperatively

Chest X-ray postoperatively. Remove the drain at 24 hours or even in the recovery room when the lung is inflated.

Complications

- Surgical emphysema
- Pneumo- or haemothorax
- Temporary (sometimes permanent) Horner's syndrome
- Potentially more dangerous than cervical sympathectomy

CERVICAL SYMPATHECTOMY (major)

Aim

To achieve permanent sympathetic blockade by division of the cervical sympathetic chain by division of the stellate ganglion below the entry of the highest white ramus communicans which arises from the first thoracic nerve. The distal division of the sympathetic chain is below the third or fourth ganglion.

Indications

Raynaud's phenomenon (syndrome), Buerger's disease, causalgia, hyperhidrosis. The technique is also of value in patients with obliterative arterial disease of the upper limb where reconstruction is not possible.

Preoperative preparations

The patient is anaesthetized and lies supine on the table with feet-down tilt. The head is turned to the opposite side.

Incision

10 cm long above the medial half or two-thirds of the clavicle.

Procedure

Deepen the incision by dividing the clavicular head of the sternomastoid and the inferior belly of the omohyoid if necessary. Identify the phrenic nerve near the medial border of the scalenus anterior. The nerve runs downwards from lateral to medial side. Mobilize it and pass a tape around it to keep it in sight at all times. The scalenus anterior muscle can now be divided from the lateral to medial side, close to the first rib, to expose the underlying subclavian artery. The subclavian vein lies in front of the muscle. Palpate the first rib and clear Sibson's fascia. Divide the fascia to expose the pleura and use blunt dissection to push the pleura down. Identify the neck of the first rib and the stellate ganglion. The cervical sympathectomy chain is palpable as a cord and the stellate ganglion can be palpated on the neck of the first rib.

Use a good spotlight and deep retractors to visualize the ganglion and chain. Pick up the chain below the level of the first rami communicantes. Dissect it distally and excise the chain from the lowest third of the stellate ganglion to an appropriate point below the third or fourth ganglion. Apply Ligaclips if it is necessary to divide intercostal veins.

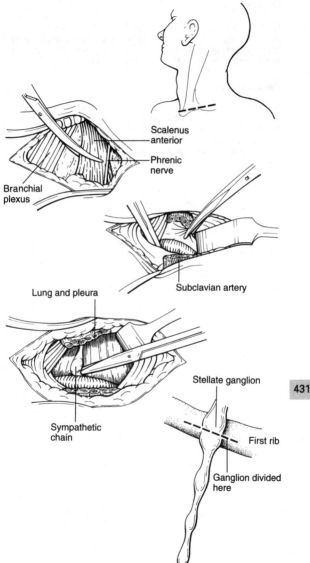

Scalenus anterior

Phrenic nerve

Branchial plexus

Subclavian artery

Lung and pleura

Stellate ganglion

431

First rib

Sympathetic chain

Ganglion divided here

CERVICAL SYMPATHECTOMY (major)
(*cont.*)

Closure

Ensure that there is no pneumothorax by asking the anaesthetist to inflate the lungs. Check for excessive bleeding and bring a suction drain through a separate stab wound. Close the wound in layers with nylon or clips to skin.

Complications

- Horner's syndrome.
- Pneumothorax (exclude with a postoperative chest X-ray)
- Neuralgia—postsympathectomy
- Excessive dryness of the affected hand (the use of hand-creams may relieve this symptom)

433

AXILLO-BIFEMORAL GRAFT (complex)

Aim

Revascularization of the lower limb(s) using flow in upper-limb arteries as the proximal input.

Indications

This is an appropriate procedure in unfit patients with aorto-iliac disease and reasonable distal run-off. It can also be carried out for patients with aneurysmal or (locally) inoperable aorto-iliac disease.

Incisions

- Bilateral groin
- Right subclavian centred on mid-clavicle about 8–10 cm long

Procedure

The groin incisions are the same as for exposure of the common, superficial, and profunda femoral arteries.

The subclavian incision may be centred over the first part of the axillary artery if it is palpable. A self-retainer is inserted and the incision is deepened between the heads of the pectoralis major until the artery is felt. Dissection then proceeds down to expose the artery, tying off its acromioclavicular branches (arteries and veins) at their exit point from the clavipectoral fascia. When this is divided, the artery is seen. Sometimes the pectoralis minor may be detached from its origin on the coracoid process to improve access. Once the artery is exposed it is controlled with slings after mobilization.

A 10 mm preclotted (reinforced) Dacron graft is then tunnelled subcutaneously to the groins using additional incisions if necessary. The graft should be sited posteriorly to prevent kinking.

The patient is then given 5000 IU heparin IV and the artery is clamped in such a way that it can be rotated to permit the anastomosis to be made to its inferior surface. Use 5/0 Prolene and make the anastomosis end-to-side. Use an over-and-over technique, starting at one corner of the back wall and progressing continuously along the front. When the anastomosis is complete clamp the graft and release the arterial clamps to restore blood flow to the arm.

Now tailor the graft to each groin, tunnelling one limb subcutaneously above the pubis. Effect the groin anastomosis end-to-side using continuous 5/0 Prolene.

At the end of the procedure release the clamps and ensure that there are no leakages.

Axillofemoral bypass graft.

434

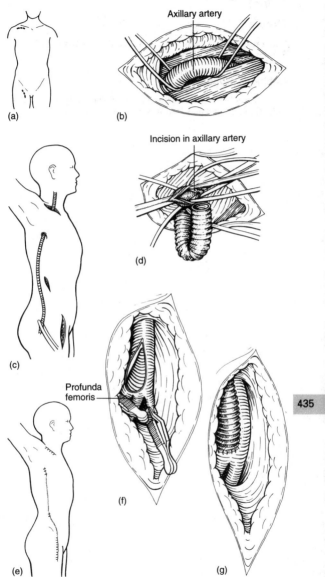

Axillary artery

(a)

(b)

Incision in axillary artery

(c)

(d)

Profunda femoris

(e)

(f)

435

(g)

AXILLO-BIFEMORAL GRAFT (complex)
(*cont.*)

Closure

Suction drains to each wound. Subcutaneous tissue in layers. Staples or nylon to skin.

Antibiotic prophylaxis

Use a broad-spectrum antibiotic prophylactically given IV at induction and at 8 and 16 hours postoperatively.

BRACHIAL EMBOLECTOMY (major)

Indications

This procedure is usually carried out in patients with uncontrolled atrial fibrillation and embolization.

Preoperative preparations

Medical control of the source of the embolus, e.g. conversion of fibrillation to sinus rhythm, if possible.

Position of patient

Supine with the affected arm extended on a board.

Incision

Longitudinal along the lower medial border of biceps. Alternatively, a lazy S incision crossing the elbow joint can give access to the medial and ulnar arteries (sometimes individually blocked).

Procedure

Deepen the incision to expose the artery. The median nerve may be in the vicinity, so take care. It sometimes lies superficial to the artery. Dissect the artery and pass loops around it proximally and distally.

Give 5000 IU heparin IV. Wait for 2–3 minutes and clamp the artery proximally. Control it distally with the loop.

Make a transverse arteriotomy and pass a size 2–3 embolectomy catheter distally. If the clot is retrieved, make sure that there is back-bleeding by releasing tension on the loop. Flush the artery distally with heparinized saline. Release the proximal clamp to ensure that there is good proximal inflow. Reapply the clamps proximally and distally, and repair the arteriotomy with 6/0 Prolene.

If there is difficulty in passing the catheter distally to the wrist make a lazy S incision across the elbow crease and expose the radial and ulnar arteries. Pass the catheter down each.

Closure

Close the wound with Nylon or staples. Suction drain.

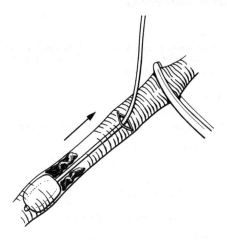

Brachial embolectomy

ESTABLISHING AN ARTERIOVENOUS FISTULA (extra-major)

Aim

To establish an arteriovenous fistula usually between the cephalic vein and radial artery at the wrist or between a femorodistal vein graft and an adjacent vein.

Indications

- Haemodialysis (cephalic vein and radial artery)
- Distension of the cephalic vein before harvesting as a vein graft
- To maintain blood flow through a femorodistal graft

Types

Side-to-side (most common) or end-to-side.

Arteriovenous fistula for haemodialysis

Vessels used
The cephalic vein and the radial artery at the wrist.

Position of the patient
Supine with the arm extended on an arm rest.

Incision
Transverse over radial artery at the wrist.

Procedure
Mobilize the artery and vein so that they will easily lie side-to-side without tension. Give the patient 5000 IU heparin IV and apply small bulldog clamps proximally and distally. Make matching longitudinal incisions in the artery and vein with a scalpel and enlarge them with right-angled scissors. These should be 4–6 mm long or about twice the width of the artery in very small vessels. Now anastomose the artery to the vein using 6/0 or 7/0 vascular sutures. Use a blunt hook to identify the cut edges, particularly of the vein, which can be gently dilated with heparinized saline. This will facilitate establishing the anastomosis which should be completed with continuous sutures on the posterior wall and interrupted on the anterior. Release the clamps. There should be an easily palpable thrill.

Closure
Close the skin wound with interrupted Nylon sutures.
  NB An end-to-side anastomosis should be established if the vessels do not lie easily together (end of vein to side of artery!). Where a distal fistula is difficult to establish or is not wanted, a side-to-side proximal brachiocephalic fistula can be established through a transverse incision above the elbow crease.

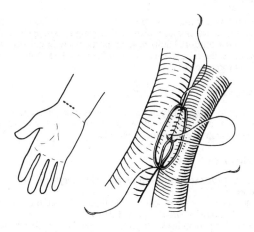

Arteriovenous fistula: side-to-side anastomosis.

LUMBAR SYMPATHECTOMY (major)

Aims

To achieve complete sympathectomy of the calf and foot by excising the second and third lumbar ganglia. The technique is used most often for limb salvage, particularly in patients with rest pain, digital gangrene, and ischaemic ulceration. Do not expect too much of the procedure.

Indications

Rest pain, digital gangrene, and ischaemic ulceration. The procedure may be carried out as an adjunct to limb salvage surgery. Do not expect too much of it.

Techniques

Phenol block (chemical blockade of the sympathetic chain)

This procedure, which is valuable in elderly patients who are anaesthetic risks, should be performed under image intensification. The patient lies on his side with the theatre table 'broken' and the side for injection uppermost. The skin is prepared with antiseptic solution and the area between the twelfth rib and the iliac crest draped. Two sites approximating the positions of the second and third lumbar vertebrae are then infiltrated with local anaesthetic a few centimetres apart at the upper edge of quadratus lumborum. After raising a skin bleb, infiltrate 5 ml deep to each. Now insert a spinal needle into one of the blebs (125 mm/18 gauge). Direct it towards the spinal column. When this is felt, 'march' the needle forwards by angling it slightly until it meets the vertebral body tangentially. The needle is now close to the sympathetic chain in the retroperitoneal space. Remove the stylet a little and place a drop of 6 per cent phenol in water on the open end. Now observe the drop of phenol. If it is in the correct space, the phenol will drop. If it is in a vessel it will rise and the manoeuvre should be repeated. Aspirate the needle. If there is no blood, inject 3–5 ml of 6 per cent phenol in water into the space, stopping for a few minutes after each millilitre injected. Check that the patient feels comfortable. Repeat this process at the other site. The successful procedure will result in a warm dry limb which is observed almost immediately. The same effect can be observed in patients kept in a warm environment, but sympathectomy makes it permanent.

Complications The most common complication is neuralgia of the groin and upper thigh. Serious dangers can be avoided by careful technique. Aortic pulsation can often be felt on the right side if the needle is misplaced. Aspiration of blood on the left may indicate that the needle is in the vena cava. It should be withdrawn slightly and aspirated again.

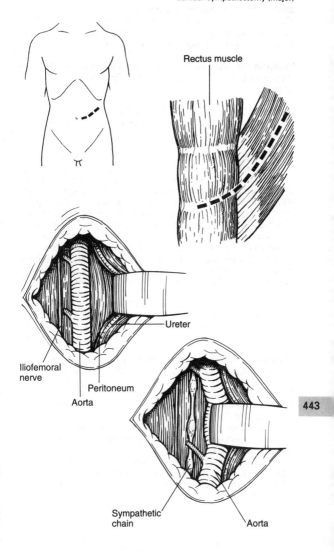

443

Lumbar sympathectomy.

LUMBAR SYMPATHECTOMY (major)

Surgical lumbar sympathectomy
This procedure can be performed transabdominally at the time of aorto-iliac surgery. It can also be performed as a separate procedure by the extraperitoneal approach.

Position of the patient The anaesthetized patient lies supine with a sandbag tucked under the side to be operated upon.

Incision Transverse from lateral rectus margin to a point about halfway between the anterior superior iliac spine and the twelfth rib.

Procedure Split the muscle fibres in gridiron fashion or divide them if the patient is well-muscled. Identify the transversalis fascia, open it, and develop the extraperitoneal space deep to it, sweeping the peritoneum forwards until you feel the definite step which is the psoas major muscle. Stay in front of the muscle. Insert two deep retractors anteriorly and superiorly, with the anterior retractor protecting the ureter.

Now feel for the sympathetic chain which lies on the anterior longitudinal ligament medial to the psoas major. It can be rolled with a pledget. Pick it up with a nerve hook and remove about 3–5 cm of chain. Control bleeding by diathermy. If lumbar vessels are in the way of your dissection, ligate and divide them.

On the left the chain lies lateral to the aorta. On the right it lies below the vena cava. Take extreme care to identify the correct structure, for the edge of the vena cava can also 'roll' to the uninitiated finger.

Closure Drain the wound with a suction drain and close it in layers using Vicryl with subcuticular Nylon to skin.

Complications
- Wound haematoma and infection.
- Injury to the ureter, vena cava, or aorta.
- Postsympathectomy neuralgia affecting the groin and antero-lateral aspect of the thigh. Treat with simple analgesia.
- Genitofemoral nerve injury.
- Sexual dysfunction occurs in about 50 per cent of males who have bilateral removal of the first lumbar ganglia.
- Gangrene may be progressive with little benefit from sympathectomy.

445

AORTIC BIFURCATION GRAFT (aorto-bifemoral) (complex)

Aims

Restoration of blood flow to the lower limbs in patients with symptomatic aorto-iliac occlusive disease.

Indications

This procedure is commonly carried out for aorto-iliac occlusive disease. The bifurcated graft can be sutured to the aorta either in an 'on-lay' fashion or by end-to-end suture after the aorta has been completely divided (with or without the aorto-iliac segment). The procedure can also be carried out in patients with abdominal aortic aneurysmal disease (see p. 434).

Incision

Long mid-line or transverse centred on umbilicus. Bilateral longitudinal groin incisions centred on mid-inguinal point.

Procedure

Expose the aorta and the aorto-iliac bifurcation (p.). Pass slings around the common iliac arteries, taking care not to damage the iliac veins. Identify the inferior mesenteric artery and its origin. Above this level the aorta is often suitable for the proximal anastomosis. Expose both common femoral arteries (p.) and their branches. Pass slings around them. Using finger dissection make retroperitoneal tunnels following each iliac artery to the common femoral in the groin.

Give the patient 5000 IU heparin IV and cross-clamp the aorta (for an end-to-end anastomosis) and the common iliac vessels. Divide the aorta. Close off the distal end or completely elevate and excise the aorto-iliac segment, ligating lumbar vessels as they appear. Carry out an end-to-end anastomosis between the divided aorta and the preclotted (if knitted) graft. A commonly used size is 10 mm × 20 mm. The anastomosis is effected by continuous 3/0 or 4/0 vascular sutures, starting on the middle of the back wall. When completed, cross-clamp the graft and release the aortic clamp slowly to check that the join is watertight. Oversew any obvious leaks.

Now tunnel the limbs of the graft retroperitoneally to the common femoral arteries and complete both distal anastomoses end-to-side with a 5/0 double-ended vascular suture. When the anastomoses are complete, release the distal clamps followed by the common femoral clamp and the clamp on the aortic graft.

For an end-to-side aortic prosthetic graft anastomosis a Satinsky clamp may be applied to a suitable portion of the aorta (usually the area involves the origin of the inferior mesenteric artery). If not, a bulldog clamp can be applied to it. The prosthetic graft is preclotted and cut obliquely so that it lies neatly on the aorta. A longitudinal incision is then made in the aorta and the debris or clot is removed. The prepared preclotted graft is then anastomosed in on-lay fashion with one continuous double-ended 3/0 or 4/0 vascular suture starting at either the heel (more common) or toe of the graft. Alternatively, separate sutures may be placed at the heel and toe of the graft. When the suture line is complete, apply a clamp across the prosthesis close to the suture line and release the aortic clamp. Complete the femoral anastomoses as described (p. 434.)

Closure

Layers. Nylon or staples to skin. Suction drains to each groin.

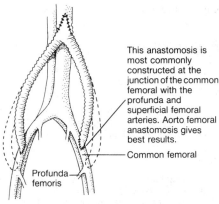

This anastomosis is most commonly constructed at the junction of the common femoral with the profunda and superficial femoral arteries. Aorto femoral anastomosis gives best results.

Common femoral

Profunda femoris

Aorto femoral bypass graft (onlay type) following atheroma

Aortic bifurcation graft.

RESECTION OF AN ABDOMINAL AORTIC ANEURYSM (complex)

Aim

Restoration of normal flow within the abdominal aorta and prevention or management of the complications associated with aneurysms: thrombosis, embolization, and rupture.

Indications

Abdominal aortic aneurysm. The procedure is best carried out electively when the operative mortality is in the order of 5 per cent. When the aneurysm ruptures, the operative mortality is in excess of 40 per cent. If left untreated, half of all patients with abdominal aortic aneurysms will die within 5 years. Even small (6 mm) aortic aneurysms have a 20 per cent rate of rupture. Therefore elective resection and grafting is indicated. Ultrasonic observation of the progression of size of small aneurysms found at screening is still under evaluation.

Preoperative preparations

Ultrasonography is accurate in assessing the size of the aneurysm and confirming the diagnosis. The patient should be as fit as possible and well advised about the implications of the procedure. Preoperative chest physiotherapy and medical control of diabetes, bronchitis, and cardiac disease should be carried out. Haematological status, biochemistry, and 4–6 units (10 units for emergencies) of blood should be available. Give prophylactic broad-spectrum antibiotics IV on induction of anaesthesia.

Position of the patient

Supine.

Incision

Long mid-line from xiphisternum to pubis, skirting the umbilicus. Insert one or two large self-retaining retractors. Alternatively, a transverse mid-abdominal incision may be used.

Procedure

Divide the peritoneum over the aneurysm. Mobilize the small bowel and pack it between moist packs either on the chest or inside the right upper quadrant. Palpate the neck of the aneurysm (usually below the left renal vein). Identify and retract the inferior mesenteric vein proximally or divide it if necessary. Dissect the common iliac vessels distally after dividing the peritoneum overlying them. Beware of damaging the ureters. Beware of the iliac veins. They may be adherent to the deep surface of the artery.

When these steps are complete, choose a suitable knitted graft (either tube or bifurcate (USCI, Meadox, Bard)). Aspirate 40 ml of blood from the inferior vena cava. Completely immerse the graft in a kidney dish in the blood until there is clot. Modern grafts do not need preclotting Then heparinize

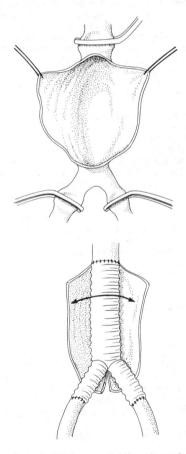

449

End-to-end anastomosis for an aortic bifurcation graft following resection of an aortic aneurysm.

the patient with IV heparin 1 unit/kg of body weight. Apply pressure to the puncture site in the vena cava, and cross-clamp the aorta proximally and both common iliac arteries. Incise the aneurysm sac longitudinally. Remove debris and thrombus.

Oversew bleeding lumbar or inferior mesenteric arteries using 3/0 vascular sutures. Identify the neck of the aneurysm (usually protruding forwards) and incise the sac on each side to give a clear view of the proximal anastomosis site. Is the bifurcation suitable as the site for the distal anastomosis? If so, use a tube graft. If not, a bifurcated graft is required.

Select a suitable graft (18–22 are most common) and make sure that it is long enough to extend from the neck of the aneurysm to both groins, if necessary. Suture it in position proximally using 2/0, 3/0, or 4/0 prolene or Ticron. When this proximal anastomosis is complete, release the aortic clamp to flush the graft and then cross-clamp the graft close to the suture line.

Now complete the lower aortic anastomosis (if a tube graft) or anastomose the limbs of the bifurcated graft into the junction of the common femoral arteries with the profunda and superficial femoral arteries (via retroperitoneal tunnels) after tying off both common iliac vessels. Alternatively, a bilateral bifurcated graft to common iliac vessel anastomoses can be carried out using 4/0 or 5/0 sutures. Before each anastomosis is complete, release the clamp on the iliac or femoral vessels to back-bleed the vessel and reclamp it. Also, release the clamp proximally to flush out clot. Then complete the anastomosis. Suture the wall of the aneurysm over the graft and close the peritoneum to prevent formation of an aortoduodenal fistula. Always ensure that the anaesthetist knows when the clamps are being released.

450 Closure

Mass with Nylon, clips or Prolene to skin.

Postoperatively

Maintain the patient's temperature using a space blanket. This prevents acidosis, peripheral vasoconstriction, and cardiac arrhythmias, all of which can result from hypothermia. Close monitoring of the pulse, CVP, blood pressure and urine output are necessary for the first 12 hours. Nasogastric suction should be monitored for 48–72 hours. Broad-spectrum antibiotics are given prophylactically for 24 hours—on induction and 8 and 16 hours postoperatively.

Prognosis

Most patients survive the operation, even for ruptured aneurysms. Deaths occur in the postoperative period owing to cardiac arrhythmias and myocardial infarction. Renal failure is a common cause of death after resection of a ruptured aneurysm. Preoperative hypertension, perioperative metabolic acidosis, and hypokalaemia are aggravating factors. The mortality rate for elective aneurysms is less than 5 per cent but is up to 50 per cent for emergency resection.

FEMORAL EMBOLECTOMY (major)

Aims

Restoration of the circulation in the femoral artery by removal of embolus.

Indications

Loss of circulation due to embolus, usually in the femoro-popliteal segment. Ninety per cent are due to myocardial disease, particularly atrial fibrillation, myocardial infarction, and rheumatic heart disease. Debris from atheromatous plaques or aortic thrombus are also common. This latter group has a poorer prognosis, and bypass grafting may be necessary as there is almost always a history of intermittent claudication or signs of ischaemia.

Preoperative preparation

Control of the primary cause includes cardiac support in the form of anti-arrhythmic drugs, diuretics, and dopamine as indicated. Careful monitoring of the patient with titration of drugs to the response, the use of analgesics, and oxygen are essential.

Anaesthetic

General anaesthetic or local anaesthetic. General anaesthetic is preferable in confused or uncooperative patients.

Position of patient

Supine.

Incision

452 Make a 12–15 cm longitudinal incision over the femoral artery from the level of the inguinal ligament. Carefully expose the common femoral artery and its bifurcation. Use sharp dissection with scissors. Pass Silastic loops round the common femoral and superficial femoral using curved forceps. Retract these tapes to expose the profunda femoris. Ligate and divide the large vein which crosses this vessel. Pass looped ligatures round small branches (particularly the posterior muscular branches).

Procedure

Heparinize the patient with 10 000 IU. of heparin IV. Control the vessels with the loops and make a 1 cm transverse arteriotomy over the bifurcation of the common femoral artery. Remove obvious clot with dissecting forceps. After checking

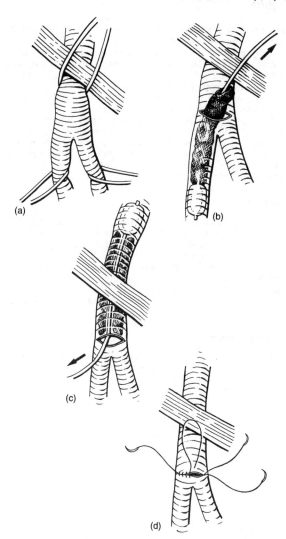

453

Femoral embolectomy.

FEMORAL EMBOLECTOMY (major)
(*cont.*)

patency, pass a number 3 or 4 embolectomy catheter, with its stillette removed, into the profunda femoris and remove any clot by inflating the balloon. Is there good back-flow after withdrawing the inflated balloon? If so instil 15–20 ml of heparinized saline (5000 IU in 500 ml) into the vessel and control it either by clamping or by means of the Silastic loops. Make several passes to ensure that all clot is removed. Repeat the technique in the superficial femoral artery.

Now pass a number 5 or 6 embolectomy catheter proximally into the aorta until good proximal flow is achieved. Control the vessel and close the arteriotomy with 5/0 or 6/0 monofilament Prolene, passing the suture from the inside to the outside of the vessel to prevent intimal damage. Use a vein patch if there is any concern about lumen size.

Closure

Bring a suction drain through a separate stab wound. Approximate the fat with interrupted Vicryl and close the skin with interrupted clips or subcuticular Nylon sutures.

A similar technique can be applied for embolectomy of the vessels of the upper limb. The use of perioperative angiography ensures patency. Conray solution (20 ml) is injected distally and the limbs screened using X-ray image intensification. If the artery is patent, close the wound. If not, repeat the embolectomy or consider bypass grafting.

Technical points

- Be gentle. The catheter can produce intimal damage. Allow the balloon to deflate a little as resistance is felt.
- If you cannot pass the catheter there may be extensive occlusive disease.

EXTRA-ANATOMICAL BYPASS FEMORO-FEMORAL CROSS-OVER GRAFT (complex)

Aims

To revascularize the lower limb in patients who have adequate circulation in one leg (due to patent iliofemoral vessels) and poor circulation in the other (due to occluded external iliac or common femoral vessels).

Indications

This operation can be done under local anaesthetic in patients with lower-limb ischaemia who would otherwise require major vascular procedure.

Preoperative preparations

Establish that there is a good femoral pulse and distal run-off on one side and none (or a markedly reduced pulse) on the other.

Exposure

Expose both the femoral arteries and their branches in the groin as described previously (p.).

Procedure

Make a suprapubic subcutaneous tunnel between the two incisions by finger dissection. Pass an 8 or 10 mm Dacron graft (woven or knitted which must be preclotted) through the tunnel from one side to the other. Give the patient 5000 IU of heparin IV. Apply clamps to the common femoral artery and its branches on the ischaemic side. Make a longitudinal arteriotomy which may extend over the origin of the profunda femoris and carry out an end-to-side anastomosis with a continuous 4/0 or 5/0 vascular suture. Now suture the other end of the graft to the common femoral artery on the other side after ensuring that the first anastomosis is sound and apply clamps to the donor side vessels and cross-clamps to the graft itself at the site of its exit from the subcutaneous tunnel. Make an appropriate arteriotomy, complete the anastomosis, and release the clamps.

Closure

Bilateral groin drains (suction) brought out through a stab wound. Close skin with Nylon sutures or staples.

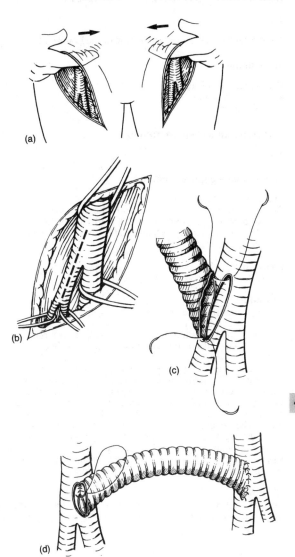

Femoro-femoral cross-over graft.

BYPASS SURGERY BELOW THE INGUINAL LIGAMENT (complex)

Aims

To re-establish the arterial circulation of the lower limb.

Indications

- Crippling claudication.
- Critical ischaemia
- Limb salvage

Femoropopliteal bypass grafting

See p. 460.

Femorodistal bypass grafting

Preoperative preparations
The saphenous vein is harvested and prepared. Alternatively, the conduit may be umbilical vein graft, a prosthetic graft (usually Goretex), or a prosthetic graft with a distal vein patch (composite graft).

Incisions
See section on access to various arteries.

Procedure
In these limb salvage procedures the anastomosis is established between the femoral vessels (usually common femoral) proximally and the anterior tibial, peroneal, or posterior tibial vessels distally. The exposure of these vessels is described on p. 408.

The conduits used may be saphenous vein (either reversed or *in situ* (see p. 466)), umbilical vein graft, or prosthetic graft (usually Goretex) in order of preference and retention of patency. The tunnels from the femoral vessels should be subcutaneous and are best established with a tunnelling instrument. The conduit can then be drawn into the tunneller to reach its target vessel, after which the tunneller is withdrawn. The anastomoses are usually established with 6/0 vascular sutures. If there is difficulty at the apex of the anastomosis, it can be completed with a few interrupted sutures.

Closure
Suction drains are brought through separate stab wounds. Staples or Nylon sutures to skin.

459

FEMOROPOPLITEAL BYPASS GRAFTING (complex)

Aims

Revascularization of the lower limb.

Indications

Atheromatous occlusion of the superficial femoral artery in patients with crippling progressive intermittent claudication (less than 100 yards) which is not improving spontaneously. It is also a limb salvage procedure for critical ischaemia.

Preoperative preparation

Attention is given to myocardial, cerebral, and renal status and the possibility of diabetes. The patient must stop smoking. Serum should be grouped and retained if needed. The leg, pubis, and lower abdomen are shaved, and if a reversed saphenous vein is to be used its course in the thigh is marked out, preferably using duplex Doppler ultrasound. Details of the extent of the disease and the feasibility of the procedure can be determined from the preoperative arteriogram and/or duplex Doppler ultrasound. On-table arteriography may be indicated.

Position of patient

Supine with the knee of the affected leg flexed to 45°. The hip is flexed and externally rotated, and the skin is prepared and draped to expose an area from groin to below the knee. The leg should also be prepared below the knee in case a more distal anastomosis has to be considered. The whole area is then covered with an adhesive incise drape.

Incisions

Expose the femoral artery in the groin and the popliteal artery above the knee through a medially placed incision between vastus medialis and sartorius tendons. Extend the incision for about 10 cm, avoiding undercutting the skin. Deepen it between the anterior border of sartorius and adductor magnus and carefully free the popliteal artery from the vein. Pass tapes around the artery. Is it suitable for distal anastomosis? If not, expose the vessel below the knee by extending the incision along the medial border of the tibia and reflect the gastrocnemius backwards. This exposes the neurovascular bundle and permits consideration of the anastomosis below the trifurcation if necessary.

Subcutaneous tunnel

This can also be made subsartorially. Start with finger dissection in the groin and distal incision. Begin the subsartorial

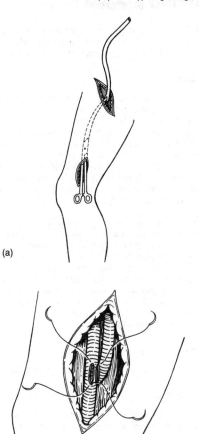

(a)

(b)

461

Femoropopliteal bypass graft for occlusive disease.

FEMOROPOPLITEAL BYPASS
GRAFTING (complex) *(cont.)*

tunnel distally. Then pass a finger under the deep fascia in front of the femoral artery. The tunnel may also be completed by using a tunnelling device such as a rigid sigmoidoscope.

Procedure

Reversed saphenous vein or 5 or 6 mm Goretex can be used (conduit). Pass the conduit through the tunnel, ensuring there are no kinks. Give 5000 IU heparin IV. Control the popliteal vessel and open it. Fashion an end-to-side anastomosis with continuous 5/0 arterial sutures. Clamp the conduit close to the anastomosis and release the popliteal clamps to check for excessive leaks. Now proceed to control the femoral artery and its branches. Fashion an end-to-side anastomosis to the common or superficial femoral artery with continuous 4/0 sutures. Release the clamps. Check the flow with arteriography or flow meter.

In situ bypass grafting is performed by exposing the long saphenous vein and anastomosing its proximal end to the common femoral artery near its bifurcation. As blood flows down the vein, puckering will appear at the site of the valves. A Hall valve stripper is then passed from below to obliterate them. Major tributaries and perforators are identified by either direct exposure or use of Doppler ultrasound and are ligated. When this has been done, the distal end is anastomosed to a suitable site on the popliteal artery or one of its three branches below the knee.

Closure

Layers. Suction drain. Clips or a subcuticular suture to skin.

Postoperatively

Check the pulses either by palpation or Doppler ultrasound. If there is evidence on arteriography of internal damage or clotting, repair or embolectomy may be necessary.

HARVESTING THE LONG SAPHENOUS VEIN FOR BYPASS GRAFTING (major)

Aim

To remove intact the required length of long saphenous vein for the bypass procedure.

Indications

- Occlusive disease of the lower limb
- Coronary artery disease
- Arterial repair and bypass in other sites

Incisions

Identify the position of the long saphenous vein and make several small skin incisions separated by bridges.

Procedure

Mobilize the vein as much as possible through each incision, ligating tributaries but being gentle to avoid damaging or stenosing the vein. In fact it is best handled with the fingers. When sufficient length of vein has been mobilized, tie both ends and remove it to prepare it for bypass grafting.

Preparation for grafting

Ask your assistant to hold the vein between finger and thumb at both ends. Reverse the vein and apply a bulldog clamp to its distal end. Now the assistant should hold the clamp and a cannula attached to a syringe containing heparinized saline can be inserted into the other end, threading the vein over it. Every 2 or 3 cm of vein can then be distended and any leaks repaired either by ligation or with a 6/0 Prolene suture. Proceed in this manner until the vein is leak proof.

If an end-to-end anastomosis is to be carried out the vein end needs no further preparation. However, if the anastomosis is to be end-to-side, the end of the vein has to be trimmed by cutting vertically down the back wall and then removing the corners.

465

IN SITU SAPHENOUS VEIN BYPASS GRAFT (complex)

For this procedure the valves of the saphenous vein must be excised individually or removed by a stripping instrument. The posterior tibial artery is frequently the recipient vessel, with the distal saphenous vein tapering conveniently to allow the narrow end to be anastomized to the artery. The exposure of the vessels proximally and distally is described on pp. 408–12.

Technique for excising the saphenous vein valves

Complete the proximal anastomosis. Note where the blood flow stops at a valve. Apply a bulldog clamp distally and control flow with a sling proximally. Make a transverse incision proximal to the valve. Grasp it with fine forceps and excise it. Repair the venous incision transversely with fine interrupted sutures. Repeat the procedure until all the valves have been removed and there is good pulsatile flow to the end of the vein. Then establish the distal anastomosis with or without an AV fistula (p. 440).

LOWER LIMB AMPUTATIONS (major)

Peripheral vascular disease accounts for 90 per cent of amputations performed in England and Wales.

Aim

- Restoration of mobility (with a prosthesis)
- Relief of pain
- To save life

Indications

Acute ischaemia
When this fails to respond to surgical or medical measures, amputation should be performed to prevent septicaemia resulting from gross tissue necrosis.

Chronic ischaemia
Patients with severe rest pain associated with ulceration, gangrene, and infection may require amputation but only after angiography when treatable lesions can be identified. Lumbar sympathectomy may improve skin blood flow and hence the viability of the flaps.

Gangrene
When gangrene is 'dry', amputation can be carried out once the line of demarcation is established. If the gangrene is 'wet', i.e. associated with putrefaction and sepsis, the risk of proximal spread and systemic sepsis is high. Preoperative control of the situation should be aimed for by the use of antibiotics, e.g. cephalosporins, aminoglycosides plus metronidazole (there are often combined aerobic and anaerobic organisms). If control is not possible, amputation may be performed anyway as a life saving procedure.

Level of amputation

Skin flaps on all amputations must be free from tension to ensure good healing.

Above knee amputation

The stump should be as long as possible, with the bone being divided at least 15 cm above the knee joint line.

Incision
'Fish-mouth' or circumferential.

Procedure
The quadriceps is divided anteriorly and the hamstrings posteriorly. Divide the sciatic nerve as high as possible to prevent postoperative entrapment. Ligate and divide the popliteal

artery and vein, and then elevate the muscles from the femur so that it can be divided at a higher level than the flap. This is performed with a saw and the femoral ends are smoothed with a file.

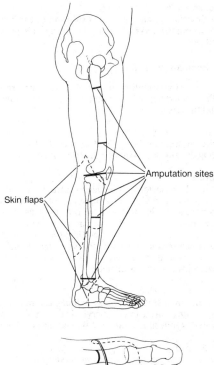

Amputation sites

Skin flaps

469

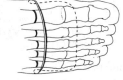

Plantar flap

Amputation sites.

LOWER LIMB AMPUTATIONS (major)
(*cont.*)

Closure
Anterior and posterior muscles are sutured with Vicryl over the femoral end. The anterior and posterior layers of the deep fascia are then closed, and the skin is sutured with interrupted Nylon. A vacuum drain should be brought out through healthy skin well away from the amputation site.

Postoperatively
Ensure that the patient practices extension of the hip joint. If the hip becomes fixed in flexion, the fitting of a prosthesis is impossible.

Below knee amputation

This is the best amputation for mobility but is contraindicated when there is extensive lower-limb sepsis or gangrene close to the tibial tuberosity.

Incision
Hemicircumferential 8 cm distal to the tibial tuberosity and extending distally as a posterior flap for a further 16 cm.

Procedure
Divide tibialis anterior and its vessels at the level of the incision. The nerve is divided at a higher level. Elevate the tibial periosteum and divide the bone with a saw 1 cm proximal to the skin incision. Bevel the tibia anteriorly with a saw and a file. Use a Gigli saw or bone cutting forceps to divide the fibula 2 cm proximal to the wound. Now expose the posterior tibial and peroneal vessels. Ligate and divide them. Taper the gastrocnemius and soleus distally.

Closure
Smooth the tibial stump and approximate the muscle and fascial flaps using interrupted Vicryl. The skin is closed with interrupted Nylon sutures and the flap is bandaged lightly.

Postoperatively
Ensure that the patient practises extension of the knee joint. Flexion of the knee makes the fitting of a prosthesis impossible.

Syme's amputation

A healthy heel is a prerequisite. The posterior flap is constructed from the heel pad and the amputation is performed through the talotibial joint. Subcutaneous tissue is dissected from the os calcis and the Achilles tendon is divided. The foot is removed and then the malleoli are divided above the line of the joint. The posterior flap is then swung upwards and sutured with Nylon. A plaster of Paris dressing is then carefully applied.

Forefoot amputation (Lisfranc)

This makes use of a short dorsal and a long plantar flap. The bones are sectioned along the base of the metatarsals. The mid-tarsal amputation is a variation of this.

Digital amputation

Toes can be amputated through a racket incision. Preservation of the base of the phalanx is preferable to disarticulation. This maintains the joint capsule with tendon attachments.

471

SURGERY FOR VARICOSE VEINS

Varicose veins occur in the long and short saphenous systems owing to valvular incompetence. They may also occur in these systems because of the incompetence of the perforating veins, usually after DVT. Surgical procedures aim to eradicate incompetence at these levels.

Preoperative preparation

The veins are marked on the skin with a marking pen before surgery. Points of control, sites of perforators, and proposed incisions should also be marked.

Trendelenburg's procedure

Position of patient
Supine with the legs abducted. The skin of the legs, groin, and lower abdomen is prepared.

Incision
Medial to the femoral pulse, 5 cm long and below and parallel to the inguinal ligament.

Procedure
The long saphenous vein is identified and all its tributaries are ligated and divided (the superficial circumflex iliac, superficial and deep external pudendal, and superficial circumflex iliac veins). The long saphenous vein is ligated and divided after identifying its junction with the femoral vein at the cribiform fascia. Use a double tie proximally and clamp the vein distally with artery forceps. A vein stripper is then passed down it distally to below the knee, cut down upon, and brought out through the incision. The vein is clamped distally, ligated, and divided.

An olive is now placed over the upper end of the stripper which is gently pulled down until it is flush with the upper end of the saphenous vein which is then ligated. The artery forceps is removed and the passage of the stripper controlled with the fingers.

Any other marked veins can now be identified through small incisions and delivered with fine mosquito forceps. Divide these veins between forceps and then gently apply traction until a segment of vein can be delivered with each forceps. Ligate and remove the veins and repeat the procedure at other sites. Close each wound with single fine Nylon sutures or Steristrips.

Close the groin wound with interrupted or cosmetic subcuticular sutures. Close the distal wound but leave the stitches untied so that the stripper can be removed. Apply crepe bandaging to the leg. Pull the stripper down (with the long saphenous vein), tie the distal sutures, apply a dressing to the wounds, and reapply further crepe bandages.

Postoperative care

Walking should begin on the first postoperative day. Supportive bandages should be worn for 2–3 weeks.

Cockett's procedure (ligation of calf perforators)

Incision

Parallel to the subcutaneous posterior border of tibia and 1 cm behind it. The incision is vertical and extended distally as required.

Procedure

Deepen the incision and divide the deep fascia in the same vertical plane. Reflect the flaps so formed until the perforators can be seen. Ligate and divide their tributaries and the perforators themselves flush with the fascia.

Closure

Close the skin with Nylon sutures. Apply a compression bandage.

Multiple ligations or multiple stab avulsions

When varicose veins are extensive they do not always communicate with the saphenous systems. In such cases they can be dealt with by making multiple incisions, delivering as much of each vein as possible, and ligating it proximally and distally. When there are perforators they should be ligated also. This may be combined with sapheno-femoral disconnection if appropriate.

An alternative to this is to make multiple incisions, raise the leg to prevent bleeding, and avulse each vein in turn, applying a pressure pad to each puncture site.

After both procedures compression bandaging should be applied, ensuring that it is not too tight.

473

12 Urology

J. R. RHIND

Circumcision	476
Pharaphimosis	478
Hydrocelectomy	480
Orchidopexy	484
Prostatectomy	486
Retropubic (Millin) prostatectomy	490
Minimally invasive surgery	494
Cystoscopy	498
Ureteroscopy	502
Urethroplasty	504
Diversions	508
Cystoplasty	514
Cystectomy	516
Pyeloplasty	520
Nephrectomy	522
Nephro-ureterectomy	526

CIRCUMCISION (intermediate)

This is the most common operation performed on children.

Indications

- Religious reasons
- Phimosis (check blood sugar in adults)—diabetes mellitus is frequently associated
- Recurrent balanitis
- Cancer of the penis affecting the prepuce

Procedure

Skin preparation. Separate all preputial adhesions. Attach two small artery forceps to the dorsum of the prepuce at the 11 and 1 o'clock positions. Make a scissor cut between the clips towards the corona but stopping 2 mm from the edge to leave some mucosa for suture. Apply a clip to hold the mucosa and dorsal skin together. Now apply a clip to the frenulum and excise each side, leaving a 3 mm fringe of mucosa. Secure haemostasis with ligatures and then suture the skin and mucosa together with chromic catgut or Vicryl type suture and apply a paraffin gauze dressing.

Postoperative analgesia

Use plain Bupivacaine hydrochloride 0.5%. Inject 5–10 ml under the symphysis pubis on either side of the bulbospongiosus. This lasts for 12 hours. An alternative is to infiltrate the remaining fringe of foreskin with Marcaine.

Complications

- *External urethral meatus stenosis* Do not carry out circumcision in the presence of inflammation.
- *Bleeding* Stop with pressure or suturing.
- *Infection* Usually superficial. Use topical antiseptics if necessary.

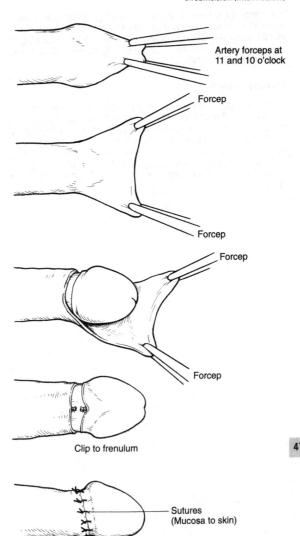

Artery forceps at
11 and 10 o'clock

Forcep

Forcep

Forcep

Forcep

Clip to frenulum

Sutures
(Mucosa to skin)

Steps in circumcision.

477

PHARAPHIMOSIS

The retracted foreskin is trapped behind the glans, particularly when the penis is erect. The result can be gangrene of the glans and so reduction is urgent. This may be by a dorsal slit (which is messy) and later circumcision, or by reduction and later circumcision (tidy).

Method of reduction

Place two gauze swabs on either side of the oedematous slippery foreskin and put the penis on the stretch. This allows the glans to decompress, and with gentle pressure on the glans it will reduce through the constriction ring and the emergency is over. Be prepared to keep the extension for up to 15 minutes, but success results in immediate relief for the patient. Circumcision can then be performed at leisure with a better cosmetic result.

HYDROCELECTOMY (intermediate)

Indications

Patients with symptomatic troublesome hydroceles.

Incision

The testicle is pushed down into the bottom of the scrotum and held with the non-dominant hand. The scrotal skin is then incised longitudinally, exposing skin, dartos muscle, and cyst covering (cremasteric muscle and connective tissue).

Procedure

The cyst covering is best pushed back with a gauze swab. This exposes the cyst which is usually blue in colour. Place two clips on the cyst wall and incise it between the clips to release the fluid. This procedure will allow a smaller scrotal incision. The testicle can then be pushed out of the scrotum. Push the cord coverings back along the cord with the gauze until the testicle and epididymis are clear of the cremasteric muscle. Parts of the cremaster may need division with scissors, but the testicle is now clear of all its coverings. The hydrocele sac can either be excised and the edge over-run with a continuous suture to stop bleeding or turned inside out (Jaboulay procedure) and the edges over-run. Bleeding vessels on the edge of the sac can be diathermized, and it is often quicker to control them with continuous sutures (e.g. continuous Vicryl or 3/0 chromic catgut). However, if the sac is very thick it is best excised or plicated using Lord's method.

Epididymal cysts (intermediate)

These require total removal of the head of the epididymis or they will recur.

Procedure

Gauze dissection with occasional scissor use towards the testis. The testicle will separate the cysts from the vessels of the cord and bring the epididymis into view. Divide this between clips. Separate the cysts and the head of the epididymis from the testicle using scissors and remove the specimen. If the cyst can be kept intact the dissection is much easier. Most bleeders are veins which can be diathermized. The artery should not be damaged.

Closure

Haemostasis is essential to avoid the use of drains which may result in infection. The Dartos muscle is closed with a continuous suture to stop any bleeding from the subcutaneous layers. The skin is then closed with interrupted absorbable sutures.

Postoperatively

The use of a scrotal support increases patient comfort and reduces the risk of bleeding. This is worn until the patient is comfortable without it.

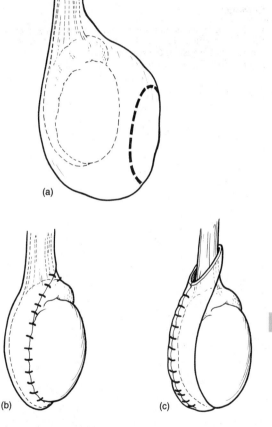

Procedures for hydrocele. (a) The sac is first incised and drained; (b) the excised sac edges can be over-run with a continuous suture, or turned inside out and sutured (c).

HYDROCELECTOMY (intermediate) (*cont.*)

Complications

- *Haematoma* This should not happen if haemostasis has been complete.
- *Infection* Unfortunately may occur and is usually treated with a broad spectrum cephalosporin. Skin scaling is an excellent indicator of the response.
- *Recurrence* When this happens re-operation is necessary. The usual finding is of a pseudocyst which should be excised, taking as much of the cyst wall as possible.

Comment

Epididymal cysts should not be removed in young men since this risks fertility. Hydroceles should only be tapped in an emergency because of the risk of either causing a haematocele or infection. Tapped hydroceles usually recur.

ORCHIDOPEXY (intermediate)

This means bringing the testis down into the scrotum.

Indications

Undescended or ectopic testicle.

Incision

Groin incision medial to the pubic tubercle.

Procedure

Use blunt dissection because the testicle may be very close to the surface. Having found the cord and testicle, make sure that there is no indirect sac. Separation of an indirect sac usually provides sufficient mobility to place the testicle in the scrotum. If still short, separate the peritoneum as much as possible. Feel for a band of tissue on the dorsum of the cord, making sure that this is not the vas deferens or the artery. Division of this may give another centimetre of length.

Dartos pouch

A finger is placed through the groin incision into the scrotum. An incision is made onto the finger, but only skin deep. Using artery forceps develop a pocket under the skin large enough to accept the testicle. Incise the tissue under the skin onto the finger and pick up the rubber of the glove with a clip. Withdraw the finger plus clip (into the groin). Attach the clip onto the loose tissue covering the testicle. By withdrawing the clip, the testicle is brought down and out through the scrotal skin into the pouch prepared for it.

Closure

The scrotal skin is closed with Dexon. The groin is closed with subcuticular Dexon or Vicryl.

Unilateral testicle

Bring it down as low as possible and reoperate at a later age. If the other testicle is normal and the undescended testicle cannot be brought down, remove it.

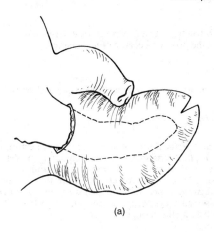

(a)

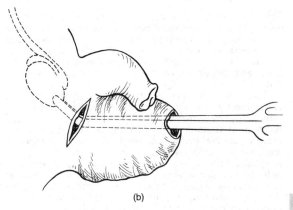

(b)

Orchidopexy and Dartos pouch.

PROSTATECTOMY (major)

Indications

- Relief of obstruction caused by prostatic enlargement.
- Removal of the prostate because of malignancy.

Approaches

Transurethral, transvesicle, retropubic (Millin), perineal, or radical retropubic.

Comment

Transvesicle and perineal prostatectomy are rarely performed in the UK. Radical retropubic prostatectomy is indicated when prostatic malignancy is confined to the gland and excision is potentially curative. Whether transurethal or retropubic prostatectomy is performed depends on the size of the prostate as assessed at cystoscopy. A prostate larger than 100 g is better removed by the retropubic route.

Transurethal prostatectomy

This is one of the most common operations performed on men and is the most common method of dealing with prostatic obstruction. Cystoscopy is performed first to assess the size of the prostate, and to exclude bladder stones and tumours. The presence of a tumour is a contraindication to prostatectomy because of the danger of implantation in the raw prostatic bed.

Modern resectoscopes are often capable of being inserted under direct vision so that only one instrument is required. If stones are present, they should be broken before the prostatic resection or vision in the bladder will be lost. The resection uses the 'cutting' current and the loop is moved backwards and forwards, removing slices of the tissue until the 'capsule' is visible. The capsule is identified by circular fibres as opposed to a cotton-wool appearance. Bleeding vessels are coagulated by placing the loop on the bleeder and pressing the coagulation pedal. (A different sound from the machine is essential to let the operator know which pedal he has pressed, and the machine must be very carefully tuned to give the correct type of current for cutting or coagulation.)

Procedure

A set plan is essential or you can become lost and either cause damage or carry out an inadequate resection. Starting at the 6 o'clock position resect the middle lobe down to the level of the veru montanum. *The veru must never be resected; it is the guide to the external sphincter.* Then turn to the 2 o'clock position and resect a channel. The veru will not be visible at this angle, so turn the instrument to 6 o'clock and check that you have not come back too far. (Err on the side of caution. You can always remove a little more, but you cannot put it back!) Continue resecting down the side of the prostate, trying to keep on the capsule and, of course, not coming further back than the veru. The prostatic lobe falls across towards the mid-line, and finally the resection is horizontal until the veru is left upstanding in the mid-line. Blood vessels can be

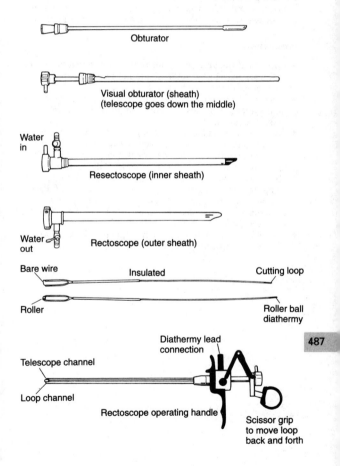

Obturator

Visual obturator (sheath)
(telescope goes down the middle)

Water in

Resectoscope (inner sheath)

Water out   Rectoscope (outer sheath)

Bare wire   Insulated   Cutting loop

Roller   Roller ball diathermy

Diathermy lead connection

Telescope channel

Loop channel

Rectoscope operating handle

Scissor grip to move loop back and forth

Resectoscope (components).

487

diathermized as they appear or left until the lobe is totally resected. Resecting between the adenoma and the capsule usually results in the final part of the resection being almost bloodless. Now turn to 11 o'clock and resect the right lobe in exactly the same way. Diathermize the bleeders and use Ellik's evacuator to wash out prostatic chips and blood clots. Make sure all chips are evacuated or they will block the catheter and keep your house-surgeon (and perhaps you too) up during the night.

Insert a catheter. This may be three-way, allowing irrigation, or two-way with a dose of frusemide to create a diuresis.

Problems?

- Lost? Find the veru or the air bubble in the bladder dome. Still lost? Insert a catheter, abandon the procedure, and try on another day.
- *Penetration of the capsule* This does not usually matter unless a large vein has been opened, in which case bleeding must be controlled.
- *Bleeding* If coagulation does not stop the bleeding, resect deeper and try again. Accuracy is essential. Is the artery spurting directly onto the lens or is it coming from a direction that you have not considered? Pull back and look about. The artery can often be seen and can be coagulated using the full length of the loop. *Still bleeding?* Pass a catheter and apply gentle traction. If this does not work, the only answer is to make a Pfannenstiel incision, open the prostatic cavity, and insert a pack.
- *You have opened the rectum!* Unfortunately this can happen. The correct procedure is a defunctioning colostomy.

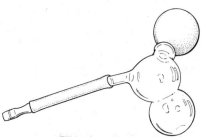

Ellick evacuator
(to wash out the bladder)

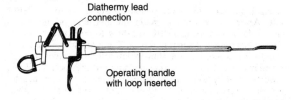

Diathermy lead
connection

Operating handle
with loop inserted

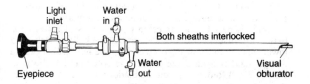

Light
inlet

Water
in

Both sheaths interlocked

Eyepiece

Water
out

Visual
obturator

Resectoscope (assembled).

RETROPUBIC (Millin) PROSTATECTOMY (major)

Indications

Benign prostatic hypertrophy.

Position of patient

Supine.

Incision

Pfannenstiel. One finger breadth above the pubic bone.

Procedure

If right handed, the operator should stand on the patient's left. After the incision is made the mid-line of the rectus sheath is picked up in a strong artery forceps and elevated. The rectus muscle is separated from the underside of the rectus sheath by sweeping the finger laterally on each side. A bleeder is usually present on each side but these can easily be diathermized by lifting up on the artery clip. The rectus muscles are then separated in the mid-line, and a sweep of the finger behind the pubis will open the retropubic space and expose the bladder and prostate (sometimes the tendinous lower inch of the rectus muscle needs to be cut vertically with scissors to its insertion onto the pubic bone to allow better exposure). A retractor is then inserted to hold the muscles apart (the Millin retractor is best for prostatectomy and a Gosset retractor is better for bladder work). The prostate, bladder neck, and lower bladder are now exposed and can be felt easily because the prostate is a hard lump with the soft bladder above it. Place a 2 × 4 folded swab on the bladder neck area and insert the middle blade of the Millin retractor. This holds the bladder away from the prostate, and also can be pressed down to show the bladder neck more easily.

Place a 2 × 4 swab on either side of the prostate. A large vein will be seen running vertically on it. Using a boomerang needle, insert no. 1 chromic catgut sutures 1 cm apart around this vessel deeply into the prostate. Tie and clip as 'stay sutures'. Using a diathermy incise the prostate horizontally to a depth of 3 mm (smoke and blood are removed by suction). The plane between the adenoma and the 'false capsule' is obvious. Open this plane with scissors and then insert the index finger cephalad into the bladder (proof that you are in the correct place). Now, mobilize the lateral lobes down to the apices by squeezing your finger between the adenoma and the false capsule. At this point the urethra is 'nipped' off by finger pressure, allowing the adenoma to be lifted out. Any connections still present at the bladder neck are either 'pinched off' or

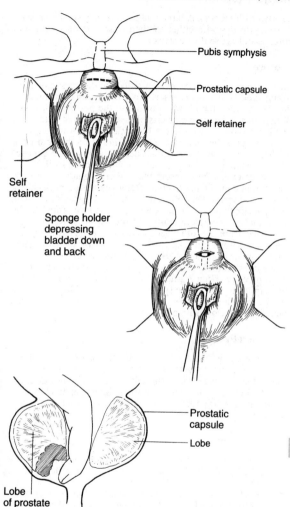

Pubis symphysis

Prostatic capsule

Self retainer

Self retainer

Sponge holder depressing bladder down and back

Prostatic capsule

Lobe

Lobe of prostate

491

Top: **Retropubic prostatectomy. Access via Pfannenstiel incision above pubis.**
Middle: **Retropubic postatectomy. Incision into the prostatic capsule.**
Bottom: **Retropubic prostatectomy. Enucleating a prostatic adenoma.**

divided with scissors. A large middle lobe may still be present. If so, grasp this with either toothed dissectors or a vulsellum forceps and excise it with scissors.

Closure

Insert the bladder-neck spreader and open the jaws to demonstrate the bladder neck. Insert no. 1 plain catgut in the midline from inside the bladder down into the posterior prostate. When this is tied, it converts the bladder neck into a V, pulling mucosa down into the prostatic cavity. An X stitch of plain catgut is then inserted on each side of the bladder neck at the 4 and 8 o'clock positions. These sutures stop 75 per cent of the bleeding, but until they are in place suction by the assistant is essential. Now insert the catheter, guide it into the bladder, and inflate the balloon. Remove the side-pack closest to you and insert a suture at the end of the capsular incision, tie, and apply a clip to the ends of the sutures (this will be your guide to complete closure of the capsule). Remove the side-pack from the other side and close the capsule with a continuous no. 1 chromic catgut, finally tying to the original suture at the end closest to you. (All these sutures are most easily inserted using a boomerang needle, and once use of this instrument has been learned you will never regret it!) Insert a pack into the retropubic space and wash any blood clots out of the bladder. Remove the pack, check for any residual bleeding, and close with a drain to the retropubic space.

Postoperatively

The catheter is managed in exactly the same way as for a transurethral prostatectomy and removed when gross bleeding and clots have cleared (usually the second day). IV fluids are discontinued as soon as normal intestinal function has returned. The drain is removed on the fifth day and the skin sutures after 7 days.

Complications

492

- *Bleeding from the drain* This should not happen if you have checked properly. If it does occur the wound needs to be reopened.
- *Urine drainage from the drain* Check that the catheter is not blocked. Provided that the catheter is clear, the leak will stop.
- *Wound infection* These patients usually have infected urine and so prophylactic antibiotics are recommended to reduce this problem.

- *Incontinence* This should not happen if you have chosen the correct operation (trying to perform a retropubic prostatectomy on a small gland has a high risk of damage to the external sphincter).

MINIMALLY INVASIVE SURGERY

Minimally invasive surgery was 'invented' by urologists when they began to break bladder stones by inserting a sound into the bladder, directing it onto the stone, and hitting it with a hammer. Another method was to insert a 'file' into the bladder and gradually grind the stone away. Modern developments with the Hopkins rod lens-telescope and fibre-optic lighting have resulted in considerable progress.

Renal calculi

Eighty-five to ninety per cent of renal stones can be dealt with by either (extracorporeal shock-wave lithotripsy) (ESWL) or percutaneous nephroscopy (PCN).

Extracorporeal shock-wave lithotripsy (major)

Shock waves are produced either by an electrohydraulic or a piezoelectric discharge. These shock waves are focused onto the stone, causing it to disintegrate. The stone particles are then passed down the ureter and into the body. The stone is localized by either X-ray or ultrasound, depending on the type of machine. The procedure requires either local anaesthetic or sedation and is performed as a day case. The patient is fit for work the next day.

Problems
- Large stones (greater than 2 cm) may require several treatments and so much debris may be released that obstruction of the lower ureter may occur (*Steinstrasse*). Large stones are better dealt with by PCN followed by ESWL.
- *Local damage* Some cases of perirenal haematoma and splenic and hepatic damage have been reported. There is evidence that renal tissue damage may also occur, as measured by tubular enzymes, but this appears to be only a temporary problem.
- Some stones are too hard.
- If there is obstruction so that the stone fragments cannot escape from the kidney or calyx, ESWL is not possible.
- *Cost* The machines are expensive to buy and run.

Percutaneous nephroscopy (complex)

Basically, this is insertion of a nephroscope into a kidney. Stones are then either removed with grasping forceps or are broken up as much as possible and the fragments removed. All this is done under direct vision.

Position of patient
Prone with table partly broken and a sandbag placed under the kidney to push it back and help to reduce movement.

Procedure
A ureteric catheter is passed into the kidney from the bladder. A syringe containing a mixture of X-ray contrast and methylene blue is attached to the end of the catheter. The patient's skin is cleaned and towels are placed. With X-ray screening, some dye is injected up the ureteric catheter to show the kidney and its pelvicalyceal system. Choose the calyx which provides the straightest route to the stone and insert a fine needle and cannula into this calyx under X-ray control. Successful puncture will be demonstrated by drainage of fluid containing methylene blue from the cannula.

Pass a guide-wire through the cannula into the renal pelvis and remove the cannula. A small incision is then made through the skin and deep fascia beside the guide-wire and dilators are passed over the guide-wire into the kidney until there is a track of 26 or 28 FR into the kidney. An Amplatz sheath (a short tube) is passed into the kidney, and the nephroscope can be inserted through this and the inside of the kidney examined. The guide-wire can be removed at this stage, but it provides a safety measure in case the Amplatz sheath becomes dislodged.

Stones can either be shattered by an electrohydraulic probe and the fragments removed using grasping forceps or eroded using ultrasound with the dust being removed by suction. Ideally, the stone should be completely cleared, but staghorn calculi may have parts which are not accessible and these may have to be left to be dealt with by ESWL.

Pelviureteric junction obstruction is managed by incision of the junction through the nephroscope and insertion of a ureteric stent down into the bladder. (There is still some argument about which size of stent should be used and how long it should be left in place.) Pelvic and calyceal tumours have been treated in this way. It is then usual to 'sterilize' the nephrostomy track with radioactive wires. (This is one way of managing a tumour in a solitary kidney.)

495

Closure
A nephrostomy tube is usually inserted at the end of the procedure and left for 48 hours. The wound is closed with interrupted Nylon.

Postoperatively
The patient can usually go home on the fourth day and be back at work in 10 days.

Complications

- *Bleeding* This is usually minor but may require exploration and removal of the kidney.
- *Perforation of the pelvis* This usually settles with nephrostomy drainage or insertion of a ureteric stent. (A stent is better since it can usually be left *in situ* for several weeks, without harm to the patient, and therefore may allow early discharge. The stent must be removed, usually about 6 weeks later.)
- *Infection* It is recommended that PCN is performed under antibiotic cover.

CYSTOSCOPY (minor)

This is the visual examination of the interior of the bladder using a cystoscope or fibre-scope.

Instruments

The cystoscope
This is a rigid instrument relying on rod lenses for vision and a fibre-optic source for light. Passage of the instrument is painful and requires general or regional anaesthesia. The patient should have reasonable hip adduction to allow introduction. Clarity of vision is excellent, and the large calibre allows a wide range of manoeuvres to be carried out through the instrument.

The fibre-scope
This is flexible and uses fibre-optics for vision and lighting. Passage of this instrument is relatively pain-free and can be done under local anaesthetic. The clarity of vision is limited, and because of the small calibre and 'bend' of the instrument limited operative manoeuvres are possible.

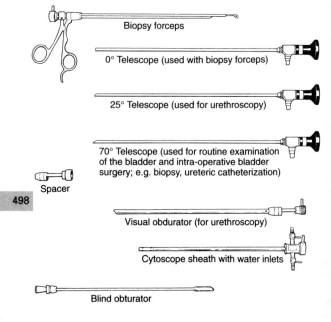

Biopsy forceps

0° Telescope (used with biopsy forceps)

25° Telescope (used for urethroscopy)

70° Telescope (used for routine examination of the bladder and intra-operative bladder surgery; e.g. biopsy, ureteric catheterization)

Spacer

Visual obdurator (for urethroscopy)

Cytoscope sheath with water inlets

Blind obturator

Cystoscopy instruments.

Uses

Diagnosis of urethral structure, bladder stones, and carcinoma of urethra and bladder. Assessment of prostatic size and normality of bladder mucosa, muscle, and ureteric orifices.

Position of patient

Lithotomy.

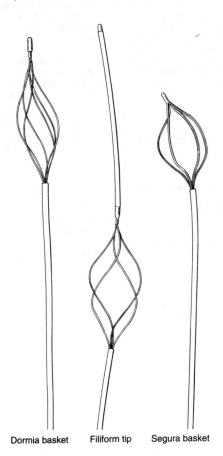

Dormia basket   Filiform tip   Segura basket

Baskets for the retrieval of stones.

CYSTOSCOPY (minor) (*cont.*)

Procedure

After cleansing the genitalia the urethra is lubricated (antiseptic in the lubricant). In the male urethroscopy should always be performed using a 0°, 25°, or 30° telescope passed with the irrigating fluid running, otherwise urethral tumours, false passages, and strictures may be missed. A forward-viewing telescope is required for assessment of prostatic size, but a 70° telescope should be used to examine the bladder. Orientation in the bladder can be difficult; the air bubble is always at the 12 o'clock position. The ureteric orifices should be at the 5 and 7 o'clock positions on the interureteric bar but may be deviated pathologically (e.g. reflux). Examine the mucosa for tumours, abnormalities of blood vessel pattern, and appearance. Check the muscle for trabeculation and the ureteric orifices for normality of position. If there are saccules or a diverticulum, record their position and check that there is not a hidden tumour. Record the size and number of stones. If in doubt about anything, take a biopsy. Always biopsy a 'first-time' tumour; never just cauterize it with diathermy.

Fibreoscopy is very similar. The instrument is forward-viewing, narrow, flexible, and has a steerable tip which often makes introduction easier than with the rigid instrument, particularly if the patient has a deformity which interferes with abduction of the hips.

Cystoscopic manoeuvres

Biopsy of suspicious lesions, diathermy of small bladder tumours or bleeding points, bladder wash-out (e.g. clot retention, small stones), catheterization of the ureter either to allow injection of radio-opaque contrast for X-ray studies or bypass obstruction, and passage of stone baskets (e.g. Dormia, Segura) to remove small stones from the lower ureter.

URETEROSCOPY (intermediate)

Ureteroscopy permits visualization of the interior of the ureter, the biopsy of ureteric lesions, removal or destruction of ureteric stones and tumours, and pushing a stone back into the kidney where it can be managed by ESWL or PCN.

Procedure

The short ureteroscope is best for lower ureteric surgery since it has a slightly tapered tip, which allows easier introduction into the ureter, and a larger operating channel. However, it cannot reach the upper ureter. A guide-wire is helpful but not essential. The ureteric orifice can be dilated with mental bougies or balloon catheters, but this is rarely necessary. This can lead to bleeding which makes it difficult to identify the orifice. Movement of the guide-wire usually opens the orifice satisfactorily.

Problems

If the ureteroscope will not enter try filling the bladder more to straighten the intramural ureter. Rotate the ureteroscope to direct the instrument lip in another direction. Pull back slightly on the guide-wire which also tends to straighten the ureter.

Ureteric perforation

If this is minor, it is not a problem. However, if it is major with substantial extravasation, a stent has to be passed over the guide-wire.

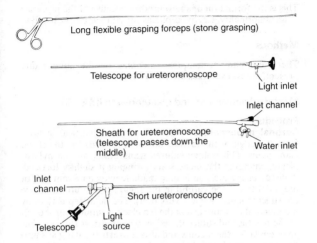

Long flexible grasping forceps (stone grasping)

Telescope for ureterorenoscope

Light inlet

Inlet channel

Sheath for ureterorenoscope
(telescope passes down the
middle)

Water inlet

Inlet channel

Short ureterorenoscope

Telescope

Light
source

Ureterorenoscope (components).

URETHROPLASTY (complex)

This is the formation of a new urethra because of the presence of an abnormality, e.g. hypospadias, stricture, multiple fistulas.

Methods

There are many techniques depending on the abnormality present. A few examples are given here.

Meatal advancement and glanuloplasty (MAGPI)

Procedure

Coronal hypospadias The first step is a vertical incision from the edge of the meatus forwards towards the tip of the glans penis. This is then sutured transversely as in a pyloroplasty, enlarging the meatus and bringing it slightly forward. A circumcizing incision is then made leaving an 8 mm cuff of preputial tissue (be careful in the region of the urethra since the subcutaneous tissue is very thin). The next step is to draw the mucosal cuff forward at the 6 o'clock position over the top of the meatus and suture the edges with mattress sutures. This gives cover for the meatus and also converts the flat glans into the more normal rounded form. If the excess preputial skin is not required to fill any skin defects, it is excised and suturing is continued as for a normal circumcision. Sutures are absorbable 6/0 (either Dexon or Vicryl). The procedure can be done as a day case, but it may be preferable to keep the child in overnight. The operation should be done before the child starts school to save embarrassment.

Subcoronal hypospadias The meatus is placed even further posteriorly, even as far as the perineum, and may be associated with a chordee (a bend in the erect penis caused by a fibrous band extending from the meatus towards the glans). If chordee is present the band must be excised, resulting in further posterior displacement of the meatus. The presence of chordee is tested by creation of an artificial erection using a tourniquet around the penis and injection of saline into one of the corpora. The gap between the meatus and the end of the glans needs to be filled by either a patch or a tube, usually the mucosal surface of the prepuce. (The skin and the mucosa of the prepuce have their individual blood supply and by separating them the mucosal surface can be swung down to provide a new urethra.) Closure over the new urethra will usually require the use of the skin part of the prepuce, but the end result should be a penis with the meatus at the end of the gland penis. Sutures are again 6/0 absorbable, and an 8 French gauge tube stent should be used with a firm dressing for 48 hours.

504

Complications

The main complication is fistula. This occurs in up to 10 per cent of cases and can be difficult to close. A flap swung across and a three-layer closure is usually successful.

Dehiscence of the closure may occur (it looks exactly the same as before), but since there is no loss of skin start again.

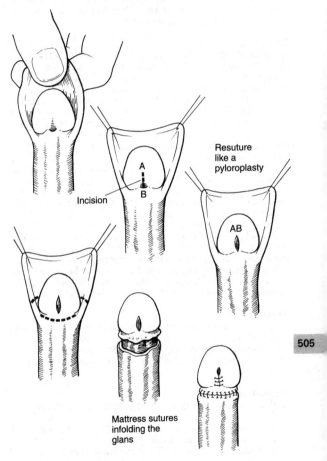

MAGPI procedure.

URETHROPLASTY (complex) (*cont.*)

Stricture

A urethrogram will give the position and apparent extent of the abnormal urethra. The urethrogram must be ascending and descending. In very tight strictures this may require a suprapubic catheter, but the upper limit of the stricture is important. The method of repair depends on whether the stricture is in the anterior (penile) or posterior (bulbomembranous) urethra.

NB The end of an abnormal urethra is always more than it looks either on X-ray or to the naked eye and so a 0.5 cm stricture often needs a 3 cm correction.

Procedure
Anterior stricture   Pass a Lister or Whyndam-Powell sound down the urethra to the stricture. Do not push the sound through the stricture (use a sound that you know is too large). Incise onto the tip of the sound and identify the urethral mucosa. Place a stay stitch through the mucosa and skin on either side. This reduces bleeding and also makes it easier to identify the urethral lumen. Using a sharp-tipped blade or fine scissors cut the urethra open through the stricture until the calibre looks normal. Stay sutures placed between the urethra and the skin again makes the procedure easier. Incise the urethra at least 1 cm into the normal-looking portion. The choice is now whether to perform a one-stage or a two-stage repair. Usually a one-stage repair can be performed by either a free scrotal graft or a pedicle graft, depending to a certain extent on the length of the defect and its position (if the defect is long, it is better to use a pedicle graft with its better blood supply). The shape of the graft is ellipsoid to replace the deficit in the urethral lumen and is sutured with 6/0 absorbable material. Subcutaneous sutures are inserted and the skin is closed, also with an absorbable suture. Some surgeons use a suprapubic diversion catheter, but a Silastic urethral catheter left in position for 48 hours may be easier.

Problems
Finding the lumen through the stricture. Use a very fine gum elastic bougie (e.g. Canne–Ryall) as a probe. Do not use metal sounds. It is too easy to make a false passage. If all fails, extend the incision further back and open the urethra in its bulbar portion.

Complications
- *Fistula* This is very rare as long as there is no distal obstruction.
- *Restricture* Since it can take at least 20 years for a stricture to form, any method must be judged accordingly. Short-term strictures can occur if the urethra has not been opened far enough on either side (3 cm is no more tedious to suture than 2 cm and does not take much longer).

Posterior stricture

These can also be repaired in a one-stage operation but since they are more complex a two-stage procedure is preferable.

First stage
A U-shaped incision is made in the perineum extending forward with the base of the U on the line between the ischial tuberosities. The incision is through skin and subcutaneous fat. This flap then strips easily backwards from the underlying tissues exposing the bulbospongiosus. It is opened with a sound in the urethra. Stay sutures picking up the urethral mucosa and the bulbospongiosus are inserted to reduce bleeding and to aid the identification of the urethral lumen. Incision of the stricture is usually into the prostatic urethra, and the Turner–Warwick retractor is very useful here. The skin flap is then sutured into the urethra with absorbable sutures, skin to mucosa. The Turner–Warwick needles make this easy for the deep parts. A soft Paul tube drain is inserted under the perineal flap and the skin to urethral mucosa sutures continued. A supra pubic or urethral Silastic diversion catheter may be inserted and left for 48 hours until oedema has settled. The drain is removed at 48 hours.

Follow-up
Patients attend for an examination under anaesthetic every 3 months. At each attendance the anterior and posterior urethral openings are checked with a 24 French gauge sound to ensure that stenosis has not occurred. If it has, the urethra needs to be opened further. Depilation of the hairy scrotal skin must also be performed. This skin is going to be used to form part of the new urethral lumen and the hairs cause irritation and also stone formation. Therefore the hair follicles in the skin to be turned in must be destroyed by electrolysis at each check-up. Three check-ups are usually adequate and the patient can then proceed to the second stage.

Second stage
A new urethra is constructed by incising the skin on either side approximately 1 cm from the mid-line of the urethra. The exact distance depends to a certain extent on the amount of normal urethral mucosa remaining. If the new urethra is too narrow, obstruction will recur. If too wide, pooling of urine and post-void dribbling will occur. The new urethra is closed with a continuous absorbable suture over an 18 French gauge Silastic catheter. Subcutaneous sutures are inserted to provide haemostasis and reduce the risk of fistula formation. The skin is closed with absorbable sutures. No drain is required and the catheter is removed at 48 hours.

507

DIVERSIONS (complex)

These are methods of urinary excretion following removal of the bladder.

Conduit

This may be either of the ileum or colon. A length of bowel is isolated with its blood supply intact. The ureters are joined onto the bowel at one end, and the other end is brought out as a cutaneous urostomy.

If the ileum is used, it is usual to perform an anastomosis which is freely refluxing so that the ends of the ureter are joined together using continuous 3/0 plain catgut either side-to-side or end-to-side. The joined ureters are then attached to the end of the ileum using continuous 3/0 chromic catgut. Stents are not essential, but infant feeding tubes can be brought through the loop and out of the urostomy. This has the advantage of making certain that neither ureteric lumen is obstructed by the anastomosis and it also allows free urinary drainage postoperatively when the loop may be atonic. Finally, the posterior peritoneum is closed around the base of the conduit so that any leakage is retroperitoneal. Indeed, if one has to re-explore the anastomosis it is easier to access.

If the colon is used, an anti-reflux anastomosis can be fashioned. The muscle of a taenium coli is incised and separated from the underlying mucosa for a distance of 2 cm. This creates a groove in which the ureter will lie and allows closure of the muscle over the top without causing obstruction. A hole is made in the mucosa at the end of the groove, and the end of the ureter is anastomosed using 3/0 plain catgut. Stents can be used as required.

Urostomy

The fashioning of the urostomy is perhaps the most important part of the diversion. It must be correctly sited (or the bag will not stay on). It should have a good spout to minimize leakage of urine and dislodgement of the flange, and the track through the abdominal muscles should be loose enough to prevent ischaemia but tight enough to prevent parastomal hernia or prolapse.

The position of the urostomy must be checked before the operation. The bag should be attached to the abdomen on the favoured side (with some fluid in the bag) and the patient should perform normal activities around the ward (walking, sitting, bending, etc.) in his usual clothes (does the belt get in the way?). The site is then clearly marked.

Procedure

Excise a disc of skin and subcutaneous fat down to the muscular fascia. Make a cruciate incision in the fascia and separate the muscles until the posterior fascia is visible. Make a similar cruciate incision into the peritoneal cavity. Pass a bowel clamp through into the abdomen and use it to replace the one on the end of the conduit which is then drawn out, making certain that the mesentery is not twisted or too tight (the length of the conduit outside the abdomen should be about 6 cm in an adult). Loosely suture the external abdominal fascia to the

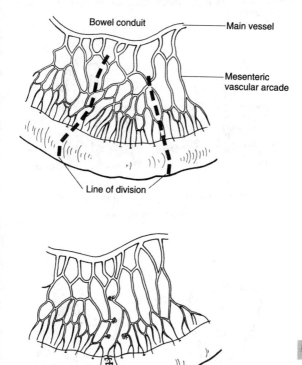

Urinary diversion.

muscle of the bowel. This should prevent prolapse and hernia-tion. Next, using a chromic catgut suture, take a bite of skin edge of the conduit wall muscle directly opposite, and then the full thickness of the end of the conduit. When this is pulled tight it everts the end into a spout. Only three or four of these everting sutures can be placed since they cannot be used on the mesenteric side of the conduit. Complete the skin-to-bowel anastomosis with chromic catgut (or Vicryl). If stents have been used, anchor them to the lip of the spout with a suture.

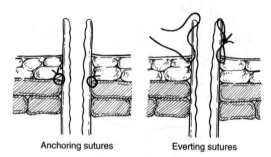

Anchoring sutures   Everting sutures

Formation of the urostomy

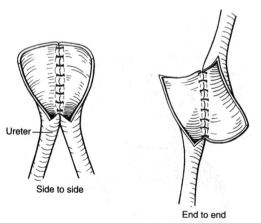

Ureter

Side to side

End to end

Methods of joining the ureters.

Complications
Immediate
- *Conduit ischaemia* Start again.
- *Stomal ischaemia* Check that the mesentery is not twisted or constricted as it comes through the abdominal wall. If it is too short, try dividing the vascular arcade. However, this may result in total loss of the conduit, so be careful.
- *Urine leak* If you have stents inserted, do not worry as it will stop.

Delayed Fifty per cent of conduits develop delayed complications such as renal failure secondary to chronic ascending infections, stones, and stomal stenosis or retraction. Ureteroconduit obstruction is less common now with the use of the end-to-end anastomosis, but it still occurs sometimes.

Ureterosigmoidostomy (complex)

In this procedure the ureters are anastomozed to the colon and urine is passed through the anus. The anastomosis is fash-

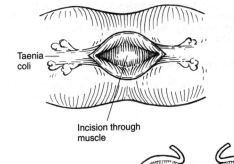

Taenia
coli

Incision through
muscle

Muscle separated from
underlying mucosa

511

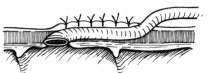

Ureter lying in a submucosal tunnel

Ureterosigmoidoscopy.

ioned in a non-refluxing way as described above. There is no need for a bowel anastomosis, and therefore the diversion is quick and has a low morbidity. However, the patient must be able to retain urine in the rectum (put 1 litre of fluid into the rectum and make the patient walk about for an hour to check continence). There is also a risk of developing carcinoma of the bowel in the vicinity of the ureterocolin anastomosis.

Complications
Include renal failure and hypochloraemic acidosis.

Neobladder

This is a false bladder which can be created by making a pouch of small bowel or caecum and stitching this onto the urethra or the prostatic capsule. Neobladder may also be attached to the skin in such a fashion that it is continent and catheterizable for emptying. Continence may be produced by an intussuscepted piece of bowel or by using the appendix as the route to the surface.

Comment
There are various methods which sound very attractive but the procedures are time-consuming. Some problems are becoming apparent, e.g. failure to catheterize, stone formation and cancer.

Ureterocutaneous diversion

This involves stitching the ureter to the skin. It is used only for very large ureters and only for a short time. These are subject to stenosis.

CYSTOPLASTY (complex)

This is augmentation or reduction in the size of the bladder.

Indications

- *Augmentation*: tuberculosis, radiotherapy, Hunner's ulcer, chronic infection, irritable detrusor
- *Reduction*: diverticulum, chronic obstruction, atony

Methods

- *Augmentation*: An isolated piece of bowel (stomach, small bowel, or colon) is sutured to the bladder
- *Reduction*: Part of the bladder (or a diverticulum) is excised

Augmentation

Incision
Lower midline.

Procedure
Expose the bladder and open it between stay sutures. Divert a segment of bowel (large or small) on its mesentery and restore continuity. Open it along its antimesenteric border and suture it to the bladder as a pouch. Use plain catgut for the inner (mucosal) layer and chromic catgut for muscle.

Closure
Close the wound in layers. Insert a tube drain which should remain in place for 5 days.

Postoperatively
Restrict oral fluids for 2 days. Solids should not be taken until about 4 days in view of the bowel anastomosis.

Reduction

The bladder is exposed and opened as above. If a simple reduction is required, free the bladder from the peritoneum and other organs and excise the excess. As long as the bladder is healthy, it is amazing how little can be left and still retain good capacity. If there is a diverticulum dissect it free and excise it with a two-layer closure of the defect. If the ureter is close pass a catheter up it to protect it.

CYSTECTOMY (complex)

This is removal of the bladder, prostate, internal iliac lymph nodes, and sometimes the urethra.

Preoperative preparations

This is a major procedure with a mortality even in the best of hands and so the patient must be as fit as possible. Four units of blood should be grouped and cross-matched. If an ileal conduit is planned, the site should be marked for the stoma and the patient should wear the bag around the ward so that it is certain the site is correct for sitting, lying, and standing.

If a ureterosigmoidostomy is planned, anal continence must be checked by instilling 1 litre of fluid into the rectum and making the patient walk about. If there is any leakage, reconsider using this form of diversion.

Position of patient

Supine with the patient catheterized. In females the vagina should be packed.

Incision

Cernay incision
This is a transverse lower abdominal incision with detachment of the rectus insertion from the pubis. It provides excellent access to both sides of the pelvis and does not encroach on the stoma site. However, it may be difficult to mobilize the bowel for the conduit.

Left paramedian incision
This is a good general purpose incision which, if long enough, allows satisfactory access to the right side of the pelvis.

Procedure

Once inside the peritoneal cavity check for metastatic spread if it has not already been established by CT or MRI scan. If there is widespread disease, the tumour may be deemed inoperable. However, if it is possible that the patient will have many problems with haematuria, frequency, and urgency, it may be possible to carry out a less radical clearance.

Identify the iliac bifurcation and divide the posterior peritoneum. Tape the ureter as it crosses the iliac bifurcation and draw it out of the way. Dissect the internal iliac artery free and ligate it in continuity. Identify the vas as it leaves the deep ring. Divide it and ligate it, but keep a long tie and clip on the bladder end. This will be a useful retractor and later a guide. With the help of the vas clear down the side of the pelvis to the internal iliac artery and then follow the artery down towards the bladder. The dissection also clears the ureter.

Once sufficient length of ureter has been cleared below the pelvic brim, it should be divided (place a stay stitch in the proximal end to make it easy to find at a later stage of the operation). Leave a long tie on the bladder end of the ureter since this is going to be your guide to the lateral side of the bladder. Continue to follow the internal iliac artery down the side of the pelvis, ligating and dividing vessels as they come off medially. Lymph nodes can be cleared at the same time. By following the artery and the ureter, the bladder is cleared down to the side of the prostate. Now the peritoneum across the front of the uterus or rectum is divided. In male patients follow the vas posteriorly to the bladder until the vesicles in the prostate are reached. Repeat the process on the other side of the pelvis.

The bladder is now held only by the prostatic attachments and the urethra. The dissection is continued anteriorly behind the pubis into the retropubic space, exposing the front of the prostate. The puboprostatic ligament and dorsal vein of the penis can be felt by finger dissection, and are best ligated in continuity and then divided (bleeding from these veins can be very difficult to control). The prostate then tilts back and the urethra is easily palpable (the catheter helps) and can be divided. It is then easy to separate the prostate from the rectum and remove the specimen. Place a large pack into the pelvis to stop any oozing and 'go and have a cup of tea'. When you return, minor bleeding will have stopped and any large vessels will be easily to deal with by either diathermy or stitches.

Variations on the above method depend on the following.
1. *How radical the clearance must be* If a total excision is required, the lateral wall of the pelvis must be cleared of all fat and connective tissue, increasing the operation time, risk of nerve and vessel injury, and postoperative morbidity. (Does the patient really require this extent of surgery?)
2. *The sex of the patient* The problem of separating the prostate from the rectum does not arise in females. The vagina (easily identified by the pack) can be entered either anteriorly or posteriorly, depending on whether the uterus is to be conserved. (A young woman requiring cystectomy for a pyocystis may still wish to have children.)
3. *The type of diversion* Neobladder connected to the urethra, intestinal conduit, rectal bladder, or ureterosigmoidosotomy?
4. *The fitness of the patient* The less fit the patient, the less you should do.
5. *Previous radiotherapy or surgery* The resultant fibrosis increases technical difficulty and bleeding, and also causes delayed wound healing and increases the risk of postoperative death.

517

CYSTECTOMY (complex) (*cont.*)

Closure

Insert a suction drain into the pelvis (to remove blood and lymph). A simple drain to the area of the ureteric anastomosis permits any urinary leakage to escape. The abdominal wound is closed usually in layers.

Postoperatively

The patient should be given IV fluids until bowel activity is back to normal and should be mobilized as soon as possible.

Complications

- *Bleeding* This should not happen if the abdomen is dry before closure. If it does, the wound has to be reopened.
- *Excessive drainage* This may be lymph or urine. Send a specimen to the laboratory for sodium and creatinine levels. The result will distinguish between urine and lymph. (Lymphatic or plasma loss can easily equal 2 litres per 24 hours but will have plasma levels of sodium and creatinine.)

PYELOPLASTY

Indications

Obstruction at the pelviureteric junction leads to renal tissue destruction with increased risk of stones, infection (pyonephrosis), traumatic damage, and hypertension.

Causes

- Neuromuscular incoordination at the pelviuretic junction (cf. Hirschsprung's disease)
- Muscular hyperplasia (cf. pyloric stenosis)
- Kinking by lower-pole vessels (30 per cent of cases)

Aims of treatment

- To improve drainage of urine
- To reduce the pelvic dead space

Position of patient

Lateral with affected side uppermost.

Procedure

There are various operations: Anderson–Hynes, Foley V-Y plasty, and Culp. The latter two procedures are only suitable for a small renal pelvis and no lower-pole vessels.

Approach

This may be via a loin or Anderson–Hynes incision. The Anderson–Hynes incision is horizontal in a line from the tip of the twelfth rib towards the umbilicus. The approach is extraperitoneal onto the ureter and the pelviuretic junction.

Advantages

Quick. Heals well.

Disadvantages

520

It is only suitable for straightforward cases. If there is doubt use the loin approach.

Method

Carry out an Anderson–Hynes pyeloplasty if the renal pelvis is large or there are lower-pole vessels only. This procedure allows the vessels to be placed behind the anastomosis after reduction in the pelvic size. If there is doubt about the viability of the suture line, use a nephrostomy (Cummings with a 'tail' down the ureter or a ureteric catheter down the ureter) to prevent obstruction while performing the anastomosis. Use plain catgut and suction drainage.

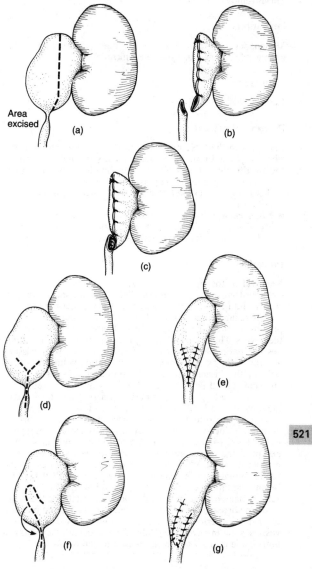

Area excised (a)

(b)

(c)

(d)

(e)

(f)

(g)

521

Pyeloplasty variations. (a)–(c) Anderson–Hynes pyeloplasty; (d) and (e) Foley V-Y plasty, (f) and (g) Culp pyeloplasty.

NEPHRECTOMY (extra-major)

This is removal of a kidney.

Indications

Malignancy, chronic infection, stone, obstruction with irreparable damage, or hypertension (rare).

Approach

Loin.

Position of patient

Lateral with the table broken to increase access between the ribs and pelvic brim. Approach is usually through the bed of the twelfth rib but may be through the eleventh if a higher approach is required, e.g. upper-pole problems.
- *Advantages* Quick; well tolerated; good access for most procedures.
- *Disadvantages* Postoperative costal nerve neuralgia may occur. Mobilization of the kidney is required before vascular control is obtained. Incisional hernias are very difficult to repair.

Procedure

Removal of the tip of the rib exposes the fat which is both extraperitoneal and perinephric. The index and middle fingers can be slid between the fat and muscles, and the muscles can be cut using either cutting diathermy or a knife. Upwards pressure of the fingers helps reduce bleeding and diathermy of the vessels. The colon and kidney are now exposed. Posteriorly lies the perinephric (Gerota's) fascia. Cut this with scissors and the kidney is available. Finger dissection below the lower pole of the kidney between the posterior muscles and the anterior fat and peritoneum will bring you to the ureter and gonadal vessels. The empty ureter is a palpably thick tube, looks white, and will demonstrate peristalsis. It is useful to place a sling around the ureter once it has been identified both as a guide and to prevent the escape of stone fragments.

The kidney is usually easy to mobilize by finger dissection, except at the upper and lower poles where scissor dissection may be required. When this is done, the kidney is free except for the renal pedicle. The vein lies anterior with the artery behind, and three clamps (Lahey) should be applied. The vessels are ligated twice proximally and once distally. A 'mass tie' of the pedicle can be carried out, but it is believed to increase the risk of arteriovenous fistula. The ligature used to tie the vessels is not important, e.g. silk, chromic catgut, Dexon (non-absorbable is probably unwise in an infected case).

Closure

A suction drain is inserted, usually away from the main wound, and the wound is then closed in layers. Each muscle layer is closed individually.

Postoperatively

There is no need for nasogastric or urethral catheters. Oral fluids can be started the next day and normal diet as soon as flatus has passed (usually the second day). The drain can usually be removed after 24–48 hours.

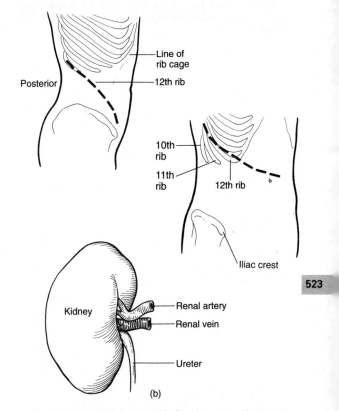

523

Nephrectomy (lateral approach); (b) Renal artery, renal vein and ureter as displayed in this approach.

NEPHRECTOMY (extra-major) (*cont.*)

Complications

- *Bleeding* The kidney has to be removed. As long as it is present it will prevent clear visualization of the surrounding anatomy and safe diathermy. Once the kidney has been removed, pack the space and 'get your breath' for a few minutes. Remove the swabs slowly and the bleeders will be easy to find. If a pedicle causes problems, pack it and wait for 10 minutes. Remove the pack slowly with a Lahey or Satinsky clamp ready and you will be surprised at how easily control can be achieved.
- *The adherent kidney* The recommended approach is to 'go under the capsule of the kidney'. However, there are problems because the kidney oozes from the denuded surfaces, increasing blood loss. When you reach the pedicle, you have to come through the capsule to identify and ligate the vessels.

NEPHRO-URETERECTOMY (extra-major)

This is removal of the kidney and ureter.

Indications

Transitional cell carcinoma of renal pelvis or ureter (not adenoacarcinoma or squamous carcinoma), associated gross hydro-ureter.

Procedure

Mobilize the kidney and divide the pedicle. Push the kidney downwards towards the iliac fossa. The loin wound is closed in the usual way and the patient then placed supine. A lower mid-line incision is made and the lower ureter is approached through the extraperitoneal route. The ureter is mobilized upwards and the kidney delivered into the wound. The ureter is then freed towards the bladder. If the indication is transitional cell carcinoma, the ureter must be mobilized through the bladder muscle and the ureteric orifice included in the specimen. This is not so important for a large ureter.

Closure

Layers. A small suction drain is brought up through a separate stab wound and can be removed on the fifth day.

13 Trauma

Vascular injuries   530
Abdominal trauma   532
Thoracic injuries   536

VASCULAR INJURIES

Ninety per cent of vascular injuries result from penetrating trauma. Vascular injury from blunt trauma may be caused by road traffic accidents or fractures. Sea-belt injuries may produce circumferential tears in the intima of the abdominal aorta. Iatrogenic causes include tight plaster of Paris splints and inadvertent intra-arterial injection of sodium thiopentone or sodium tetradecyl sulphate during injection of varicose veins. Prompt diagnosis and treatment are required to save life or limb.

Types of injury

Punctures, contusions, lacerations, or transection. Punctures and lacerations usually contine to bleed. Contusions may lead to occlusion of a vessel due to intimal dissection flaps. Transection injuries may stop bleeding owing to vessel retraction.

Venous injuries may follow penetrating trauma or the vessel may be compressed by surrounding haematoma or soft tissue swelling. Oedema and distal venous congestion will cause gangrene. If there is arterial and venous injury, an arteriovenous fistula may develop.

Assessment of the patient

Examination of traumatized patients *must* be meticulous. The state of the peripheral circulation must be established and frequently reassessed—peripheral pulses, temperature, colour, capillary and venous return. Note absent distal pulsation or pulsating haematomas. If there is swelling make use of the Doppler probe. This can produce false positives. In shocked patients carry out repeated assessments after resuscitation. If there are signs of impaired circulation carry out *arteriography*.

Principles of management

- Control bleeding by direct pressure.
- Relieve shock by resuscitation.
- Evaluate the peripheral circulation. Is there ischaemia? Perform angiography unless obvious fracture is present.
- Formally explore puncture wounds. This requires expertise with wide exposure of the vessels proximally and distally to secure control.
- Reduce fractures and dislocations.

Complications of vascular injury

Early
- Haemorrhage
- Thrombosis
- False aneurysm

Late
- Secondary haemorrhage
- Arteriovenous
- False aneurysm
- Vascular insufficiency
- Ischaemic muscle contracture

Indications for surgery

Signs of vascular insufficiency, continuing bleeding, expanding haematoma, vascular bruit.

Surgical procedures

- Punctures and clean lacerations—primary closure
- Ragged lacerations and intimal flaps—excision and reconstruction with venous patch or excision with anastomosis
- Intramural haematoma, vascular wall disruption, intimal disruption, excision and interposition, graft

  NB Irrigate the distal vascular tree with heparinized saline. Interposition grafts are necessary if the repair causes tension or stenosis, or there is extensive local sepsis.

ABDOMINAL TRAUMA

Causes

- Blunt: road traffic accidents, industrial injuries, sporting accidents
- Penetrating: stab wounds, low- and high-velocity missile injuries

NB Resuscitation may have to be carried out concurrent with examination.

History

Trauma of sufficient force. Ask about shoulder tip pain (splenic injury). Ask about the position of the victim at the time of injury, if penetrating.

Examination

Is the patient shocked? Note the presence of patterned bruising suggestive of severe pressure. Measure the abdominal girth and mark the site for future measurements. Note whether there is distension, localized tenderness, guarding, or rigidity. 'Spring' the pelvis. Perform a rectal examination. Is there blood on the finger? Ask the patient to pass urine if conscious. Failure may imply urethral injury. Are there associated injuries, e.g. head, rib, cervical spine, etc.

Investigations

- Chest X-ray (erect if possible): look for diaphragmatic injury, rib fracture near the spleen, subphrenic air suggestive of ruptured viscus.
- Erect and supine abdominal X-ray: look for splenic or renal shadows, the position of the gastric bubble, and whether it is displaced. Look for the psoas shadow. Is it obscured by haematoma? Look at the pelvis. Is it fractured?
- Peritoneal lavage is an accurate method of establishing the presence of bleeding.
- A four-quadrant tap with a no. 1 needle has a high false-positive rate and is not so valuable.
- IVU, contrast radiography, arteriography, and CT scans are occasionally indicated.

Indications for laparotomy

- Eviscerations
- Gunshot wounds (90 per cent have intra-abdominal damage)
- Copious blood on peritoneal lavage
- Patterned abrasions or shoulder tip pain
- Continuing shock despite resuscitation
- Subphrenic gas
- Signs of spreading peritonitis

Laparotomy

Use a vertical midline incision. Make it separate from any stab wound. Examine every organ in order (see laparotomy). Note your findings. Remember that often more than one organ is damaged. When the peritoneum is opened, you may encounter massive haemorrhage. Be prepared by having blood ready. Deliver the small intestine. Evacuate clot. If bleeding is rapid, pack with large gauze packs. Remove them slowly and control each bleeding point in turn.

Management of specific injuries

Spleen
Remove completely if it is shattered. If it is not extensively damaged, try to preserve it by repair, partial splenectomy, or enclosing the organ in a mesh sac.

Liver
Drain small lacerations with closed suction drains or a soft corrugated drain brought out through a single opening in the abdominal wall below the level of the laceration so that dependent drainage occurs. Explore deep lacerations and suture or ligate bleeding points. Then drain. If unsuccessful, suture or apply an omental pack into the laceration and suture the edges with catgut. If none of these is possible, hepatic lobectomy or segmentectomy should be undertaken. Temporary control of bleeding can be achieved by clamping the free edge of the lesser omentum (Pringle's manoeuvre). If haemorrhage is due to hepatic vein fracture, proximal and distal control of the vena cava may permit haemostasis by identification of the veins from within the liver substance.

Kidney
If pulped, carry out a nephrectomy? Did the IVU confirm function on the other side? If possible, repair or perform only a partial nephrectomy.

Bowel
Close small bowel injuries with a single layer of interrupted sutures. If the mesentery is injured, repair the defect and resect compromised bowel with end-to-end anastomosis. Mobilize the duodenum if injury is suspected. Perforations are easily missed in the extraperitoneal part. Perform a feeding jejunostomy if it has to be repaired. Convert caecal injuries into a caecostomy. In other sites the injured bowel should be exteriorized and a double-barrelled colostomy fashioned. Resect massive injuries. Bring out a proximal colostomy if there is doubt about the anastomosis.

533

ABDOMINAL TRAUMA (cont.)

Stomach

Close wounds with Vicryl or PDS. Pass a nasogastric tube.

Pancreas

Resect a damaged tail and drain the area. Emergency pancreaticoduodenectomy may be required for injuries to the head.

References

Bewes, P. C. (1983). Open and closed abdominal injuries. *British Journal of Hospital Medicine*, **29** (5), 402–10.

Blumgart, L. H. (1980). Hepatic resection. In *Recent advances in surgery*, Vol. 10 (ed. S. Taylor), Ch. 1, pp. 1–26. Churchill Livingstone, Edinburgh.

Odling-Smee, W. (1984). Abdominal injuries. *Surgery I*, **15**, 348–53.

THORACIC INJURIES

Thoracic injury accounts for 25 per cent of deaths from trauma. Fifty per cent of patients who die from multiple injuries also have a significant thoracic injury. Open injuries are caused by penetrating trauma from knives or gunshot. Closed injuries occur after blasts, blunt trauma, and deceleration. Road traffic accidents are the most common cause.

Open injuries

Complications are pneumothorax, haemothorax, intrathoracic visceral, and arterial damage and infection.

Management guidelines
Aim to establish an airway, stop bleeding, and restore the circulation.
- Take a brief history
- Establish pulse, blood pressure, and two IV lines for rapid fluid replacement
- Determine haemoglobin, haematocrit, blood gases, group, and cross-match
- Examine the chest back and front. Are there associated injuries?
- Cover or close sucking chest wounds. If breath sounds are absent on the side of the injury and the patient is unstable, drain the chest
- Record the drainage. It is often considerable initially, but slows down as the lung expands
- When the patient is stable obtain an erect posteroanterior chest X-ray
- Persistent shock or bleeding are indications for thoracotomy
- Aortography, Gastrografin swallow, or peritoneal lavage may be indicated

Closed injuries

Complications are rib fractures, flail segment, injury of the aorta and its branches, myocardial contusion or rupture, ruptured diaphragm, or oesophagus. Blast injuries are associated with intra-alveolar haemorrhage, pulmonary haematoma, and hypoxia.

Management guidelines
536 Establish the airway, assess ventilation, and correct blood loss.
- If the patient remains persistently shocked despite attempts at resuscitation, thoracotomy or laparotomy are indicated.
- Diaphragmatic rupture can occur immediately or at any time up to weeks after injury. Look for bowel (stomach or colon) in the chest. Examine the diaphragm at all laparotomies for trauma.

- Suspect oesophageal rupture if there is deep subcutaneous emphysema from the mandible to the clavicle or mediastinal emphysema on the chest X-ray.
- Blunt cardiac injury can lead to tamponade or ECG changes from contusion which can mimic infarction. If tamponade is suspected (blood pressure down, JVP up, QRS changes on ECG) carry out pericardial aspiration to confirm the diagnosis and buy time until thoracotomy. Most cases are due to a tear in the right atrium. Consider bypass surgery.
- Flail chest and pulmonary contusion. Many patients develop hypoxia and will need mechanical ventilation. Others can be treated with blood volume replacement with whole blood or fresh frozen plasma, IV diuretics (20 mg frusemide every 12 hours for 72 hours), methylprednisolone (30 mg/kg for 72 hours), frequent aspiration of pulmonary secretions, and early ambulation.
- Use aortography to diagnose vascular injury in stable patients. Thoracotomy is indicated if the patient is unstable.
NB All patients with chest injuries need adequate analgesia. Use intermittent morphine administration or intercostal blocks.

References

Trinkle, J. K. and Richardson, J. D. (1981). In *Thoracic injuries in trauma* (ed. D. Carter and H.C. Polk), pp. 66–98. Butterworths, London.

14 Operative orthopaedic surgery

C. M. E. LENNOX, G. PACKER, and
G. BANNISTER

Introduction   542

Basic Principles

Tourniquets and tourniquet time   546
Fracture reduction   548
Application of plaster cast   550
Open reduction and internal fixation—
     general principles   552
Cast bracing   558
Prevention of venous thrombosis   560
Infection in orthopaedic surgery   562
Compound fractures   564
Management of peripheral nerve injuries   566
Bone grafts   568

The Upper Limb
Adults
Decompression of tennis elbow   572
Trigger finger decompression   574
Median nerve decompression   576
Ulnar nerve decompression at the elbow   578
Rotator cuff tears   580
Acromioclavicular dislocation   582
Dislocation of the shoulder   584
Fractures of the proximal humerus   586
Fractures of the shaft of the humerus   590
Fractures of the distal humerus   592
Fractures of the olecranon   594
Fractures of the radial head   596
Fractures of the shafts of radius and ulna   598
Monteggia and Galeazzi fracture
     dislocations   600
Barton's fracture   602
Colles' fracture   604
Smith's fracture   606

Hand Injuries
Principles of treatment 610
Peripheral nerve dysfunction after a fracture
    or dislocation 614
Infections in the hand 616
Fracture dislocations of the carpus 618
Fractures of the hand 622
Flexor tendon injuries 630
Extensor tendon injuries 634
Ligament injuries 636
Finger-tip injuries 638

Children
Introduction 642
Fractures around the shoulder 644
Fractures of the distal humerus 646
Injuries of the proximal radial epiphysis 652
Juvenile Monteggia and Galeazzi fractures 654
Fractures of the shafts of radius and ulna 656
Displaced fracture of the distal radius 658

The Lower Limb
Total hip replacement 662
Total knee replacement 664
Keller's arthroplasty 666
Mitchell's osteotomy 668
Reduction of a dislocated hip 670
Internal fixation of a subcapital fracture of
    the neck of the femur 672
Dynamic hip screw for fractured neck of femur 674
Hemiarthroplasty for fractured neck of
    femur 676
Dynamic hip screw for subtrochanteric
    fracture of the femur 678
Intramedullary nailing for fracture of the
    shaft of the femur 680
Skeletal traction for fracture of the shaft of
    the femur 682
Dynamic condylar screw for
    supra/intracondylar fracture of femur 684

Repair of rupture of the quadriceps tendon 686
Tension band wiring of the patella 688
Patellectomy for fracture of the patella 690
Repair of rupture of the patellar tendon 692
Examination under anaesthetic and
  arthroscopy of the knee joint 694
Internal fixation of fractures of the tibial
  condyle 696
Fractures of the shaft of the tibia 698
Intramedullary nailing of fractures of the
  tibia 700
External fixation for tibial fracture 702
Open reduction and internal fixation of ankle
  fractures 704
Repair of rupture of the Achilles tendon 708

INTRODUCTION

For each of the operative procedures described the following
general principles apply.

- A full history and examination has been taken and associated injuries excluded.
- Informed consent has been obtained from the patient or his parent or guardian.
- The position of the patient is supine upon the operating table, unless stated otherwise.
- The operation may be performed under a general anaesthetic or regional anaesthesia as appropriate.
- A tourniquet is applied for operations to the upper and lower limbs where appropriate.
- The complications common to all orthopaedic operations which are described in the introductory section apply and only complications specific to the procedure are described.
- Operations which include the insertion of prosthetic material require the administration of antibiotics (typically a cephalosporin) on induction and at 8 and 16 hours postoperatively.

BASIC PRINCIPLES

This section begins with a description of some of the general techniques in orthopaedic and traumatic surgery.

TOURNIQUETS AND TOURNIQUET TIME

Indications

The three indications for the use of a tourniquet are:
- Haemostasis in the presence of uncontrollable distal bleeding.
- A bloodless field for reconstructive surgery.
- Isolation of the circulation to allow distal infusion of local anaesthetic for intravenous regional blocks.

Special indications

Patients of Mediterranean, African, or Indian subcontinent origin should be screened for haemoglobinopathies as these may cause sludging of red cells under ischaemic conditions. African patients should be tested for sickle cell, Indians for HbE, and Mediterranean patients for thalassaemia. These conditions are relative contraindications to the use of a tourniquet. If the operating surgeon feels that a tourniquet is essential, the limb should be exsanguinated prior to inflation of the tourniquet.

Methods of application

Haemostasis
Before application of the tourniquet:
- The limb should be elevated.
- Local pressure should be applied.

The tourniquet should be placed proximal to the bleeding point only if the two previous methods have failed. Once applied, it should be released for at least 15 minutes every 90 minutes

Bloodless field
A tourniquet should be placed as proximal as possible to afford maximum surgical access and ensure that the pressure is distributed over the more muscular parts of the limb. Plaster wool should be placed around the limb, which should be exsanguinated by elevation (for 2 minutes) or by a Rhys–Davies exsanguinator or an Esmarch bandage.

A tourniquet should be inflated to twice systolic blood pressure for the upper limb and three times systolic blood pressure for the lower limb (add 50 mmHg for obese patients).

Intravenous regional anaesthesia
This is applicable to the upper limb, as the pressures required for the lower limb render it too uncomfortable for routine use. The procedure should not be undertaken unless two doctors are present, at least one of whom is skilled in intubation and resuscitation in the event of leakage of local anaesthetic into the systemic circulation.

Technique

- Intravenous access to both upper limbs.
- Exsanguination.
- Cuff inflation.
- Injection of 40 ml of 0.25 per cent Prilocaine into the IV cannula in the exsanguinated limb.
- If a double cuff is used, the more distal cuff should be inflated when the pressure in the more proximal cuff causes discomfort.
- Regardless of the length of the procedure, the tourniquet should be left in place for 20 minutes to prevent release of local anaesthesia into the systemic circulation.

Duration of application of tourniquet

- In elective procedures on limbs of normal vasculature, 2 hours
- After trauma or in limbs of poor vasculature, 1 hour.

Complications

- Ischaemia after prolonged application.
- Cutaneous bruising under the tourniquet (rare).
- If the limb is prepared with an alcoholic preparation, alcohol may be absorbed by the wool and may cause skin damage or may even ignite if diathermy is used. A waterproof seal, e.g. with Sleek, may prevent this.

FRACTURE REDUCTION

Definition

Reduction is the lessening of deformity and is a relative term. If the reduction is 'anatomical', alignment is perfectly restored. The vast majority of closed reductions are relative and non-anatomical.

Aims of reduction

- Reduction must be anatomical in intra-articular fractures and long bones of the forearm as differential shortening disrupts the radio-ulnar joint.
- Relative reduction of the humerus, femur, and tibia should incorporate rotational alignment identical to that of the opposite limb, coronal and saggital displacement within 5° of neutral, and shortening of not more than 1 cm.

Manipulative reduction

An assistant applies counter-traction and the surgeon first increases the deformity of the fracture. Longitudinal traction is then applied, the deformity is over-corrected, and a well-padded cast is applied using three-point traction to maintain the intact periosteum under tension.

Postoperative care

Exposed digits should be tested every 4 hours for sensation, active, and passive movement, and capillary return by staff experienced in the care of fractures. If the patient is nursed in conditions other than these, a 1 inch strip should be taken from the plaster cast longitudinally throughout its length and down to skin.

Complications

Compartment syndrome

If the patient complains of increasing pain in an adequately immobilized limb after adequate analgesia (morphine 15 mg for a 70 kg man), a compartment syndrome should be suspected. The plaster should be bivalved and if symptoms do not settle fasciotomy should be performed (preceded by measurement of compartment pressure if available).

Loss of reduction as fracture swelling diminishes

An X-ray of the fracture should be taken 1 week after surgery to ensure that alignment has been maintained. Loss of alignment is an indication for remanipulation or internal fixation.

Duration of immobilization

The 'rule of fives' can be applied. This entails 5 weeks immobilization for cancellous bone fractures of the upper limb doubling to 10 weeks for those of cortical bone and the spine. Cortical bone of the lower limb requires a further doubling of the period to 20 weeks. The exceptions to the rule are the clavicle (3 weeks), the scaphoid (6 weeks), and the ankle and foot (6–8 weeks).

Rehabilitation after removal of plaster

In general an equivalent period of time to that spent in plaster is required to rehabilitate fractures fully. Thus a wrist fracture is rehabilitated after 10–12 weeks and a femoral shaft fracture, treated conservatively, after 9 months.

APPLICATION OF PLASTER CAST

Aims

- To provide stability after fracture or soft tissue injury.
- To maintain the position of the joint after traumatic or paralytic conditions so that if stiffness does occur maximum use of the limb is retained.

Position of the joint

The joint should be immobilized as close as possible to the position of ankylosis so that if stiffness results the limb remains functional. These positions are as follows.

- Spine: straight
- Shoulder: 45° abduction, 45° flexion
- Elbow: 90° flexion, neutral rotation
- Wrist: neutral rotation, neutral flexion
- Hip: 15° abduction, 15° flexion
- Knee: 0–30° flexion
- Ankle: neutral plantar dorsiflexion, varus–valgus
- Forefoot: neutral plantar/dorsiflexion

Preparation

Plaster may be applied:

- When the limb is stable following a minor fracture or a more severe fracture has become sticky
- When an unstable fracture has been reduced.

In the former situation a better-fitting lighter and stronger cast can be applied using plaster rolls. In the latter, slabs can be used as they can be applied quickly, minimizing the risk of loss of reduction and requiring less skilled assistance. Slabs can be reinforced later.

Method

Plaster rolls

Type of plaster	No. of rolls	Size
Colles	2	4 in
	1	3 in
Forearm	5	4 in
	1	3 in
Long-leg cylinder	8	6 in
Below knee	6	6 in
Long leg	9	6 in

Procedure

- Limb is held in correct position by an assistant
- Powder limb
- Apply stockinette, leaving 3 inches proximal and distal to be folded back over the wool and plaster.

- Apply wool as a single layer over muscular areas and as a triple layer over bony areas
- Dip plaster in to cold water until bubbling stops after about 45 seconds. Water is squeezed from the peripheral 1 cm to ensure that the plaster roll does not fall off the spool, but retaining water to allow working time.
- Apply plaster at the rate of three turns at the end to every one in the centre.
- Roll back stockinette over the plaster
- Smooth wet plaster in a rotatory fashion initially, and then longitudinally to give a strong aesthetically satisfactory cast.

Slabs

- Fracture reduction is held by surgeon.
- Prepare slab by measuring length on normal limb as follows:

Fracture	Slab	Size
Wrist	Single layer	6 in (with hole for thumb)
Elbow	Backslab	6 in
Tibia	Double slab	8 in
	U-slab	8 in
Ankle	Double slab	8 in
	U-slab	8 in

- Apply wool.
- Dip slab in hot water to speed setting.
- Apply slab and hold until adherent.
- Apply cottonoid bandage.
- Hold plaster until solid.

Postoperative care

As for following the reduction of a fracture. Application of plaster often occurs on an out-patient basis, and written instructions should be provided on the care of the plaster. More importantly, the patient should be instructed to return if the pain increases or swelling occurs.

The slab can be completed when the swelling has subsided (approximately 48 hours) or, more usually, after a check X-ray at 1 week.

Complications

The two main complications are vascular occlusion, leading to a compartment syndrome, or local pressure on skin and nerves.

Local pressure under the cast should be suspected if the patient complains of pain under the plaster. The cast should always be windowed over the site of the pain.

OPEN REDUCTION AND INTERNAL FIXATION—GENERAL PRINCIPLES

Background

Internal fixation of fractures has had a chequered history because technical failure often resulted in infection and fixation devices were mechanically unsound.

Whilst the vast majority of fractures could be satisfactorily treated by plaster of Paris or traction, prolonged immobilization sometimes caused joint stiffness and retarded rehabilitation. In addition, it was often impossible to maintain the anatomical reduction required in intra-articular and forearm fractures using conservative means. For this reason a group of Swiss surgeons formed an association to standardize the operative technique and instrumentation. The initial aim of the group was rigid internal fixation. There has been some change in objectives over the last 30 years with advances in the knowledge of fracture healing. The principles of this group of surgeons have been partially adopted in trauma management and their instrumentation has been almost universally adopted, and a basic understanding of these is a prerequisite to operative intervention in fractures.

Principles of the technique

- Preservation of the soft tissues
- Anatomical reduction
- Rigid internal fixation of bone by restoring anatomy and compression of the fracture

Types of bone healing

The use of AO (Arbeitsgemeinschaft für Osteosynthese fragen) techniques has altered the type of bone healing seen in clinical practice. There are four types of bone healing, of which two occur in closed techniques and two predominate in a rigidly fixed fracture.

Creeping substitution

Healing of cancellous bone is by creeping substitution. The bone dies back for 2 mm and then revascularizes, causing union with minimal external callus.

Callus formation

In cortical bone the periosteum is stripped away from the fracture edges. This forms a cuff of new bone, or callus, around the fracture site, which itself does not remodel until bone rigidity has been re-established. Once remodelling of the cortical bone has taken place, the callus reabsorbs. In practice, this takes place within 2–3 years in children and almost never completes its course in adults.

Primary remodelling

If a plate is used to achieve cortical rigidity, there is no stimulus to callus formation and remodelling takes place primarily. However, this only occurs if the fracture edges are opposed within micrometres of each other, and in practice only in part of a plated fracture if at all. Primary remodelling is difficult to monitor as the sole radiological index is gradual loss of definition of the fracture site. Union is less strong than healing by callus, and premature plate removal may result in refracture.

Gap healing

More commonly, a sluggish periosteal response from the side of the fracture that is not plated spreads across the fracture site. Again, this is difficult to monitor as the surgeon has to rely on loss of radiological definition of the fracture.

Complications of AO techniques

The main complication is infection, which may be as high as 10 per cent in tibial fractures even in expert hands. Complications in 2 per cent of tibial platings, are recorded in even the most expert centres.

Screws and plates

AO techniques achieve compression with screws and plates.

Objectives

To maintain fracture fixation after reduction.

Indications

- Intra-articular fractures
- Forearm fractures
- Spiral/oblique or segmental long-bone fractures

Procedure

Plates may be of two types, neutralization plates or dynamic compression plates (DCPs). A DCP can be used as a neutralization plate. If it is used for this purpose, the screw should be inserted in an offset position.

Screws may be self-tapping or round-ended. Self-tapping screws have sharp ends. AO screws are cylindrical. Wood screws, which are conical, are no longer used in bone fixation. The grip of a screw depends on the amount of bone engaged. This in turn relates to the width of the thread and the gap between the threads (pitch). The core of the screw corresponds to the drill size that should be used. The screws may be partially or fully threaded. Partially threaded screws compress bone between the screw head and the thread. AO screws are either cortical or cancellous. Only cancellous

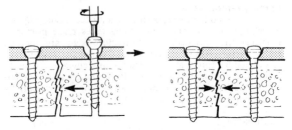

Dynamic compression achieved by offsetting holes in plate.

screws can be partially threaded. The core diameter of AO large fragment screws is 3.2 mm and that of small fragment screws is 2.5 mm.

Preoperative preparation

Radiographs should be carefully examined for potential comminution or bone loss. Any loss of the cortex must be made good by autologous bone grafting. Extreme comminution is a contraindication to plate fixation as surgical exposure tends to devitalize bone fragments. Fixation technique should be planned and discussed with the theatre staff and assistants before commencing.

Positioning

Patients should be positioned to allow access to both the fracture and potential bone-grafting sites. Remember that intraoperative radiographs or image intensification may also be required.

Incision

Skin incisions should be fasciocutaneous. The surgical approach should aim to expose the fracture with the minimum of dissection.

Reduction and fixation

The fracture should be fully visualized with the minimum of soft tissue dissection, temporarily held with reduction forceps, and if possible stabilized with a compression (lag) screw. In cancellous bone a partially threaded screw is used. In cortical bone it is necessary to overdrill the near cortex with a 4.5 mm drill whilst the thread engages in the tapped far cortex. In transverse fractures compression using an offset screw and a DCP is indicated. The plate can be placed either on or beneath the periosteum. An X-ray of the fracture is taken, the tourniquet is released, and haemostasis is achieved. Muscle and skin are closed in layers. A splint is applied to maintain adjacent joints in the position of function.

554

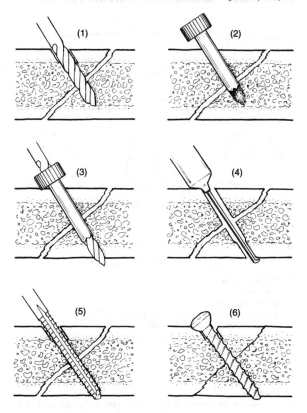

Lag screw techinque.
(1) 4.5 mm drill to proximal cortex.
(2) 4.5 mm sleeve to proximal cortex.
(3) 3.2 mm drill to distal cortex.
(4) Depth gauge for screw length.
(5) 4.5 mm tap to distal cortex.
(6) After countersinking screw-head, lag screw inserted compressing potential surfaces.

Postoperative care
- Antibiotic prophylaxis for 24 hours
- Elevation of the limb
- Drains removed after 24 hours
- Active movement can be commenced when pain allows but the joint should be splinted at night

555

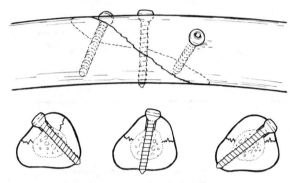

Triple lag screw fixation of spiral fracture.

- Sutures removed after 10–14 days
- Check X-ray as clinically indicated

Complications
- Infection
- Delayed union
- Avoidance of full weight-bearing for 6–10 weeks
- Possible removal of metalwork

The patient should be advised of these complications prior to surgery.

External fixation

Indication
Comminuted or open fractures that cannot be controlled in plaster or where soft tissue injury requires treatment.

Types of fixator
There are two generic types of fixator.
- Uniaxial: single-bar frame, e.g Orthofix
- Multiaxial, e.g. Hoffman, Ilizarov

Complications
Pin-track problems are the most common complication of external fixators. Delayed union may result, particularly if very rigid frame configurations are used.

Postoperative care
Pin sites should be cleaned daily and extended if there is any impingement of skin against the pins.

CAST BRACING

Background

Cast bracing evolved from a patellar-tendon-bearing below-knee prosthesis developed in the United States. The principle was initially applied to tibial shaft fractures using a well-moulded cast around the tibial tuberosity and the subcutaneous triangular anatomy of the proximal tibia. By resecting the plaster proximal to the patella and in the popliteal fossa, it was possible to retain rotational control whilst allowing knee flexion and weight-bearing. This obviated knee stiffness that resulted from prolonged immobilization of tibial shaft fractures in a long leg cast. The principle was then applied to the femur, forearm, and humerus.

Mode of action

Control of the fracture by cast bracing is achieved by compression of the soft tissues around the fracture site, rather than the effects of unweighting it. Indeed weight-bearing enhances callus formation.

Timing of cast bracing

A cast brace should be applied when a fracture is sticky and swelling has subsided. In general terms this may be after 10 days for a Colles' fracture, 4–6 weeks for a tibial fracture, and 6–8 weeks for a femoral shaft fracture.

Materials

Plaster of Paris, light-weight acrylics, and thermoplastic materials can all be used with equal success. It is not possible to bear weight on a plaster of Paris brace until 48 hours have elapsed to allow it to dry.

Subsequent care

Varus deformity is a particular problem in mid-shaft femoral fractures and a check radiograph should be performed weekly for 2 weeks and then after a further 2 weeks when the femur has been braced.

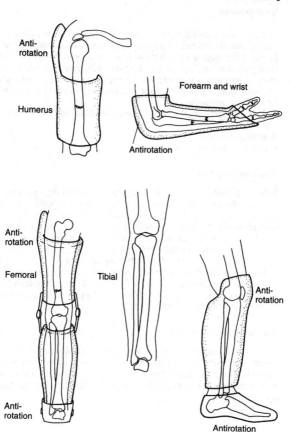

Cast bracing.

PREVENTION OF VENOUS THROMBOSIS

Background

Orthopaedic patients with lower-limb fractures or disorders of the hip are at high risk of deep venous thrombosis. Radioactive-labelled fibrinogen studies show that as many as 70 per cent of such patients develop venous thrombosis. Approximately 1 per cent of patients who undergo hip replacement die as a result of pulmonary embolism from (usually undetected) proximal venous thromboses.

Two principle methods have been used to reduce this complication:
- anticoagulation
- enhancement of venous return

Anticoagulation

Full anticoagulation with warfarin undoubtedly prevents venous thrombosis but carries with it the complications of haemorrhage. For this reason partial anticoagulation with subcutaneous heparin has been employed. This reduces the incidence of DVT in hospital. Subcutaneous heparin is less effective in orthopaedics than in abdominal surgery. Low-dose warfarin is not effective in hip replacement.

Low-molecular-weight heparins reduce the incidence of in-patient venous thrombosis by a factor of 3. Bleeding complications have been reported, although they are less frequent and severe than in full warfarinization.

Enhanced venous return

This is most simply achieved with compression stockings and more effectively with a foot pump. The best results in the prevention of venous thrombosis, both by anticoagulation and by enhancing venous return, have been found following the use of a foot pump.

INFECTION IN ORTHOPAEDIC SURGERY

Background

The implants used in orthopaedic surgery act as adjuvants for any organisms that gain access during an operation. Experimentally 100 000 organisms are required to cause osteomyelitis, whereas in the presence of methylmethacrylate bone cement as few as 10 are sufficient.

The consequences of infection in orthopaedics may be catastrophic as implanted material may have to be removed, tissue healing is indolent, recovery is prolonged or partial, and the functional result is inferior to an uninfected case.

Principles of prevention of infection

Except for open fractures, 90–95 per cent of organisms gain access to wounds in operating theatres. A very small proportion gain haematologenous access from remote sites of sepsis later. The principal source of infection in theatre is the air. Air contamination relates directly to the number of personnel and the degree to which the air is exposed to the contents of their groins, axillae, and noses. Patients are an additional source of bacteria.

Five principles can be employed in reducing infection:

Theatre practice and clothing
- Theatre staff should be kept to a minimum.
- Nasal organisms should be restricted with masks. Axillary and perineal organisms should be restricted by tight occlusive clothing with elasticated cuffs around the neck, arms waist, and feet.
- Patients should bathe in chlorhexidine preoperatively.

Clean air
Organisms in theatre air can be reduced by:
- Increased filtration, e.g. Charnley Howarth enclosure
- Ultraviolet light (UVC)

Enhanced host resistance
Host resistance can be enhanced by using prophylactic antibiotics. These must be given preoperatively and, if a tourniquet is used, sufficiently early to allow access to tissues. Most cephalosporins require between 10 and 30 minutes to gain satisfactory tissue levels, and if given intravenously perioperatively should be administered before anaesthetic agents to allow satisfactory uptake. The main action of the agent used should be antistaphylococcal, and 24-hour cover is the minimum effective in orthopaedic surgery.

Removal of organisms
Thorough lavage with a needle and syringe removes 25 per cent of organisms from a wound at the end of the procedure.

Disinfection

Hydrogen peroxide and Povidone-iodine are inactivated by plasma
proteins, but chlorhexidine 0.05 per cent kills organisms in solution.

Recommendations

As many of the available techniques as possible should be used. All are cost effective. Antibiotic prophylaxis reduces infection by a factor of 3 and clean air by a factor of 2.

Precautions against HIV and hepatitis

It is now recommended that extra precautions be taken where it is considered that HIV or hepatitis is a potential risk, e.g. in the treatment of compound fractures or when using power tools or lavage which might cause splashing or aerosol formation.
Precautions include:
- wearing double gloves
- face protection by means of goggles or a visor
- use of impervious gowns and drapes
- the surgeon should pick up the scalpel rather than have it passed by the scrub nurse

COMPOUND FRACTURES

Classification (Gustillo)

Classification is based upon the size of the wound and the amount of soft tissue injury.

Type	Size of wound	Other factors
I	<1 cm	Low energy, usually from inside out
II	<10 cm	Moderate energy
III	>10 cm	High energy, high-velocity Gunshot wounds, barnyard injuries, segmental fractures, neurovascular injuries

Type III fractures are further classified as follows:

IIIA	Adequate soft tissue coverage
IIIB	Massive soft tissue destruction, bony exposure
IIIC	Fractures associated with repairable vascular injury

Principles of management

- Prevention of contamination
- Removal of dead and contaminated tissue
- Stabilization of the fracture

Technique

Infection is prevented by rapid coverage of the wound with an iodine-soaked swab. A Polaroid photograph prevents the need for this to be disturbed prior to theatre. Prophylactic antibiotics and cover for tetanus are applied. The wound is extended under a tourniquet and the bone ends are explored and curetted. The fracture is reduced and stabilized. In type I and II fractures it is permissible to use plaster of Paris or intramedullary nailing. In type III fractures an external fixator or an unreamed nail is used. Except for type I fractures, primary plating carries an unacceptable risk of infection.

The wound should be left open and delayed primary closure performed after 3–4 days. Exceptionally, type I fractures may be closed primarily provided that apposition can be obtained without tension. Open wounds should be dressed with several layers of paraffin gauze to prevent drying. In type III wounds the aim is to produce a clean area of healing tissue which can then be reconstructed either by skin graft or plastic flaps. Plastic surgeons should be involved early (within 12 hours) in the treatment and management of a type III fracture.

MANAGEMENT OF PERIPHERAL NERVE INJURIES

Classification

- **Neuropraxia**: nerve concussion sustained by blunt trauma or mild traction. Recovery 6–12 weeks.
- **Axonotmesis**: traction injury in which the axon is ruptured but the nerve sheath remains intact. Degeneration takes place as far as the proximal node of Ranvier following which the axon regrows. The axon will continue to regrow at a maximum rate of 1 mm/day, but if muscle power has not returned within 18 months it is unlikely to do so because the end-plates will have degenerated within that time.
- **Neurotmesis** occurs when the nerve is severed or totally avulsed as in brachial plexus injuries. Unless the nerve is reopposed, axons from the proximal end form a neuroma and there is no recovery. Neurotmesis should be suspected in sharp injuries and should be repaired. Even with the use of an operating microscope, there is only partial recovery following neurotmesis. Recovery is better in pure motor or sensory nerves than in a mixture of the two.

Principles of treatment

- Sensory protection
- Splintage of paralysed muscles in their position of contraction and physiotherapy to maintain passive joint movement
- Exploration of sharp injuries and those showing no evidence of recovery after 6–8 weeks

Signs of regeneration

- Changing sensory level
- Distally advancing Tinel's sign
- Electrophysiological evidence

BONE GRAFTS

Classification

Bone grafts can be obtained from three sources.
- From the patient himself—**autograft**. This is usually taken from the iliac crest. There is a greater abundance posteriorly than anteriorly. In addition, pure cancellous bone can be taken from the trochanters, the femoral condyles, or the proximal tibia.
- From a member of the same species—**homograft** or **allograft**. This comprises either femoral heads taken during hip arthroplasty or entire bones harvested at the time of organ donation.
- From other mammals—**xenograft**. This is deproteinized bone taken from either oxen (Kiel) or sheep (Oswestry).

Autograft is by far the best material. If allograft or xenograft is used, its osteogenic potential can be enhanced by the addition of autologous marrow.

UPPER LIMB

Adults

DECOMPRESSION OF TENNIS ELBOW (intermediate)

Indications

Symptoms of tennis elbow resistant to physiotherapy and injections.

Incision

A curved incision over the lateral epicondyle.

Procedure

The fascia is divided, and the lateral epicondyle and the common extensor origin are exposed. Using sharp dissection the origin is elevated, taking care not to enter the elbow joint.

Closure

Vicryl to subcutaneous tissues. Interrupted or continuous sutures to skin.

Rehabilitation

A wool and crepe dressing is applied. The elbow is mobilized once sutures have been removed after 14 days.

Complications

The patient must be warned that the operation is only approximately 60 per cent successful.

TRIGGER FINGER DECOMPRESSION (intermediate)

Indications

Triggering of the flexor tendon in its sheath.

Incision

A transverse incision at the level of the triggering, usually just proximal to the proximal finger crease.

Procedure

The incision is deepened until the flexor tendon and its sheath is exposed. The triggering is confirmed and the flexor tendon sheath is divided to allow the tendon to run freely.

Closure

Interupted sutures to skin.

Rehabilitation

The finger is mobilized immediately.

Complications

- Recurrence of the triggering
- Damage to the digital nerves

MEDIAN NERVE DECOMPRESSION (intermediate)

Indications

Carpal tunnel syndrome not responding to conservative measures.

Incision

The incision is made over the carpal tunnel in line with the ring finger ray. The incision should not extend proximal to the distal wrist crease.

Procedure

The incision is deepened until the flexor retinaculum is exposed, the most distal part of the retinaculum is divided, and a McDonald dissector is inserted deep to the ligament to protect the nerve whilst the remainder of the ligament is divided.

Closure

Interrupted sutures to skin.

Rehabilitation

The fingers and hand are mobilized immediately.

Complications

- Incomplete division of the retinaculum, particularly proximally
- Damage to the median nerve
- Damage to the superficial palmar arch

ULNAR NERVE DECOMPRESSION AT THE ELBOW (intermediate)

Indications

Ulnar neuritis affecting the ulnar nerve at the elbow.

Incision

A curved incision over the medial epicondyle, extending for approximately 5 cm proximally and distally.

Procedure

The fascia is divided and the ulnar nerve is identified posterior to the medial epicondyle. The nerve is freed from any adhesions. The nerve is explored proximally and particularly distally to ensure that it is not compressed between the two heads of flexor carpi ulnaris.

Closure

Vicryl to subcutaneous tissues plus skin sutures.

Rehabilitation

A wool and crepe dressing is applied. Mobilization of the elbow is encouraged.

ROTATOR CUFF TEARS (major)

Indications

In patients aged over 40 years moderate trauma may cause a tear of the rotator cuff if it is already degenerate. Pain may result in an inability to abduct the arm actively. If this persists following an injection of local anaesthetic a complete rupture of the rotator cuff may be present.

Position

Supine. Use of a head-ring and the beach chair position facilitates exposure. Alternatively, a sandbag between the shoulder blades is helpful.

Incision

Anterior commencing just lateral to the coracoid process and extending proximally above the clavicle and distally in line with the deltopectoral groove (sabre cut incision).

Procedure

Identify the deltopectoral groove and use an osteotome to detach the deltoid from its origin with a sliver of bone. Perform an anterior acromionectomy using an osteotome sufficient to excise a wedge-shaped sliver of bone detaching the coraco-acromial ligament. This should expose the supraspinatus part of the rotator cuff and the tear can be inspected. After abrading the edges of the tear, draw them together with non-absorbable sutures and, if necessary, anchor the insertion of the tendon to the humeral head through drill holes.

Closure

Reattach the deltoid using drill holes into the acromion and a no. 1 Vicryl suture. Subcutaneous Vicryl and continuous Nylon to skin.

Rehabilitation

The shoulder may require to be immobilized in abduction to protect the repair. Physiotherapy to regain shoulder movements may be required.

Complications

Beware of injury to the axillary nerve.

ACROMIOCLAVICULAR DISLOCATION (intermediate)

Indications

Most acromioclavicular injuries are treated conservatively with a good functional result. However, in some grade III injuries surgery may be indicated for pain and deformity.

Position

Supine, utilizing a head-ring or sandbag between the shoulder blades.

Incision

As for rotator cuff repair.

Procedure

Retract the deltoid muscle to expose the coracoid process. Clean the articular surfaces of the clavicle and the acromion, including the intra-articular disc of cartilage. Identify the remains of the coraco-acromial ligaments. If they are adequate, insert mattress sutures into them to tie into drill holes on the lower surface of the clavicle. If the coraco-acromial ligaments are not well preserved, substitute a graft (e.g. a strip of fascia lata or a prosthetic graft such as Dacron). Stabilize the acromioclavicular joint by two stout K-wires. For ease of insertion pass the wires in a retrograde fashion through the articular surface of the acromion and out through the skin on the point of the shoulder. Reduce the joint and then pass the wires medially into the clavicle.

Closure

In layers. Vicryl to subcutaneous layer, Nylon to skin.

Rehabilitation

Immobilize the arm in a sling for 2 weeks and then allow gradual mobilization. Remove the wires at 8 weeks.

Complications

Ensure that the K-wires are left outside the skin with a right-angled bend as they have a propensity to migration at this site.

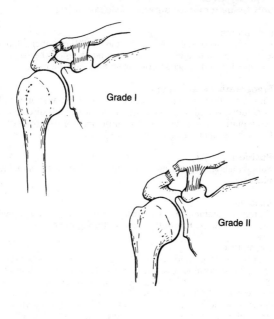

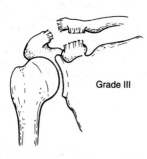

Grades of dislocation of acromioclavicular joint.

DISLOCATION OF THE SHOULDER

Soft tissue repair for anterior dislocation (major)

Indications
Recurrent dislocation of the shoulder. The number of dislocations permitted before surgery depends upon the surgeon and the demands placed upon the shoulder by the patient.

Preoperative assessment
This is required to ensure that the shoulder dislocation is unidirectional (in this case anterior) rather than multidirectional. Examination under anaesthetic, shoulder athroscopy, and a CT arthrogram of the shoulder are all useful.

Position
Supine, using a head-ring or a sandbag between the shoulder blades.

Incision
Anterior, commencing just lateral to the coracoid and extending distally in the line of the deltopectoral groove.

Procedure
Identify, protect, and retract the cephalic vein which runs in the deltopectoral groove. Retract the deltoid muscle laterally. Secure haemostasis at all stages. Osteotomize the coracoid process, having first predrilled the coracoid to allow its subsequent reattachment. The coracoid and its attached muscles are reflected downwards allowing exposure through the clavipectoral fascia of the muscle belly of the subscapularis muscle. Insert stay sutures into the subscapularis and then incise it close to the lesser tuberosity. This exposes the anterior capsule which is divided longitudinally at its medial edge to expose the Bankart lesion (anterior detachment of the labrum).

Reattach the detached labrum (suture anchors facilitate this) using non-absorbable sutures. Repair the capsule and double-breast it if lax. Reattach the subscapularis.

Closure
In layers over a suction drain.

Rehabilitation
Immobilize the arm by means of a body bandage or splint for 3 weeks and then commence mobilization.

Complications
Beware of injury to the musculocutaneous nerve when the coracoid is mobilized.

Bristow procedure

The Bristow procedure is an alternative method of preventing

recurrent dislocation using a sling as a dynamic stabilizer. It
has the advantage that it does not limit external rotation.

Procedure
The coracoid is predrilled and that part of the coracoid to
which the short head of the biceps and the coracobrachialis
attach is osteotomized. A transverse muscle splitting incision
is made in the subscapularis muscle to allow exposure of the
antero-inferior portion of the neck of the glenoid. The cortical
bone of the neck is roughened to encourage union with the
coracoid which is then attached using a cancellous screw.

Closure
As above.

Complications
Care must be taken that the screw does not penetrate the
joint surface.

Rehabilitation
As above.

FRACTURES OF THE PROXIMAL HUMERUS

A four-part fracture with or without a dislocation of the humeral head is the most common reason for internal fixation of shoulder fractures. Comminution in this injury may be severe because the muscle attachments of the tuberosities may cause them to become widely displaced. This may make accurate fixation of these fractures difficult.

Internal fixation of these fractures is described, but a hemi-arthroplasty may be more suitable in certain patients, particularly the elderly.

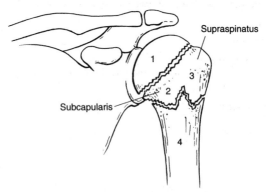

Four-part fracture of proximal humerus. The four parts of the injury are widely separate because of the muscle attachment.

Reduction and internal fixation of a four-part humeral fracture/fracture dislocation (major)

Indications
Young patients or those without severe comminution or osteoporosis.

Position
Supine with the head on a head support to facilitate intra-operative X-rays.

Incision
Sabre cut as previously described.

Procedure
The approach is through the deltopectoral groove taking care to protect or ligate the cephalic vein. The medial fibres of deltoid are detached from the clavicle using diathermy.

Through the clavipectoral fascia, identify the tendon of the long head of the biceps which will lie between the fragments of the greater and lesser tuberosities. Draw these fragments together, identify their origins on the humeral head (having reduced the head into the glenoid if dislocated), and use a wire-box suture to secure all three fragments. An AO T-shaped plate is usually the best means of attaching the humeral head to the shaft.

Closure
Reattach the deltoid using Vicryl sutures. Close in layers over a suction drain.

Rehabilitation
The aim is to commence active movement as soon as possible, but this depends upon the degree of comminution and the fixation obtained.

Complications
The main risk is of avascular necrosis of the humeral head, particularly if it has been dislocated. If the fragments are detached from their soft tissues, consider a hemiarthroplasty.

Hemiarthroplasty for shoulder fractures (major)

Indications
Elderly patients or those unsuitable for internal fixation.

Incision
As above.

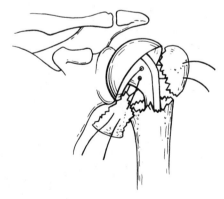

Hemiarthroplasty.

FRACTURES OF THE PROXIMAL HUMERUS (cont.)

Procedure
The articular fragment is removed. A variety of prostheses are available, of which the Neer is the best known. Select a prosthesis of suitable size and insert it into the humeral shaft with 35°–40° of retroversion, protecting the long head of biceps. Draw the tuberosity fragments together under the lip of the prosthesis and hold with a wire suture. Reduce the prosthesis and suture the defect in the rotator cuff (Vicryl), replacing the long head of biceps. Perform a partial subacromial decompression to prevent postoperative impingement.

Closure
As above.

Rehabilitation
Passive and active shoulder movements are commenced under physiotherapy supervision.

Complications
- Impingement
- Dislocation of the prosthesis

FRACTURES OF THE SHAFT OF HUMERUS

Most fractures of the shaft of the humerus are treated by conservative means, usually with a 'hanging cast'. Operative treatment may be indicated for transverse fractures which may be unstable and go on to non-union.

Treatment may be by means of open reduction and internal fixation with a plate, usually accompanied by bone grafting or intramedullary fixation.

Internal fixation of fractures of the shaft of the humerus (major)

Indications
Non-union of humeral shaft fracture.

Incision
The anterolateral approach gives good exposure of most of the humeral shaft. The incision starts proximally in line with the anterior border of the deltoid muscle from a point midway between its origin and insertion, distally to the level of its insertion, and then along the lateral border of the biceps to within 7.5 cm of the elbow.

Procedure
The fascia is divided and the deltoid is retracted laterally and the biceps medially to expose the humeral shaft. The brachialis muscle is exposed distal to the insertion of the deltoid and split longitudinally to bone. The two halves are retracted subperiosteally. This is made easier by relaxing the brachialis muscle (elbow flexion).

The fracture is reduced and temporarily held by bone clamps whilst a broad DCP is applied. Compression is used, and if there is comminution or if the operation is for non-union, cancellous bone graft is packed around the fracture.

Closure
In layers over a suction drain.

Rehabilitation
Mobilization of the shoulder and elbow under physiotherapy supervision.

Complications
The radial nerve should be protected by the lateral part of the brachialis muscle but in acute fractures it may be involved in the fracture site. If there is a radial nerve palsy, a posterior incision exposing the radial nerve should be employed.

The humerus experiences large degrees of torque and it is essential that rigid fixation is achieved. For this reason a *broad* DCP should be used and bone grafting should be employed if there is comminution.

Intramedullary fixation of humeral shaft fractures

Intramedullary fixation of humeral shaft fractures avoids the exposure required for internal fixation and, as the fracture heals with callus, avoids the problems of plate failure. However, there are difficulties associated with the insertion of these devices and with their proximal and distal locking.

Procedure
Nails can be inserted in an antegrade or retrograde fashion. The technique of locking varies with the particular nail and the mode of insertion, and is outside the scope of this book.

FRACTURES OF THE DISTAL HUMERUS

The mechanism of injury is usually a fall on the outstretched arm, or a glancing blow (the 'side-swipe' injury). If the fracture is very comminuted, early mobilization with no attempt at reduction (bag-of-bones technique) is an alternative to inadequate internal fixation. The neurovascular status of the arm requires careful assessment.

Internal fixation of fracture of the distal humerus (major)

Indications
Fractures of the distal humerus with displacement of the articular surface.

Preoperative investigations
Good radiographs are essential in the planning of this operation. It may be necessary to repeat the radiographs with traction and closed reduction of the fracture prior to the skin incision.

Position
Lateral position with the affected arm uppermost and resting in a support or over a padded bar.

Incision
Mid-line incision centred over the olecranon and extending proximally and distally.

Procedure
The triceps tendon may be reflected as a strip to expose the fracture or when there is a large intra-articular component the olecranon may be osteotomized. The ulnar nerve is identified and preserved. The fracture is reduced. The key to reduction is to reduce the articular surface of the humerus first and then to reduce the shaft of humerus onto this. The reduction of the articular surface is maintained by a cancellous screw. The condyles are reattached to the shaft using well-contoured DCP plates (or pelvic reconstruction plates if available).

Closure
The triceps flap is repaired using Vicryl sutures if the olecranon was osteotomized. It is replaced using a tension-band wire technique.

Rehabilitation
Active mobilization of the elbow is commenced as soon as possible.

Complications
- Failure of fixation
- Injury to the ulnar nerve

FRACTURE OF THE OLECRANON

The mechanism of injury is a fall onto the outstretched hand. As this is an avulsion injury, a tension-band wire technique is used which relies on early active movement to achieve compression at the fracture site.

Tension-band wiring of the olecranon (major)

Indication
Fracture of the olecranon with displacement.

Position
Supine with the arm across the chest.

Incision
An incision curved around the olecranon and extending distally parallel to the ulna for 5 cm.

Procedure
The fracture ends are cleaned using a curette and the fracture is reduced and held with sharp bone-reduction forceps. Two parallel 2 mm K-wires are inserted using a mini-driver and the AO parallel guide. A 2 mm drill is used to make a hole in the ulna approximately 10 cm from the fracture and a stout flexible wire is passed through this hole and deep to the triceps incision and the K-wires. The wire is tightened with a twist on either side to achieve compression of the fracture. Active flexion of the elbow achieves even more compression.

Closure
Vicryl to subcutaneous tissues. Clips to skin.

Rehabilitation
Early active mobilization of the elbow.

Complications
Failure of fixation.

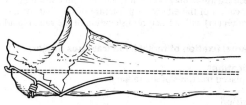

Lateral view

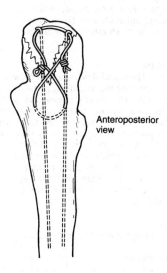

Anteroposterior
view

Tension-band wiring of fracture of the olecranon.

FRACTURES OF THE RADIAL HEAD

These fractures may occur in isolation or in combination with dislocation of the elbow, or a fracture of the shaft of the ulna (Monteggia) with a fracture/dislocation of the radial head.

Internal fixation of radial head fractures (major)

Indications
Displaced fractures of the radial head.

Position
Supine with the arm on an arm-board.

Incision
With the forearm pronated, make an oblique incision from the lateral epicondyle of the humerus downwards and backwards to the subcutaneous border of the ulna 5 cm below the olecranon.

Procedure
Incise the fascia and dissect between the origin of the extensor carpi ulnaris and the anconeus, retracting the proximal border of the supinator distally. Incise the joint capsule in a line which is parallel to but proximal to the course of the posterior interosseus nerve. If most of the radial head is comminuted, conservative treatment with early movement may encourage union in a reasonable position. If there is wide displacement, excision of the whole head preserving the annular ligament is performed via this approach. If internal fixation is to be performed, a 2.5 mm mini-screw as a lag screw is usually appropriate. The screws are inserted parallel to the articular surface of the radius.

Closure
Vicryl to the capsule. Nylon to skin.

Rehabilitation
Early active mobilization of the elbow.

Complications
The posterior interosseous nerve may be damaged by the incision if continued to distally. More commonly, a neuropraxia from retraction can occur.

FRACTURES OF THE SHAFTS OF RADIUS AND ULNA

Plaster fixation is unlikely to provide adequate control if both bones of the forearm are fractured. There is a high incidence of malunion, malrotation, and cross union. The resultant deformity is due to the many opposing forces which act on each of the fractured ends of both bones.

Open reduction and internal fixation of fractures of the radius and ulna (major)

Know your anatomy well to avoid damaging neurovascular structures. It is wise to expose both fractures and to attempt to reduce both before fixing one or the other rigidly. If you apply a compression plate to one of the fractures and subsequently turn your attention to the other you may find it impossible to reduce the second.

Incision

The surgical approach to the shaft of the ulna is usually straightforward since it is subcutaneous throughout its length and dissection is relatively easy. However, approach to the shaft of the radius is hazardous and sound knowledge of anatomy is essential.

Surgical approach to the distal radius Make a longitudinal anterolateral incision (Henry). Identify the medial border of the brachilradialis muscle and its tendon, under which lies the radial nerve which must be carefully protected as the fracture is exposed.

Surgical approach to the proximal radial shaft If the fracture of the radius is higher than mid-shaft, the anterior approach is more difficult because of the risk to damage to the posterior interosseus nerve and branches of the median nerve. By identifying the insertion of the supinator muscle and dividing that insertion and by subperiosteal exposure of the proximal shaft of the radius, the posterior interosseus nerve should be protected.

A posterior incision (Thompson) is a slightly safer alternative, particularly for injuries of the proximal radius. Make a skin incision over the proximal third of the radius with the arm in pronation. The incision should be parallel to the shaft of the radius. Dissect between the muscle bellies of the extensor digitorum comminus and the extensor carpi radialis brevis. The supinator muscle lies in the base of the approach and should be elevated or divided provided that the posterior interosseus nerve is first identified and protected.

Alternative Boyd approach to the proximal third of the radius and ulna Make a skin incision parallel to the radial border of the ulna from the tip of the olecranon distally. The

598

supinator origin is incised from the sharp border of the ulna and lifted forward by subperiosteal dissection in one sheet, thus protecting the posterior interosseus nerve. This provides good access to the radial head and neck and proximal ulna (e.g. in a high Monteggia fracture).

Procedure
Once the fractures have been exposed, they are reduced and the reduction is maintained by small DCPs with interfragmentary compression with or without lag screws.

Closure
Vicryl to subcutaneous tissues and Nylon to skin

Rehabilitation
Active movements of the elbow, wrist, and hand are commenced immediately.

Complications
A compartment syndrome of the forearm may occur. The radial nerve is most at risk in exposure of the shaft of the radius, and the importance of knowing the anatomy of the region cannot be overemphasized. Non-union of one or more bones may occur after plating. If there is comminution at the time of surgery or a fracture gap persists following fixation, bone graft should be used.

MONTEGGIA AND GALEAZZI
FRACTURE DISLOCATIONS

As the bones of the forearm act as a parallelogram and are connected by joints at each end, when there is a fracture of only one of the bones or the forearm the possibility of a disruption of the superior or inferior radio-ulnar joints must be excluded. The exception to this is a direct blow, usually to the ulna (the nightstick injury), which may result in a transverse fracture.

The Monteggia fracture is fracture of the proximal ulna with dislocation of the radial head. The Galeazzi fracture is fracture of the shaft of the radius with a dislocation of the distal ulna.

Treatment consists of open reduction and internal fixation of the fracture, which usually results in reduction of the dislocation. Occasionally open reduction or stabilization of the joint is required.

BARTON'S FRACTURE (major)

This is a marginal fracture where the anterior lip of the articular surface of the radius is displaced in a volar direction and the carpus slides forward in the same direction, resulting in deformity and distortion of the articular surface of the distal radius. This injury usually requires internal fixation to achieve and maintain reduction.

Incision

A longitudinal incision on the radial side of the anterior aspect of the distal forearm.

Procedure

Dissection is between the tendon of flexor carpi radialis and the palmaris longus. By dividing the insertion of the muscle fibres of pronator quadratus from the radial shaft, the fracture is exposed. Clean the fracture ends with a small curette. Reduce the fracture under direct vision and maintain reduction by applying the buttress plate which is contoured and positioned in such a way as to prevent the anterior and proximal drift of the fracture. The proximal part of the plate is screwed onto the radius. It is not always necessary to insert screws into the distal part of the plate.

Closure

Vicryl to subcutaneous tissues. Nylon to skin.

Rehabilitation

Early active movement of the wrist is encouraged.

Complications

Injury to the median nerve. If screws are inserted into the distal fragment, care must be taken that the joint is not penetrated.

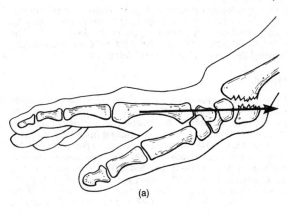

(a)

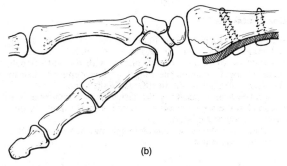

(b)

Barton's fracture.(a) Anterior marginal fragment and carpus slide proximal with dorsiflexion of the wrist. (b) Application of buttress plate.

COLLES' FRACTURE (intermediate)

This very common pattern of injury involves a non-articular largely transverse or slightly oblique fracture, which may be comminuted dorsally, within 2.5 cm of the distal radius. The resulting deformity involves dorsal tilting of the articular surface and the classical 'dinner fork' deformity.

Procedure

Under general anaesthetic or a Biers block, or occasionally under a haematoma (local anaesthetic instilled directly into the fracture site) block, the fracture is first disimpacted by longitudinal traction whilst an assistant maintains counter-traction. Then the deformity is increased dorsally to allow the posterior cortices to hitch together. Still maintaining traction, the wrist is brought down into a slightly flexed position with ulnar deviation. A check radiograph should show that the slightly volar orientation (10°) of the articular surface of the radius has been restored. A Colles' backslab is then applied with moulding.

Rehabilitation

A check radiograph is taken after 1 week and the plaster is then completed. The plaster is removed after 5 weeks.

Complications

Ensure that traction is maintained on the fingers during reduction rather than by grasping the four metacarpals together as application of the plaster with the metacarpals bunched together limits the range of movements possible in the plaster and may result in stiffness of the hand.

Numbness in a median nerve distribution is common. If it does not settle with elevation, an acute carpal tunnel decompression may be required.

Rupture of the extensor pollicis longus may occur at a variable time after this injury.

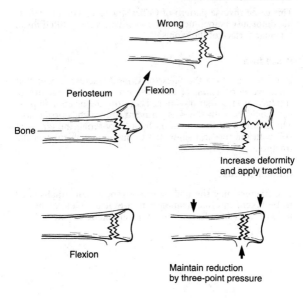

Reduction of Colles' fracture.

SMITH'S FRACTURE (intermediate)

This is the reverse pattern of Colles' fracture, with the resulting deformity being due to an excessively volarly tilted distal articular surface of the radius.

Procedure

Reduction is along the lines for Colles' fracture except that excessive dorsiflexion of the wrist can allow the fracture to slip further in a volar direction. Therefore the position in plaster should be with the wrist in neutral or slight dorsiflexion. The arm is held in supination by incorporating the elbow at 90°, with the forearm supinated to maintain reduction of the fracture.

Complications

The fracture may slip and therefore repeat radiographs need to be taken. Internal fixation with a buttress plate along the lines described for Barton's fracture should be considered.

Hand Injuries

PRINCIPLES OF TREATMENT

Particular principles are appropriate to the treatment of hand injuries.

- Do not underestimate the effect of an injury, however apparently minor.
- Swelling and or stiffness lead to loss of function.
- Oedema of the hand behaves like glue. Therefore (1) high elevation and (2) early, active movements are essential.
- Inadequate treatment of a minor injury may result in stiffness of the whole hand.
- Know your anatomy and apply it when assessing an injury.
- Record in detail the findings at the initial examination.
- Rehabilitation requires a team approach involving patient, surgeon, physiotherapist, and hand therapist.
- Digits should be referred to by name not number.

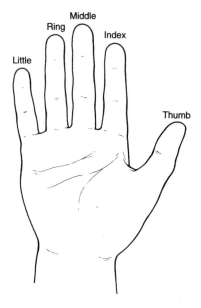

Digit names.

Splints

If splints and bandages are required, never immobilize the hand with the metacarpophalangeal joints in extension. The 'position of function' maintains some flexion of these joints to prevent stiffness.

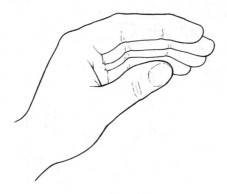

Position of function.

Surgical incisions in the hand

- Never create an incision that crosses a skin crease.
- When repairing a wound which crosses a skin crease, incorporate Z-plasties to prevent contracture of the scar.

Anaesthesia

The patient's age and personality and the nature of the injury influence the choice of anaesthesia which may be:
- Local anaesthesia by ring block (with 1 or 2 per cent Xylocaine *without* adrenaline)
- Regional block by Bier's block technique or brachial plexus block
- Local nerve blocks of radial, ulnar, or median nerves depending on the site of the injury
- General anaesthesia

Tourniquet

Digital or upper arm.

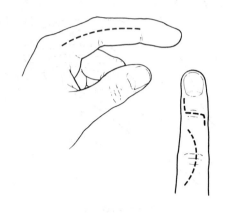

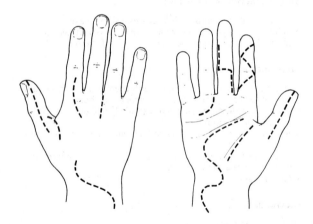

Correct incisions.

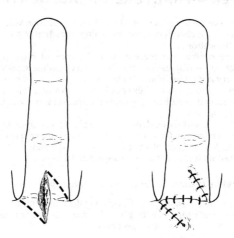

Z-plasty closure of laceration crossing a flexor crease.

PERIPHERAL NERVE DYSFUNCTION AFTER A FRACTURE OR DISLOCATION

Indications for surgical exploration include the following.
- If nerve function is compromised after reduction of a fracture or dislocation.
- Nerve dysfunction present from the time of blunt injury, fracture, or dislocation, may be observed while signs of recovery are taking place. If there is no evidence of recovery, nerve conduction studies should be performed. The longer the delay in repair the poorer is the recovery, particularly of motor nerves.
- Extensive soft tissue damage at the site of a compound fracture requires exploration to exclude damage to nerves.
- Complete division of a nerve in an incised wound.
- Neuroma formation or scarring around a nerve.

Operative technique for primary nerve repair

Identify the cut ends and perform an end-to-end suture without tension. The suture may be placed epineurally or perineurally.
The type of suture depends upon:
- The size of the nerve
- The experience of the operator
- The time available (if other injuries are likely to take a long time to repair, secondary nerve sutures may be preferable).
Orientate the cut ends by using landmarks such as small surface vessels and the size of the individual fascicles.

Techniques of secondary nerve repair

- Perform a neurolysis to free the cut ends.
- Excise any neuroma formation.
- Cut both ends of the nerve back until a bundle pattern is visible.
- Free or transpose the nerve proximally or distally to allow anastomosis without tension.
- If end-to-end anastomosis is not possible without tension, insert cable grafts from lengths of sural nerve.

INFECTIONS OF THE HAND

Whitlow

This is a tense collection of pus under the nail-fold which may cause extreme pain.

Procedure
Evacuate pus either by a short incision over the point of maximum fluctuation or by raising the nail-fold with the points of a pair of scissors. Alternatively, remove the base of the nail itself, allowing pus to drain.

Pulp abscess

This is usually the result of a penetrating injury. Because of the tough septae between the skin and the underlying phalanx and because the hand is densely innervated with sensory endings a pulp abscess is usually extremely painful and requires urgent decompression.

Procedure
Drain the abscess through a fish-mouth incision. Leave the incision open until it heals.

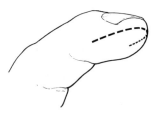

Fish-mouth incision of finger pulp.

Suppurative tenosynovitis

Infection within a flexor tendon sheath may be caused by a penetrating injury or by haematogenous spread. The finger is held stiffly, splinted by the tense collection within the sheath, and there is palpable or visible swelling of front of the finger. Any attempt to extend the finger passively causes extreme pain.

Procedure
616 Open the sheath at its proximal and distal ends and thoroughly irrigate with normal saline and an antibiotic. An intravenous cannula is an ideal size through which to inject directly into the sheath. This procedure may need to be repeated two or three times before the infection heals.

Rehabilitation
Intensive physiotherapy is required to achieve optimal function.

Palmar space infection

This is also an extremely painful condition. There are three spaces in the palm surrounded by vertical septae. Since the palmar skin is tough, the swelling is often most obvious on the dorsum of the hand or initially presents as a web-space swelling.

Procedure
If the web space is the site of the abscess, make anterior and posterior incisions rather than dividing the web space itself. Take care to look for extension of the abscess via the lumbrical canal into the palmar space.

Human bite injury

Beware this classic injury—a puncture wound over the knuckle caused by the clenched fist striking an opponent's teeth—the infection is often due to anaerobic organisms from the mouth.

Procedure
Open the joint surfaces by an S-incision and thoroughly lavage the area. Leave the wound open.

Postoperatively
Elevate the hand and encourage early active movements.

High-pressure nozzle injury

Oil or paint forced through the skin from a high pressure jet spreads widely through the subcutaneous tissues causing severe irritation, oedema, and tissue necrosis. The injury may present initially with only a small puncture wound but with pain out of proportion to the injury.

Procedure
Lay open the digit using a Brunner incision (p. 610). Excise all the contaminated tissue. After releasing the tourniquet and achieving haemostasis, leave the wounds open and apply dressings. Arrange frequent changes of dressings and repeat debridement in theatre as required.

617

Postoperatively
Elevate the limb postoperatively, administer analgesia, and encourage early active function. Close the wounds when the swelling has gone if possible. If not, apply a skin graft.

FRACTURE DISLOCATIONS OF THE CARPUS

Mechanism of injury

Hyperextension is the usual method of injury, causing fracture of the scaphoid with or without dislocations around the mid-carpal joint. The scaphoid straddles the mid-carpal joint. This may cause a fracture of the waist of the scaphoid and a variety of other patterns of injury depending on which part of the complex absorbed the force of the injury—the trans-scaphoid perilunate dislocation is the extreme result. If the scaphoid does not fracture, the scapholunate ligaments may tear and the resulting instability is difficult to diagnose or demonstrate radiologically.

- Beware the isolated anterior dislocation of the lunate.
- Be suspicious if the arcs of the articular surfaces of the capitate, lunate, and radius are not concentric on the radiograph.
- The median nerve may be compromised.

If the injury includes a fracture of the waist of the scaphoid, internal fixation of the fracture will help to restore the mid-carpal stability. An isolated fracture of the waist of the scaphoid will usually unite after 2 or 3 months in plaster of Paris, but if there is any original displacement of the fracture, or if there is no sign of union progressing after 4–8 weeks in plaster, consider internal fixation.

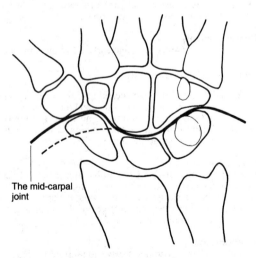

The mid-carpal joint

Carpal bones: the mid=carpal joint and the line of the trans-scaphoid perilunate dislocation.

Internal fixation of fracture of waist of scaphoid (major)

Position
Supinate the forearm on a hand table.

Incision
A volar incision on the radial side of and parallel to the tendon of flexor carpi radialis. Distal to the insertion of the flexor carpi radialis, the incision curves in line with the thumb.

Procedure
Incise the joint capsule avoiding the deep branch of the radial artery. Expose the scaphoid and demonstrate the fracture by ulnar flexion of the wrist. Fix the fracture either with an AO small-fragment screw or a Herbert screw (using the jig supplied).

Rehabilitation
A plaster of Paris back-slab is applied and the wrist mobilized once the wounds have healed.

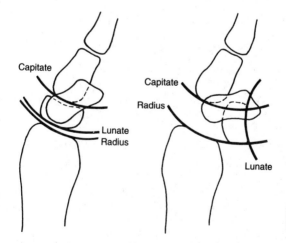

Lateral view of carpal bones indicating loss of concentricity in lunate dislocation.

FRACTURE DISLOCATIONS OF THE CARPUS (*cont.*)

Reduction of a dislocated lunate (major)

Procedure
First attempt a closed reduction by dorsiflexion and direct pressure. If this is not possible, perform an open reduction through a curved anterior incision and divide the flexor retinaculum (this also allows decompression of the median nerve). Open the anterior joint capsule, reduce the dislocation, and close the capsule.

Rehabilitation
Immobilize the wrist in a plaster cast for 4 weeks and then allow active movement.

FRACTURES OF THE HAND

The principles applied to the management of long-bone fractures elsewhere are equally applicable to the hand. Rigid fixation of long-bone fractures allows early movement of the hand as a whole functional unit. Wherever possible, intra-articular fractures should be reduced adequately and held securely by internal fixation.

Finger fractures

Mechanism of injury
Crush injury of the finger tip is common, e.g. a direct blow from a hammer or catching the finger in a door. Crush injuries of the finger tip may cause comminution of the 'tuft' of the terminal phalanx. These usually heal well without specific treatment. Direct your attention to the associated soft tissue injury.

Proximal and middle phalanx

Mechanism of injury
Crush injuries can cause comminuted fractures, whereas twisting injuries cause fracture patterns very similar to those of the tibial and femoral shafts, i.e. transverse, oblique, spiral displaced, or spiral undisplaced depending on the violence of the twisting force. Be on the look-out for associated injuries to the tendons or the skin.

Treatment
Splint the inherently stable fractures by strapping to the neighbouring digit and encourage active mobilization. Avoid malrotation. Neighbour strapping and early movement keeps the fracture in correct rotation.

Indications for surgery
Unstable fractures.

Internal fixation of middle and proximal phalangeal fractures (major)

Incision
Mid-lateral incision.

Procedure
Attempt to achieve closed reduction by manipulation and stabilize the fracture with percutaneous K-wires with the aid of an image intensifier. Using AO mini-screws and plates is technically demanding, but the techniques are similar to those employed in the treatment of fractures elsewhere. Open reduction may be required, particularly for fractures involving the articular surfaces

Closure
Nylon to skin.

Rehabilitation
Early active movements to prevent stiffness.

Complications
Stiffness due to joint contracture or adherence of tendons, particularly the extensor apparatus.

Comminuted and/or compound fractures of the finger (major)

Mechanism of injury
Usually a crushing force. External fixation is a very useful technique for these injuries.

Procedure
A commercial fixator can be used or a fixator can be fashioned from K-wires and cement.

Clean and trim the wound thoroughly. Insert the K-wires percutaneously into uninjured bone proximal and distal to the fracture. Prepare a lump of bone cement and mould it across the wires, having bent the ends in order to provide a more secure fixation within the cement. While the cement is hardening, adjust the fracture position as required by viewing the position on the image intensifier.

Rehabilitation
Dress the wounds as appropriate. The wires will control the fracture. Encourage early active movement.

Intra-articular fractures

Fractures of the base or the middle phalanx or the condyle of the proximal phalanx may result in unacceptable angulation of the joint. Reduce the fracture accurately and hold together with two K-wires or a mini-lag screw.

Fracture dislocations in the fingers

A fracture dislocation of the base of the middle phalanx is a very difficult injury.

Procedure
Reduce the fracture through a mid-lateral incision. If the anterior fragment is large enough, it may be possible to fix the fragment with a tiny lag screw, but of course this necessitates elevating the flexor sheath and tendons. It is safer to perform a ligamentotaxis procedure, i.e. external fixation using two wires

623

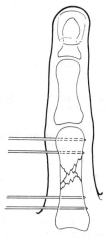

K-wires and bone cement acting as external fixation of comminuted fracture of proximal phalanx.

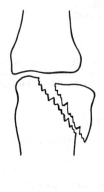 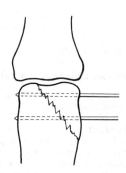

K-wires transfixing condylar fracture of proximal phalanx.

and cement with distraction across the joint to encourage reduction of the fracture.

Complications
This fracture rarely heals well enough to restore normal function, and it is important to warn the patient of this before surgery.

Metacarpal fractures

Mechanism of injury
This usually results from a twisting injury and rarely from a direct blow. Metacarpals may fracture at the neck, shaft, or base. Treatment is influenced by other associated injuries, by

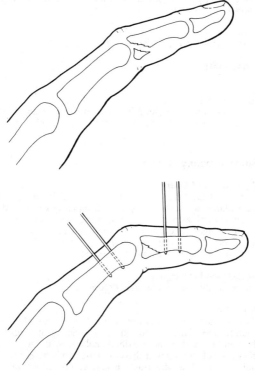

625

**K-wires and bone cement acting as external fixation of a fracture/
dislocation of the base of the middle phalanx.**

age, and by occupation. Fracture of a single metacarpal shaft usually does well and heals without malunion because of the splinting effect of the neighbouring metacarpals. The exception is the little finger, where significant angulation may result in an unacceptable cosmetic result.

Reduction and fixation of a metacarpal shaft fracture (major)

Incision
Dorsal incision in line with the affected metacarpal or between the metacarpals if more than one is fractured.

Procedure
The fracture is reduced and the reduction is temporarily maintained by reduction forceps whilst a small fragment plate is applied.

Closure
Vicryl to close the periosteum. Nylon to skin.

Rehabilitation
Early active mobilization.

Complications
Stiffness of the hand and adherence of the extensor tendons to the plate (hence the need to close the periosteum over the plate).

'Boxer's fracture' (intermediate)

Mechanism of injury
Fracture of the neck of the fifth metacarpal is very common and is due to a direct blow, usually from using a clenched fist. When angulation is not severe, treatment is by simply strapping the finger to its neighbour and encouraging early active movement. Malrotation is the greatest complication. Splints, bandages, and plaster should be avoided.

Indications for surgery
Severe angulation or rotational deformity.

Procedure
Closed reduction is performed by flexing the MCP joint (metacarpophalangeal) to 90° and pushing it backwards through the shaft of the proximal phalanx. With image intensifier control, use a power driver to pass two K-wires proximal and two distal to the fracture and secure either with the cement technique or by advancing wires into the neighbouring metacarpals.

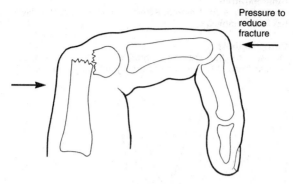

Fracture of the neck of a metacarpal.

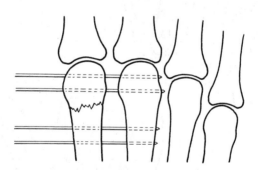

Trans-metacarpal K-wires for stabilization of a fracture of the neck of the little finger metacarpal.

Rehabilitation
Encourage early active mobilization and remove the wires at 4 weeks.

Bennett's fracture (intermediate)

This is a fracture dislocation at the base of the thumb metacarpal which is inherently unstable.

Procedure
The fracture is reduced by traction and extension of the thumb, and a K-wire is inserted under image intensifier control either to transfix the fracture or more usually just distal to the fracture and into the adjacent metacarpal to maintain the reduction.

627

FRACTURES OF THE HAND (*cont.*)

Rehabilitation
Plaster of Paris for 1 month. Remove the wires once the plaster has been removed.

Complications
Damage to the cutaneous branch of the radial nerve, osteoarthritis of the carpometacarpal joint of the thumb.

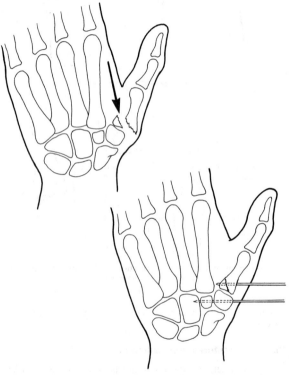

Bennet's fracture of the bone of the first metacarpal with K-wires either transfixing the fracture or inserted proximally to act as a buttress.

FLEXOR TENDON INJURIES (major)

The integrity of the flexor tendons can be restored using sutures. However, the technique required must be meticulous to restore normal function. The *flexor digitorum sublimis* (FDS) and *flexor digitorum profundus* (FDP) within the flexor tendon sheath slide over each other and under the pulleys of the flexor sheath which must be preserved during repair. This particularly applies to repairs in 'no man's land'.

Incision

Brunner incision (p. 610).

Procedure

The incisions are extended proximally and distally until the cut ends of the tendon are identified. Preserve the flexor tendon sheath and in particular the pulleys. A technique of tendon suture is the Kessler stitch using a non-absorbable suture augmented by a continuous circumferential suture. Where possible attempt to preserve both the FDP and the FDS to maintain the vascularity of both.

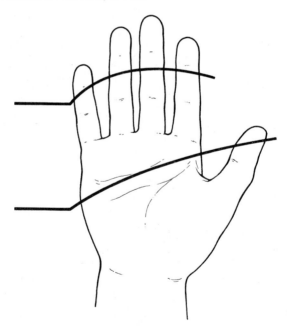

No-man's land.

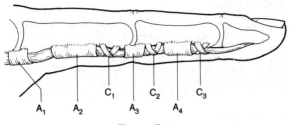

Flexor pulleys.

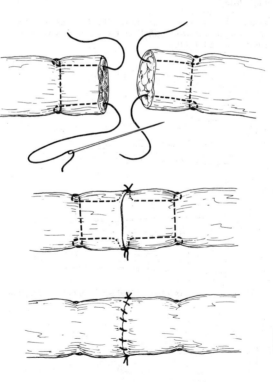

631

Kessler suture and circumferential stitch.

FLEXOR TENDON INJURIES (major)
(*cont.*)

Rehabilitation

Controlled tendon movement is required to get the balance between mobilization to prevent adhesions and the risk of rupture. A Kleinert splint is a dynamic splint attached to the finger-nail on elastic, tethered at wrist level to a volar slab. Apply a dorsal slab of plaster of Paris with the MCP joints in flexion. Active flexion of the whole hand can then be encouraged. This arrangement should be maintained for 4–6 weeks.

Complications

Tendon rupture or adhesions of the tendon.

Repair of laceration or avulsion of FDP at its distal insertion

Use the incisions as shown on p. 610. Reattach the tendon to the base of the distal phalanx by a stainless steel pull-out suture over a button.

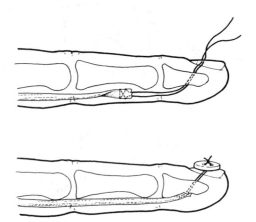

Pull-out suture to tether the Profundus tendon to the distal phalanx.

EXTENSOR TENDON INJURIES

Indications for surgery (intermediate)

An extensor tendon divided at the level of the neck of the metacarpal or more distally should be repaired to restore MCP joint extension.

Incision

Extend the laceration proximally and distally.

Procedure

Repair the extensor tendon, which is ribbon-shaped at this level, using interrupted or continuous sutures.

Rehabilitation

Protect the hand in a dorsal plaster hood for 3–4 weeks.

Boutonnière deformity (intermediate)

Indications for surgery
A Boutonnière deformity results from division of the extensor apparatus (the central slip) over the dorsum of the PIP joint.

Incision
An S-incision over the PIP joint.

Procedure
Extend the laceration to expose the injured central slip of the extensor apparatus and suture it back into position or pass the suture through the drill hole in the base of the middle phalanx.

Closure
Nylon to skin.

Rehabilitation
Protect the finger with the PIP joint in extension for 6 weeks.

Complications
The main complication is joint stiffness.

Mallet finger (intermediate)

Indications for surgery
If the extensor tendon has been avulsed from its insertion into the distal phalanx without a bony fragment, splint the DIP joint in extension for 6 weeks. The results are often disappointing. Internal fixation is indicated if a large fragment of the base of the distal phalanx has been avulsed.

Incision
An S-incision over the DIP.

Procedure
Replace the fragment of bone and hold it with either a mini-fragment screw or a K-wire.

Rehabilitation
Mobilize the hand if a K-wire has been used. Remove it at 3 weeks.

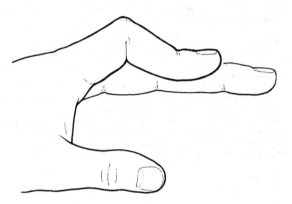

Boutonnière deformity.

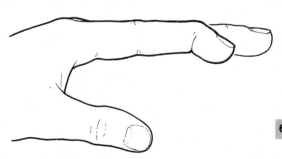

Mallet deformity.

LIGAMENT INJURIES

Ruptures of the collateral ligaments of the PIP joints of the fingers are common but rarely require repair. They may be associated with a dislocation. Treatment consists of neighbour strapping and early mobilization.

Rupture of the ulnar collateral ligament of the thumb MCP joint

This is a common injury and has become more so with the popularity of dry ski slopes.

Preoperative investigations
Clinical examination may demonstrate instability, but the thumb may be too painful to examine. Stress radiographs may demonstrate instability.

Incision
Longitudinal over the ulnar border of the thumb MCP.

Procedure
The ruptured ligament cannot be replaced because of the interposed tendon of the adductor muscle. Divide the adductor tendon to allow replacement of the ligament. The position of the ligament can be maintained by suture to bone (a suture anchor may be of benefit) or, if the bony fragment is large enough, by a K-wire, a mini-fragment screw, or a tension-band wire technique. The thumb adductor is then repaired.

Closure
Nylon to skin.

Rehabilitation
Protect the repair in plaster of Paris for 3 weeks.

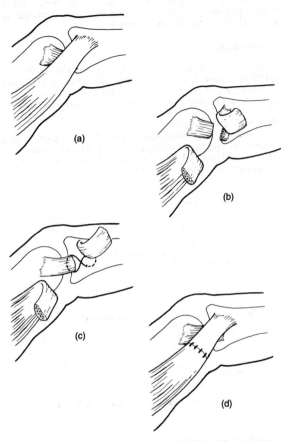

Ruptured ulnar collateral ligament (UCL) of MCP joint of thumb: (a), (b) division of adductor pollicis tendon reveals rupture of UCL; (c) repair of ruptured UCL by figure-of-eight wire; (c) repair of adductor tendon.

FINGER-TIP INJURIES

The choice of treatment for loss of tissue (pulp, bone, or nail-bed) from the finger tip depends upon the age, sex, occupation, personality, and which finger is involved.

Young children

If there is no bone exposed, finger-tip injuries in this age group are treated with a non-adherent dressing. Healing is often remarkable. If bone is exposed, cleaning, trimming, and application of a dressing under general anaesthetic is required.

Nail-bed 'dislocation'

This is usually associated with an underlying terminal phalanx fracture or epiphyseal injury in children. The nail needs to be cleaned and reduced under the nail-fold by manipulating the epiphyseal separation into place.

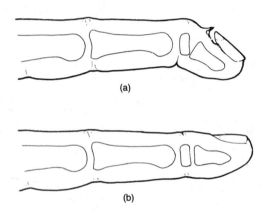

Dislocation of nail base:(a) dislocated; (b) reduced.

Adults (intermediate)

Where there is significant loss of bone and pulp, choose between formal terminalization and procedures to preserve the length of digits. In a manual worker the quickest way to achieve return to normal hand function is to terminalize the digit. Preserve the length of the thumb at all cost.

Procedure

Excise the damaged skin edges and trim down to the bone until the skin flaps can be closed across the end of the digit without tension. If the amputation is at the level of the DIP joint, remove the articular surface of the joint and round off the shoulders of the middle phalanx. Identify the digital nerve and dissect it proximally, as far as possible, in order to avoid painful neuroma formation in the tip of the stump. If the amputation is proximal to the DIP joint, tether the cut end of the FDP tendon to the flexor sheath in order to prevent the development of an 'intrinsic plus' deformity caused by the pull of the lumbrical muscle which results from the proximal retraction of the FDP from which the lumbrical takes origin.

Closure
Interrupted Nylon sutures to skin.

Rehabilitation
Early active mobilization of the hand.

Indications for procedures to preserve digit length
Preservation is indicated for cosmetic reasons in all the fingers or where the injury involves the thumb. Split-thickness or full-thickness grafts can be used as well as advancement flaps.

Children

INTRODUCTION

Children's fractures behave rather differently from those of adults.

Greenstick fractures involve buckling of a long bone rather than a complete fracture. Clinically significant angulation in a greenstick fracture should be corrected by manipulation.

Complete fractures in children tend to heal quickly because of the tough periosteum which is often not completely torn so that subperiosteal bone is laid down rapidly. Careful review of these fractures over the first few weeks is vital to recognize and treat the deformity before the fracture begins to unite, after which further manipulation is very difficult, if not impossible.

Epiphyseal fractures and separations are described according to the Salter–Harris classification which is very useful for providing a prognosis. Types IV and V may result in premature fusion of the epiphysis and subsequent deformity.

Most fractures in children can be treated conservatively by closed manipulation under radiographic control. However, there are notable exceptions.

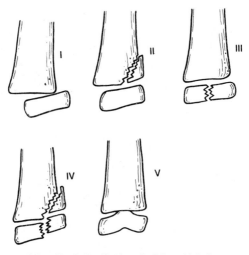

Salter–Harris classification of epiphyseal injuries.

FRACTURES AROUND THE SHOULDER

Salter–Harris type I and II injuries of the proximal humeral epiphysis are not uncommon. If they are badly displaced, closed manipulation is usually sucessful. Fractures of the proximal shaft of the humerus usually unite rapidly because of the strong periosteal sleeve which remains intact.

FRACTURES OF THE DISTAL HUMERUS

Supracondylar fracture

Introduction
This is a common injury caused by a fall onto the outstretched hand. It is infamous for its association with ischaemic contracture of the forearm muscles caused by contusion or intimal damage of the brachial artery (although the incidence is only 0.5 per cent) and with a cubitus varus (gunstock deformity). There are three components to this: coronal tilting, rotation in the horizontal plane, and backward angulation. If closed manipulation is to be successful, all three components must be corrected. Undisplaced fractures can be treated conservatively by a collar and cuff.

Closed manipulation is performed under general anaesthesia applying gentle traction to the elbow in only slight flexion and with direct pressure over the point of the olecranon, pushing forwards whilst the elbow is flexed and the forearm pronated. At just beyond 90° flexion, the sling effect of the triceps complex should maintain reduction.

Radiographs are difficult to achieve, particularly in the AP plane as the fracture position may be lost if the elbow is extended beyond 90°.

If the fracture is more significantly displaced, closed manipulation may be unsuccessful, particularly if there is associated massive swelling which is often the case. In these injuries there may be compromise to the circulation of the distal arm, and so a period of traction is wise whilst the swelling is reducing, keeping a close eye on the distal circulation during this time.

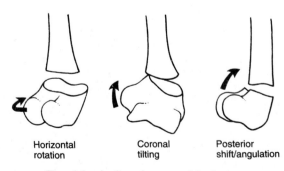

| Horizontal rotation | Coronal tilting | Posterior shift/angulation |

Three deforming forces in supracondylar fracture.

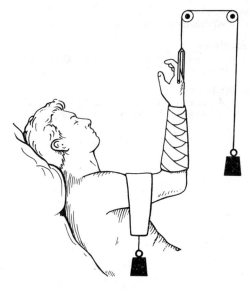

Supracondylar traction.

Closed reduction/internal fixation of a supracondylar fracture of the humerus (major)

If a closed manipulation is unsuccessful perform an open reduction.

Position
Prone.

Incision
Mid-dorsal skin incision.

Procedure
Either split triceps in the line of the muscle fibres or reflect a tongue of triceps down to expose the fracture. Clean the fracture ends and, in particular, disimpact the spike which is the cause of failure to reduce the fracture. Percutaneous wires can then be inserted under direct vision taking care to avoid the ulnar nerve medially.

647

FRACTURES OF THE DISTAL HUMERUS (*cont.*)

Closure
Vicryl to subcutaneous tissues and Nylon to skin.

Complications
Injury to the ulna or residual defomity are the most common complications.

Rehabilitation
Apply a plaster of Paris slab for 3 weeks until the wires are removed and gentle mobilization is commenced.

FRACTURES OF THE DISTAL HUMERUS (*cont.*)

Radiographs may be misleading because the fragment is often much larger than it appears on X-ray, as the distal humerus is largely cartilaginous in a child. Failure to recognize, reduce accurately, and hold these fractures may result in non-union or malunion or disturbance of the epiphyseal plate.

Fractures of the medial epicondyle

This is usually an avulsion injury which may appear as a very small fragment on radiographs. In fact the avulsed segment is quite large and contains the origin of the flexor mass. Occasionally the displacement may take the fragment into the elbow joint itself. Suspect this injury if an AP radiograph fails to confirm the presence of the medial epicondyle in a child more than 6 years old. A radiograph of the opposite elbow may be helpful.

Internal fixation of the medial epicondyle (major)
Incision A longitudinal incision on the medial side of the elbow, identifying and protecting the ulnar nerve.

Procedure Pulling on the flexor mass by extending the wrist may help to identify the epicondyle. Prepare the site of avulsion from the distal humerus. Clean the fragment and hold it with two percutaneous K-wires or a small fragment screw.

Closure Vicryl to subcutaneous tissues and Nylon to skin.

Rehabilitation Apply a plaster back-slab with the elbow at 90°. Allow gentle mobilization at 2–3 weeks or when the wires are removed at 4 weeks.

Complications Injury to the ulnar nerve.

Fracture of the lateral condyle

This injury may occur as part of a fracture dislocation of the elbow, and is usually a Salter–Harris type II injury. Accurate reduction and fixation are very important to avoid a cubitus valgus deformity and secondary ulnar nerve tension.

Open reduction and internal fixation of a lateral condyle fracture (major)
Incision A longitudinal incision on the lateral aspect of the elbow which does not extend beyond the level of the radial neck.

Procedure Identify the avulsed fragment. The fracture surfaces are cleaned and the fracture reduced (it is usually rotated because of the pull of the extensor mass) and held with percutaneous K-wires or with a cancellous screw depending on the age of the child.

Closure Vicryl to subcutaneous tissues and Nylon to skin.

Rehabilitation Apply a plaster back-slab for 2–3 weeks with the elbow at 90°. Follow this with gentle mobilization, removing the K-wires at about 6 weeks.

Complications The posterior interosseous nerve is at risk if the incision extends beyond the radial neck.

INJURIES OF THE PROXIMAL RADIAL EPIPHYSIS

Salter–Harris I and II injuries of the radial head are common. A tilt of less than 30° is usually treated conservatively. A tilt of greater than 30° should be corrected initially by closed manipulation under general anaesthesia, applying a varus stress across the extended elbow while pronating/supinating the forearm with direct pressure over the radial head with a thumb.

Open reduction of a displaced radial head fracture (major)

Incision
Make a short oblique incision proximal to the level of the radial neck.

Procedure
Split the muscle in line with its fibres and thus expose the head of the radius which can be reduced under direct vision. If it is not completely stable, a percutaneous K-wire can be inserted through the back of the elbow joint, across the capitellum, and longitudinally into the radius with the elbow flexed to 90°.

Closure
Vicryl to subcutaneous tissues and Nylon to skin.

Rehabilitation
Immobilize the elbow with a plaster back-slab for 3 weeks until the wire is removed.

Complications
The posterior interosseous nerve is at risk if the incision is extended beyond the radial neck.

JUVENILE MONTEGGIA AND GALEAZZI FRACTURES

These fractures are described in the adult section but are more common in children and may be stable after closed manipulation if the shaft fracture is greenstick in nature.

Internal fixation of an anterior Monteggia fracture dislocation (major)

Incision
A Boyd approach is used (see p. 598).

Procedure
The radial head is reduced and the annular ligament is repaired if necessary. The proximal ulnar fracture is stabilized with a small DCP. If the radial head is unstable, a percutaneous K-wire can be inserted through the back of the elbow across the capitellum and into the radial head with the elbow flexed to 90°.

Rehabilitation
The elbow is immobilized until the K-wire is removed at 3 weeks.

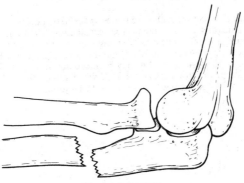

Monteggia fracture

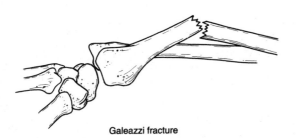

Galeazzi fracture

Monteggia and Galeazzi fractures.

FRACTURES OF THE SHAFTS OF RADIUS AND ULNA

If closed reduction in theatre under anaesthetic fails to reduce this injury or if the reduction is extremely unstable, fix the fractures internally after performing open reduction using the surgical approaches described for the equivalent adult fractures. In the young child it may be more appropriate to hold the fractures with percutaneous K-wires rather than plates. Beware a compartment syndrome in this injury.

DISPLACED FRACTURE OF THE DISTAL RADIUS (major)

Attempt a closed manipulation of this injury, but it must be done in an operating theatre with radiographic control in case closed manipulation is unsuccessful. Failure to reduce this injury is usually due to interposed fibres of pronator quadratus.

Incision

Make a longitudinal incision parallel to the distal radius just lateral to the radial artery.

Procedure

Retract the artery medially and expose the pronator quadratus muscle which will be interposed between the fracture ends blocking fracture reduction. Divide the pronator quadratus from its insertion into the radius in line with the skin incision. This will allow the fracture to be reduced and held with two crossed K-wires inserted percutaneously. The protruding end of the wires should be bent to prevent proximal migration.

Rehabilitation

Apply a plaster back-slab. Remove the wires and mobilize the wrist at 3–4 weeks depending on the age of the child.

The Lower Limb

TOTAL HIP REPLACEMENT (major)

There are a variety of hip prostheses and approaches to the hip, and thus the operation described will vary from surgeon to surgeon.

Indication

Osteoarthritis or rheumatoid arthritis affecting the hip.

Position

Supine on the table. A sandbag may be used under the ipsilateral buttock.

Incision

Centred over the greater trochanter, straight distally and curved posteriorly proximally.

Procedure

The fascia lata is divided longitudinally and a Charnley incisional retractor (north–south retractor) is inserted. The tendon of the gluteus medius muscle is detached from the greater trochanter together with the proximal part of the vastis lateralis muscle and retracted. The capsule of the hip joint is divided and excised, and the leg is adducted to allow the hip to dislocate. The leg is externally rotated until the tibia is horizontal to the floor and the head is removed using a power saw. The leg is internally rotated and a Charnley east–west retractor is inserted. The remaining capsule is excised and the acetabulum is cleared of any soft tissues. The acetabulum is prepared by removing any remaining articular cartilage using cheesegrater reamers until subchondral bone is exposed (as shown by punctate bleeding). Keyholes are prepared using a suitable drill and a trial prosthesis is inserted. A definitive prosthesis is then cemented in using gentamicin-loaded cement.

The east–west retractor is then removed and the femur is prepared. The leg is externally rotated until the tibia is horizontal to the floor. Adduction of the leg facilitates the exposure. The femoral canal is prepared using reamers and a trial prosthesis is inserted. The hip is reduced (a swab around the neck of the prosthesis facilitates later dislocation) and the stability of the hip is assessed. The hip is then dislocated and the trial prosthesis is removed. A cement restrictor is inserted into the femoral shaft and the definitive prosthesis is inserted, again using gentamicin-loaded cement. The hip is reduced.

Closure

The gluteus medius is reattached using a no. 1 Vicryl suture and the fascia lata is repaired with no. 1 Vicryl. Two suction drains are used.

Rehabilitation

A check radiograph is taken and the patient is mobilized.

Complications

The sciatic nerve is at risk during this procedure, particularly if there is preoperative shortening. Penetration of the acetabulum may result in damage to the pelvic organs. The prosthesis may dislocate in the immediate postoperative period.

TOTAL KNEE REPLACEMENT (major)

Even more than for a hip replacement, the procedure for knee replacement is dependent on the particular prosthesis used as the operator is required to follow a series of jigs. Thus this description needs to be read in conjunction with the manufacturer's instructions.

Indications

Osteoarthritis and rheumatoid arthritis of the knee.

Incision

A mid-line incision is used, extending from the quadriceps muscle over the front of the knee to the tibial tubercle.

Procedure

The knee is entered by a medial parapatellar incision. The infrapatellar fat pad is excised and the patella rotated through 180° so that its articular surface faces upwards. The meniscal remnants are excised and the femoral and tibial surfaces prepared using the jigs supplied. The definitive components are inserted using gentamicin—loaded cement after a suitable trial reduction. The patella is trimmed, and if it has a tendency to sublux on flexion of the knee a lateral release is performed.

Closure

The capsule and extensor apparatus are closed using interrupted sutures over two drains.

Rehabilitation

The knee is mobilized once the drains have been removed and the postoperative radiograph seen. The patient is mobilized with weight-bearing as able.

Complications

The posterior structures of the knee and in particular the popliteal artery are at risk during this operation.

KELLER'S ARTHROPLASTY (major)

Indications

Osteoarthritis of the MTP joint of the hallux.

Incision

Dorsal incision centred over the MTP joint of the hallux.

Procedure

The incision is deepened to the capsule which is divided in line with the skin incision. The bunion is exposed and removed using an osteotome. The proximal phalanx is dissected free and divided so that 50 per cent of its length is removed using a bone cutter. The proximal phalanx is then removed, taking care to preserve the flexor tendon. The extensor tendon can be elongated in a Z fashion if necessary.

Closure

The capsule is repaired using Vicryl and the skin is sutured.

Rehabilitation

A Zimmer splint can be used to maintain the position of the toe for a period of 2 weeks.

Complications

The dorsal branch of the digital nerve may be divided with resulting painful neuroma formation. The flexor tendon must be preserved to prevent dorsiflexion of the toe.

MITCHELL'S OSTETOMY (major)

Indications

Adolescent hallux valgus, or hallux valgus at any age where the MTP joint is well preserved.

Incision

A dorsomedial incision centred over the MTP joint of the hallux.

Procedure

The capsule of the joint is exposed and a Y-shaped incision is made in the capsule over the bunion and down the shaft. The bunion is excised using an osteotome. The distal part of the shaft is exposed taking care not to strip the periosteum from the lateral aspect of the metatarsal head. Two drill holes are made and a step osteotomy is performed. The osteotomy is displaced and the position maintained with a no. 1 absorbable suture.

Closure

The capsule is closed in a Y to V fashion to maintain position. The skin is closed with interrupted sutures.

Rehabilitation

A Zimmer splint is applied for 2 weeks until the wounds have healed followed by plaster bootees for a further 4 weeks.

Complications

Avascular necrosis of the metatarsal head may occur if the periosteum is stripped from the lateral part of the metatarsal head. There may be non-union at the osteotomy site, particularly if the osteotomy is in the cortical bone of the shaft. Damage to the dorsal branch of the digital nerve with subsequent neuroma formation may occur.

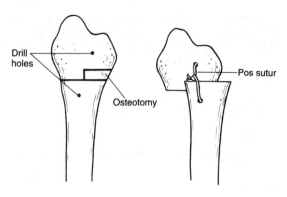

Mitchell's osteotomy.

REDUCTION OF A DISLOCATED HIP (major)

Reduction of a hip dislocated as a result of trauma is a surgical emergency because of the risk of avascular damage to the femoral head. The sciatic nerve is also at risk. Failure to obtain reduction is an indication for open reduction of the hip.

Indication

Traumatic dislocation of the hip with or without an associated fracture of the acetabulum.

Position

Supine. Reduction may be facilitated by placing the patient on the floor.

Procedure

Reduction is achieved by traction on a flexed hip facilitated by an assistant stabilizing the pelvis. Reduction is usually obvious. An acetabular fracture may prevent reduction by interposition.

Postoperatively

Nurse the patient flat in bed on skin traction for 6 weeks.

Complications

The sciatic nerve may be damaged, usually as a result of a neuropraxia. Avascular necrosis of the femoral head may occur up to 3 years after the dislocation and may predispose to osteoarthritis.

INTERNAL FIXATION OF A SUBCAPITAL FRACTURE OF THE NECK OF THE FEMUR (major)

A variety of devices are available. Most are based on the insertion of parallel screws over guide-wires. The insertion of AO cannulated screws is described.

Indications

Subcapital fractures of Garden grades I or II in the elderly. All subcapital fractures in the young.

Position

Supine on a fracture table. The reduction needs to be checked using an image intensifier prior to draping the patient.

Incision

Lateral incision 7 cm long, starting 2 cm distal to the greater trochanter and extending distally.

Procedure

Divide the fascia lata in line with the incision and divide the vastis lateralis to expose the lateral cortex of the femur. Pass a guide-wire by hand over the front of the femoral neck to indicate the neck alignment. Using the parallel guide provided insert three screws in a triangular pattern. Use the image intensifier to confirm the position of the screws in both AP and lateral screening.

Remove the guide-wire. For each screw, measure the screw length required using the direct measure, and then drill, tap, and insert a screw of the correct length. Use a washer and ensure that the threads of the screw are distal to the fracture site to allow compression (lag screw). Check the screw position using the image intensifier. Remove the guide-wires.

Closure

Interrupted Vicryl sutures to the fascia lata. Continuous or interrupted sutures to skin.

Rehabilitation

Check radiographs. Mobilize as soon as the radiographs are seen and the drains removed. Mobilization without weight-bearing is ideal, but is often impractical in the elderly. Remove sutures at 14 days.

Complications

- Avascular necrosis of the femoral head
- Implant failure

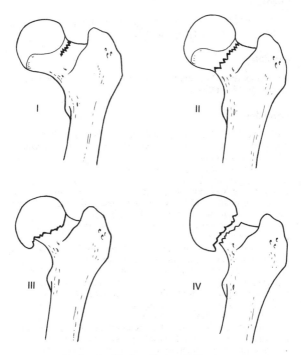

Garden classification of subcapital fracture.

DYNAMIC HIP SCREW FOR FRACTURED NECK OF FEMUR (major)

Extracapsular fractures of the neck of the femur, e.g. basal cervical and trochanteric fractures.

Position

Supine on a fracture table. Use an image intensifier to check reduction prior to draping the patient.

Incision

Lateral incision 2 cm distal to the tip of the greater trochanter, extending 15 cm distally.

Procedure

Incise the fascia lata in line with the skin incision. Detach the origin of the vastis lateralis from the femur and strip distally using a periosteal elevator.

Pass a guide-wire by hand over the femoral neck to ascertain its alignment. Using a guide (usually 135°), pass a guide-wire into the neck parallel to the first wire in the lateral plane. Check the position of the guide-wire using the image intensifier. The ideal position is in the subchondral bone of the femoral head, central in the neck and slightly towards the calcar in the AP view.

Remove the guide and measure using the direct measuring device. Subtract 5 mm from the measurement, set the cannulated reamer to the final measurement, and select a dynamic hip screw of the same length. Ream the femoral neck and then insert the hip screw using the introducer. Check the position of the screw using the image intensifier once it is inserted to between the first and second marks on the introducer. Remember to ensure that the notch on the introducer points proximally and that the handle is parallel to the femoral shaft so that the plate alignment is correct. Remove the introducer and pass the barrel of the plate over the hip screw. Use the impactor to apply the plate to the femoral shaft (usually a four-hole plate) and insert four screws in the usual AO fashion. Check the position of the plate on the image intensifier.

Closure

Vicryl to the fascia lata. Interrupted or continuous suture to skin.

Rehabilitation

Mobilize with full weight-bearing when radiographs have been seen and the drains removed.

Complications

Implant failure.

HEMIARTHROPLASTY FOR FRACTURED NECK OF FEMUR (major)

Indications

Displaced subcapital fractures of the femur (Garden grades III and IV). A range of devices are available. A bipolar device such as Monk's prosthesis probably reduces acetabular wear but is more expensive than an Austin Moore prosthesis. If the patient is young, consider a primary total hip replacement.

Position

Supine on the table. A sandbag under the affected buttock aids exposure.

Incision

15 cm long centred over the greater trochanter, with the proximal incision curved backwards to facilitate reaming of the femur.

Procedure

Divide the fascia lata in the line of the incision and insert a Charnley north–south retractor. Identify the plane between the gluteus medius and gluteus minimus, and then detach the medius from its insertion on the lateral border of the femur using cutting diathermy. This exposes the capsule of the neck which is incised in a T fashion. This is accompanied by release of haematoma from the fracture site. Expose the femoral neck so that it can be trimmed using a saw. The angle of the cut is obtained by crossing the leg over the other so that the tibia is at 90° to the floor and using a trial prosthesis as a template. Next, having brought the leg back, remove the femoral head by screwing a corkscrew into the head until it spins in the acetabulum. Pull to remove the head. Measure the femoral head using callipers and select a prosthesis of the same size (if the size does not match completely, choose a prosthesis one size smaller). With the leg crossed over and the tibia at 90° use a box chisel to enlarge the lateral portion of the femoral canal. Insert a blunt bone spike down the shaft to start the tract for reaming and enlarge this by means of broaches. Insert the prosthesis into the femoral shaft, ensuring that it is seated on the calcar. Check that the acetabulum is clear of any debris and reduce the prosthesis by traction in the line of the femur. A skid placed over the head and into the acetabulum facilitates reduction. Check the stability of the prosthesis.

Closure

Reattach the gluteus with Vicryl sutures. Vicryl to fascia lata. Interrupted or continuous skin suture.

Rehabilitation

Mobilize with full weight-bearing.

Complications

- Dislocation of the prosthesis
- Splitting of the femur at operation
- Erosion of the acetabulum by the prosthesis.

DYNAMIC HIP SCREW FOR SUBTROCHANTERIC FRACTURE OF THE FEMUR (major plus)

Indications

Fracture of the subtrochanteric region of the femur.

Position

Supine on a fracture table. Check the position of the fracture using an image intensifier before draping patient.

Incision

Starting 2 cm distal to the greater trochanter, the distal extension depends upon the fracture.

Procedure

Incise the fascia lata in line with the incision and detach the vastus lateralis from its origin, using a periosteal elevator to strip muscle from the fracture site. Reduce the fracture by means of reduction forceps and maintain the reduction with lag screws, ensuring that they will not interfere with subsequent application of the plate. Insert the dynamic hip screw in the normal fashion. The length of plate used depends upon the fracture. Ensure that there are eight cortices distal to the fracture line. It may be possible to insert lag screws through the plate. If there is comminution, consider bone grafting. Check the position of the plate with the image intensifier.

Closure

Vicryl to fascia lata. Interrupted or continuous suture to skin.

Rehabilitation

Mobilize the patient with partial weight-bearing using crutches once the radiographs have been seen.

Complications

Implant failure.

INTRAMEDULLARY NAILING FOR FRACTURE OF THE SHAFT OF THE FEMUR (extra-major)

Indications

- Absolute: neurovascular injury
- Relative: multiple injury

Intramedullary nails allow early mobilization and this prevents the problems of conservative treatment such as malunion and the problems of prolonged recumbency.

Position

Insert a Steinman pin into the distal femur to facilitate reduction of the fracture. Use an image intensifier to ensure that the pin is placed as distally as possible to avoid interference with the nail. Attach the pin via a Bohler's stirrup to the traction table and check reduction using the image intensifier. The unaffected limb is flexed and abducted (in a suitable support) so that screening of the whole femur can be performed.

Incision

The incision extends from the tip of the greater trochanter proximally.

Procedure

Use scissors to split the glutei and insert a self-retaining retractor. Palpate the greater trochanter and insert the starting broach into the piriform fossa. Insert a hand reamer into the hole made and pass down the femur, checking position on both AP and lateral screening. Remove the hand reamer and insert an olive-tipped guide-wire. Pass this across the fracture site (an assistant may be required to manipulate the fracture) and into the distal fragment. Ensure that the tip of the guide-wire lies in the centre of the femoral condyles and check the position using the image intensifier. Ream the femoral canal by passing the flexible reamers over the guide-wire in turn. Use a skin protector and Kocher's forceps to prevent removal of the guide-wire during reaming. Continue reaming, increasing the size of the reamer until medullary bone is removed and the reamer just begins to bite against the cortex. Select a width of intramedullary nail 0.5 mm less than the size of the final reamer. Using a guide-wire of the same length, measure the amount of guide-wire protruding to estimate the length of the nail required. Having ascertained the length, attach the nail to the insertion jig provided. Insert the plastic tube over the olive-tipped guide-wire. This prevents loss of the reduction whilst the guide-wire is replaced with a non-olive-tipped wire. Remove the plastic tube and recheck the position of the wire in the distal fragment. Insert the nail over the guide-wire and by means of gentle taps with a hammer pass the nail across the fracture site. Use the image intensifier to check the position of both the proximal and distal ends of the nail. If the fracture is non-comminuted and mid-shaft, it can be left unlocked.

To lock the nail proceed as follows. To lock the proximal part use the jig provided to pass a drill through the proximal femur and the nail, measure the length of the screw required, and insert the screw, checking position on the image intensifier. To insert the two distal locking screws first ensure that the image intensifier is situated so that a true lateral view of one of the holes is obtained. Make a stab incision in the skin over the hole and position the drill so that it lies in the centre of the hole in the lateral view. Ensure that the drill lies in the same plane as the arm of the image intensifier and drill through the lateral cortex of the femur, the nail, and the medial cortex of the femur. Insert a screw of the correct length and repeat the process for the other screw hole, checking the position of the screws using the image intensifier.

Closure

Vicryl to fascia. Interrupted or continuous sutures to skin. Remove the traction pin from the distal femur.

Rehabilitation

Check radiographs. Mobilize the patient with partial weight-bearing when radiographs have been seen and drains removed.

Complications

Implant failure. If there is evidence of delayed union, the nail can be dynamized by removal of the locking screws from the end of the nail furthest from the fracture site.

SKELETAL TRACTION FOR FRACTURE OF THE SHAFT OF THE FEMUR (intermediate)

Indications

Conservative treatment of a fracture of the shaft of the femur. Skin traction and a Thomas splint can be employed as a temporary measure (e.g. prior to intramedullary nailing), but skeletal traction using a Denham pin inserted into the tibia is required in order to maintain reduction of conservatively treated femoral fractures.

Position

Supine on a traction bed.

Procedure

An assistant holds the foot to ensure that the leg lies with the patella horizontal to the floor. The site of insertion is 1 cm distal to the tibial tubercle and 2.5 cm behind the anterior border of the tibia. The pin should be inserted from the lateral to the medial border of the tibia to minimize risk of injury to the common peroneal nerve. Make a stab incision over the point of insertion on the lateral cortex. Select a Denham pin of the required size and load into the hand chuck. Insert the pin into the tibia by an oscillating motion, ensuring that it is inserted at right angles to the long axis of the limb and parallel to the underside of the patella. Insert the pin until it passes through the medial cortex. Then continue gentle insertion until the pin just begins to dent the skin. Make a second stab incision over this point and continue insertion until the threads of the pin reach the lateral cortex. At this point change the oscillating motion to rotation of the pin so that the threads engage the cortex. Seven complete turns of the pin are required. If necessary enlarge (or make cruciate) the skin incisions to ensure that there is no tension on the skin as this predisposes to pin infection. Attach a Bohler's stirrup to the pin and protect the pin ends with shields. Manipulation and the application of traction can then be performed.

Rehabilitation

Regular cleaning and dressing of the pin sites.

Complications

Pin-tract infection or loosening of the pin.

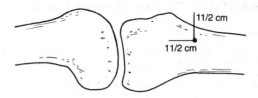

Site of insertion for skeletal traction.

DYNAMIC CONDYLAR SCREW FOR SUPRA- OR INTRACONDYLAR FRACTURE OF THE FEMUR (extra-major)

Indications

Supracondylar fractures of the femur are difficult to treat by conservative means because of the difficulty of maintaining the reduction. Intracondylar fractures need to be anatomically reduced to allow early mobilization of the knee joint.

Position

Supine on the table or on a fracture table.

Incision

Lateral skin incision extending proximally from the lateral condyle of the femur. The limit of the proximal extension depends upon the particular fracture.

Procedure

Incise the fascia lata in the line of the skin incision to expose the vastus lateralis. Strip this muscle using a periosteal elevator to expose the fracture. If the fracture is supracondylar, reduce the fracture using bone clamps. Reduction can be maintained by lag screws if suitable. Two guide-wires are then inserted to identify the plane of insertion of the screw. The first is passed percutaneously across the knee joint from lateral to medial to indicate the angle of the condyles. The second is passed under the patella to indicate the angle of inclination of the condyles. A mounted guide-wire is inserted across the condyles, ensuring that it is parallel to the two wires. The point of insertion is shown in the figure. This guide-wire must also be in the longitudinal plane of the femur so that the plate can be applied. By using the direct measure and subtracting 5 mm a screw of the correct length can be selected. The dynamic condylar screw (DCS) reamer is set to length of the screw chosen and the condylae are reamed over the guide-wire. The screw is then inserted using the introducer, the image intensifier may be used to check the screw length and position. A DCS plate of the required length, i.e. allowing eight cortices proximal to the fracture, is selected and applied. The plate is fixed using appropriate screws. The position of the plate and screws is checked on the image intensifier.

Closure

Vicryl to fascia. Continuous or interrupted sutures to skin.

14 Operative orthopaedic surgery
Dynamic condylar screw for supra- or intracondylar fracture of the femur
(extra-major)

Rehabilitation

The patient is mobilized after a check radiograph, with the amount of weight-bearing depending on the individual fracture.

Complications

- Residual knee stiffness
- Osteoarthritis of the knee
- Implant failure

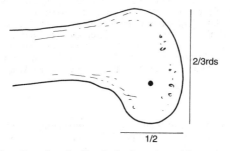

Site of insertion of guide-wire for dynamic condylar screw.

REPAIR OF RUPTURE OF THE QUADRICEPS TENDON (major)

Indication

Acute rupture of the quadriceps tendon.

Incision

A mid-line incision centred over the upper pole of the patella.

Procedure

The incision is deepened through the retinaculum and the rupture is confirmed. The knee joint is washed out with normal saline. The quadriceps tendon is repaired using interrupted sutures of no. 1 Vicryl. Often the rupture occurs at the insertion of the tendon onto the patella, and drill holes into the patella facilitate reattachment. These holes should be drilled obliquely to avoid penetrating the articular surface of the patella.

Closure

Vicryl to subcutaneous tissues. Interrupted or continuous sutures to skin. A well-padded plaster of Paris cylinder is applied.

Rehabilitation

The patient is mobilized with partial weight-bearing on crutches. The plaster is removed at 6 weeks and the knee is mobilized.

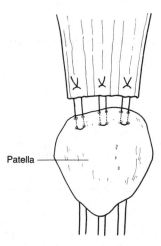

Patella

Method of reattachment of quadriceps tendon.

TENSION-BAND WIRING OF THE PATELLA (major)

Indication

Transverse fracture of the patella with displacement.

Incision

Mid-line over the patella.

Procedure

The fracture is exposed and the knee joint washed out with saline to remove the haemarthrosis. The fracture is reduced and held with sharp reduction forceps, ensuring that the articular surface is accurately reconstructed. Two stout parallel K-wires are inserted from the proximal to the distal border of the patella, making sure that they do not impinge on the articular surface. A figure-of-eight loop is formed around the wires and the loops are tightened. The proximal K-wires are bent through 180° and the excess removed with wire cutters. A punch is used to embed these wires in the proximal patella over the wire loop. The distal part of the K-wires is trimmed and bent slightly (excessive bending hinders later removal) to prevent them appearing through the skin. The tension band is then tested by flexing and extending the knee. If the procedure is performed for a comminuted fracture, a further circumferential wire can be used to help contain the fragments.

Closure

Vicryl to close the patella retinaculum. Continuous or interrupted sutures to skin. Plaster wool and crepe bandage.

Rehabilitation

Mobilize the knee and allow the patient to mobilize with partial weight-bearing when comfortable.

Complications

- Patellofemoral osteoarthritis
- Implant failure

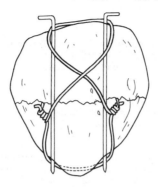

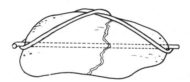

Tension band wiring of patella.

PATELLECTOMY FOR FRACTURE OF THE PATELLA (major)

Indications

Comminuted fractures of the patella. However, partial patellectomy plus tension-band wiring of the larger fragments is often performed instead of total patellectomy.

Incision

A mid-line incision centred on the patella.

Procedure

The fracture is exposed and the fragments of patella are removed by sharp dissection, keeping close to bone to prevent further damage to the extensor mechanism. The joint is washed out with normal saline. The quadriceps mechanism is reconstructed using no. 0 Vicryl mattress sutures.

Closure

Interrupted or continuous sutures to skin. A plaster of Paris cylinder (well padded) is applied with the knee extended.

Rehabilitation

Mobilize the patient with non-weight-bearing on crutches. At the end of 3 weeks remove the plaster and start straight raising and gentle knee flexion.

Complications

- Failure to regain full flexion
- Extensor lag

REPAIR OF RUPTURE OF THE PATELLAR TENDON (major)

Indications

Disruption of the patellar tendon requires repair to allow early mobilization of the knee joint.

Incision

Mid-line incision extending from the patella to the upper tibia is used.

Procedure

The rupture is confirmed and the joint is washed out with normal saline. The patella tendon is repaired using no. 1 Vicryl mattress sutures. If necessary, holes are drilled into the lower pole of the patella to attach the sutures. The repair is protected by means of a figure-of-eight wire around the patella. A hole is drilled into the upper tibia distal to the tibial tubercle for the lower loop of the wire. The wire is tightened and the tension tested by flexing and extending the knee.

Closure

Vicryl to subcutaneous tissues. Interrupted or continuous sutures to skin. Wool and crepe dressing.

Rehabilitation

Mobilize the knee and allow the patient to mobilize with partial weight-bearing.

Complications

Re-rupture of the tendon.

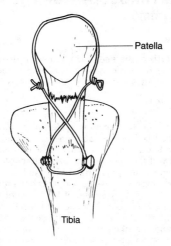

Figure-of-eight wire loop to protect patellar tendon repair.

EXAMINATION UNDER ANAESTHETIC AND ARTHROSCOPY OF THE KNEE JOINT (major)

Indications

Haemarthrosis of the knee joint and when the knee is locked due to a bucket-handle tear. Early diagnosis and treatment of acute knee injuries may improve the prognosis.

Procedure

Examination of the knee is undertaken with the patient anaesthetized before the tourniquet is applied. Examine for medial and lateral ligament laxity. Use the Lachmann test to detect laxity of the anterior cruciate ligament. A tourniquet is then applied to the upper thigh. With the knee flexed to 90° a vertical stab incision is made, one thumb-nail proximal to the lateral tibial condyle, just lateral to the patella tendon. The tract into the knee joint is made with the blunt arthroscopy introducer. Once the knee joint has been entered, the knee is extended and the blunt introducer is removed. If there is a haemarthrosis, no attempt is made to inspect the knee but the irrigation fluid is attached and the knee joint is washed out (introduction of a separate drain into the suprapatellar pouch may be necessary). When the fluid obtained from the knee becomes clear (this usually requires 1.5–2 litres of normal saline), insert the 30° arthroscope and perform a diagnostic arthroscopy. Meniscal tears are resected or consideration is given to meniscal repair.

Closure

Steristrips or sutures to skin.

Rehabilitation

The nature of the rehabilitation depends upon the findings of arthroscopy and examination under anaesthetic.

Complications

A compartment syndrome may result from extravasation of fluid if the haemarthrosis is not contained within the knee joint, most commonly in association with a complete rupture of the medial ligament.

Arthroscopy for acute knee injuries in the presence of a haemarthrosis is technically difficult. If the patient continues to complain of symptoms, a repeat arthroscopy under more favourable conditions is advised.

INTERNAL FIXATION OF FRACTURES OF THE TIBIAL CONDYLE (major plus)

Indications

Fractures of the tibial condyle with disruption of the articular surface of the knee.

Incision

The incision used depends upon the particular fracture. A mid-line incision gives good exposure and may be utilized if later arthroplasty is required. Usually, however, an incision centred over the tibial tubercle and curved over the affected condyle is used. When both condyles are involved, a mid-line or 'goblet' incision may be used. Ensure that the incision extends proximal to the knee joint.

Procedure

The incision is deepened to the fracture and the knee joint is entered. The knee joint is washed out and the meniscus elevated. Occasionally it may be involved in the fracture site. The defect in the articular surface of the condyle is reconstructed. This often leaves a defect in the cancellous bone of the condyle which needs to be replaced by bone graft. The bone graft is usually taken from the iliac crest. Once the articular surface has been accurately reconstructed the fracture is fixed, usually temporarily by means of a K-wire and then by two screws. These cancellous screws are inserted by standard AO techniques. The position of the screws is checked on an image intensifier. If the fracture extends onto the tibial shaft, a buttress plate may be applied in addition, with the condylar screws being inserted through the plate.

Closure

The knee joint is closed with Vicryl. Vicryl sutures to the subcutaneous tissues and interrupted or continuous sutures to skin.

Rehabilitation

Mobilization of the knee is commenced immediately if a continuous passive motion machine is available and is followed by active knee mobilization. The patient is mobilized with non-weight-bearing on crutches for 6 weeks.

Complications

Intra-articular fractures of the knee may predispose to later degenerative arthritis. Stiffness of the knee may occur.

FRACTURES OF THE SHAFT OF THE TIBIA

The main methods of treatment of fractures of the shaft of the tibia include external bracing (e.g. plaster of Paris), open reduction and internal fixation, intramedullary nailing, and external fixation. The method used for a particular fracture is very much a personal decision, although each method has advantages in particular circumstances.

Open reduction and internal fixation (major)

Indications
Internal fixation by means of plate and screws is most suitable for spiral fractures where one or more lag screws can be inserted and a neutralization plate applied. It is particularly suitable for fractures close to the metaphysis where intramedullary and external fixation is technically difficult. Grade I compound fractures can be treated by internal fixation.

Incision
The incision centred over the fracture site is curved to the lateral side of the lower leg to avoid the subcutaneous border of the tibia. The fracture site is exposed and periosteal stripping is kept to a minimum to preserve the blood supply. The fracture is reduced and temporarily held by means of a reduction clamp until a 3.2 mm lag screw is inserted. A neutralization plate (a narrow DCP) is selected to allow six cortical fixations, both proximal and distal to the fracture. The plate is contoured and affixed to the medial border of the tibia without stripping the periosteum to preserve the blood supply. The position of the plate is checked using an image intensifier.

Closure
Vicryl to subcutaneous tissues. Interrupted sutures to skin. Plaster wool and crepe.

Rehabilitation
The knee and ankle are mobilized immediately on a continuous passive motion machine if available, and then actively. The patient is mobilized with partial weight-bearing on crutches.

Complications
Implant failure due to the slow union rate is the most important complication.

INTRAMEDULLARY NAILING OF FRACTURES OF THE TIBIA (extra-major)

Indications

Intramedullary nailing of the tibia is particularly suited to transverse or comminuted fractures. Grade I compound fractures are suitable.

Position

An os calcis pin is inserted to allow traction on the affected limb. The patient is placed on the fracture table, the knee is flexed to 90° over a well-padded bar, and traction is applied through the os calcis pin. In order to allow radiography of the tibia the unaffected limb is flexed and abducted at the hip and placed into a well-padded support. Position the image intensifier so that the whole length of the tibia can be screened.

Incision

An incision is made over the middle of the patella tendon.

Procedure

The incision is deepened through the patella tendon to expose the upper border of the tibia. The pad of extra-articular fat over the upper border of the tibia is retracted and the entry point in the middle of the tibia is identified. The starter broach is used and an olive-tipped guide-wire is passed across the fracture site into the distal tibia. The tibia is then reamed to a size 1 mm larger than the diameter of the nail. The upper locking screws are inserted using the jig and the insertion of the distal locking screws is facilitated by raising the foot-piece attached to the os calcis pin so that the tibia is horizontal. The traction should be reduced prior to insertion of the distal locking screws so that the fracture is not distracted.

Closure

Vicryl to repair the patellar tendon. Interrupted sutures to skin. Plaster wool and crepe dressing.

Rehabilitation

The patient is mobilized with partial weight-bearing on crutches.

Complications

Compartment syndrome. If there is evidence of delayed union the nail can be dynamized by removal of either the proximal or distal locking screws (those furthest from the fracture site).

EXTERNAL FIXATION FOR TIBIAL FRACTURE (major)

Indications

Comminuted fractures of the tibia, grade II and III fractures, and fractures complicated by soft tissue or bony loss.

Procedure

The exact procedure depends upon the fixator used. If the fixator is to be employed on a closed fracture, use of an os calcis pin and setting up on the traction table as for an intra-medullary nailing aids reduction. If the AO fixator is used, the fracture is first reduced and if necessary held with a bone clamp. Usually two screws above and two screws below are employed, and are inserted into the medial border of the tibia. A stab incision is made over the first insertion site and the guide provided is used. The near cortex is drilled with a 4.5 mm drill and the far cortex with a 3.2 mm drill. The measuring device is used to select a screw of the correct length and this is inserted. The double frame is then assembled and clamped to this screw. The other three screws are then inserted in a similar fashion using the frame and the drill guide. The reduction of the fracture is confirmed on an image intensifier. If there is a compound wound, it is debrided, thorough lavage with saline is performed, and the wound is left open.

Rehabilitation

The pin sites are dressed daily. When the soft tissue problems are resolved the external fixator can be dynamized.

Complications

Pin-tract infection is the most common complication. Non-union may occur if dynamization is not performed.

OPEN REDUCTION AND INTERNAL FIXATION OF ANKLE FRACTURES (major)

The fixation employed in the treatment of ankle fractures depends upon the nature of the fracture and preoperative planning is invaluable. Fractures of the posterior malleolus require fixation if they involve more than 30 per cent of the articular surface of the tibia. If the fracture of the fibula is proximal, e.g. an AO type C fracture, a three-cortex screw across the diastasis may be employed instead of direct reduction and plate fixation. Comminuted fractures involving the articular surface (pylon fractures), may require bone grafting as well as plate fixation.

Indications

Unstable fractures of the ankle and intra-articular fractures.

Incision

An incision just anterior to the fibula is used, together with a curved incision centred over the medial malleolus if required.

Procedure

The fibular fracture is exposed if there is a posterior malleolus fracture. This is fixed first. The fibular fragment is externally rotated so that the articular surface of the tibia is exposed. The fracture of the posterior malleolus is reduced and held with a bone clamp. A stab incision is made anteriorly and a small-fragment cancellous screw of suitable length is inserted after drilling, measuring, and tapping. The fracture of the fibula is reduced and held with a bone clamp. A small-fragment lag screw is inserted in the usual fashion and then a 1/3 tubular (fibular plate) of suitable size (usually five or six holes) is applied. The position of the screws is checked on an image intensifier and the ankle is stressed to ensure that no diastasis persists. If diastasis is still present, one of the screws in the plate is removed and replaced by a three-cortex screw. As its name suggests, this passes across the two cortices of the fibula and the lateral cortex of the tibia. When drilling the hole for this screw, it is important to angle the screw 20° anteriorly to enter the tibia. This drill hole is tapped so that excessive compression across the screw cannot occur.

If there is no fracture of the medial malleolus but rupture of the medial ligament, the medial side does not require exploration provided that the image intensifier confirms that the ankle is reduced. Occasionally a flap of medial ligament remains trapped within the joint, and this is an indication for reduction and repair using Vicryl sutures. If there is a fracture of the medial malleolus, the fracture is exposed and reduced

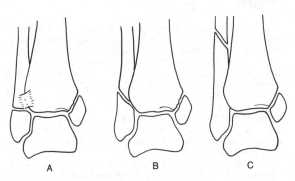

AO classification of ankle fractures.

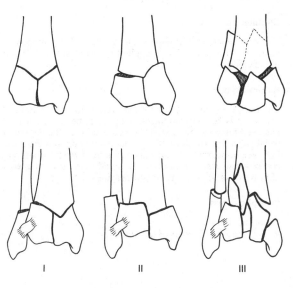

Classification of Pylon fractures.

OPEN REDUCTION AND INTERNAL FIXATION OF ANKLE FRACTURES (major)

and held first with a bone clamp and then with a 2 mm K-wire. This K-wire should be inserted at right angles to the fracture line, ensuring that it does not enter the ankle joint. The parallel guide is passed over the wire and a 2 mm drill hole is made parallel to the wire. A small-fragment half-threaded cancellous screw of suitable length (usually 35–40 mm) and a washer are inserted into this drill hole. If the fragment is very small, the K-wire can be left after being trimmed, but usually the wire is removed and another cancellous screw and washer of similar length are inserted. This ensures that the screws inserted are parallel. The position is checked on an image intensifier.

If the fracture is of a Pilon type, the articular surface of the tibia is exposed by means of an incision which commences over the anterior border of the tibia and curves towards the medial malleolus. Bone grafting may be required and a suitable plate (e.g. a clover-leaf) applied.

Closure

Vicryl to subcutaneous tissues. Interrupted sutures to skin. A paster of Paris back-slab is applied with the ankle in 90° of dorsiflexion.

Rehabilitation

The back-slab and suction drain are removed at 24 hours and the ankle is actively mobilized. Once dorsiflexion to neutral has been regained, the patient is mobilized with the degree of weight-bearing (usually 10 kg) depending on the fracture. Full weight-bearing is usually allowed after 3 weeks. If a three-cortex screw has been inserted, it should be removed (usually after 6 weeks) before any weight-bearing is allowed.

Complications

- Implant failure
- Degenerative arthritis of the ankle joint

REPAIR OF RUPTURE OF THE ACHILLES TENDON (major)

Indications

Acute rupture of the Achilles tendon.

Position

Prone.

Incision

An incision is made over the medial border of the Achilles tendon curved distally away from the calcaneum.

Procedure

The incision is deepened through the paratenon and the tendon rupture is exposed. The repair is performed with a no. 1 PDS suture using a Kessler–Mason–Allen repair. A 2/0 continuous suture is also used. The paratenon is repaired with a 2/0 Vicryl suture.

Closure

Interrupted or continuous sutures are used to skin and well-padded below-knee plaster of Paris is applied with the ankle in equinus.

Rehabilitation

The patient is mobilized with non-weight-bearing on crutches. The plaster is changed after 3 weeks and the sutures removed. The plaster is removed after 6 weeks, although a 2.5 cm heel raise is worn on the affected side for a further month.

Complications

- Wound infection or breakdown
- Re-rupture of the tendon

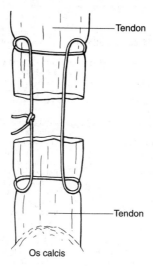

Tendon

Tendon

Os calcis

**Repair of Achilles tendon rupture using a
Kessler–Mason–Allen suture.**

Index

abdominal aorta
  exposure, and iliac bifurcation
    408
  resection of aneurysm 448–51
  trauma to 530
abdominal incisions
  oblique 166–7
  transverse 164–5
  vertical 162–3
abdominal surgery, second-loop
    340
abdominal trauma 532–4
abscess
  antibiotics 80
  breast 376
  ischiorectal 298
  pelvic 75
  perianal 298
  pulp 616
abscess surgical set 96–7
ACE inhibitors 25
Achilles tendon repair 708–9
acromioclavicular dislocation
    582–3
acupuncture 51
Addison's disease 11
adrenalectomy 322–3
adrenaline 55
adult respiratory distress
    syndrome (ARDS) 45
airway management 33–5
alcoholism 12
alfentanil 25
allergic reactions
  anaesthetic agents 12, 24, 40
  aspirin 25
allograft (homograft) 568
alpha-adrenergic agents 48, 55
American Society of
    Anesthesiologists (ASA)
    classification 16
aminoglycosides 11
amputation
  foot 471
  lower limb 468–71
amputation surgical set 98–9
anaemia 9, 11, 12
anaesthesia
  airway management 33
  balanced 21–2
  biochemical mechanisms 20
  conduct 32–9
  crisis 36
  hand injuries 611
  maintenance 36–7

monitoring 37–8
  reversal 38–9
  sequence 20–1
  total intravenous 20
anaesthetic agents
  allergic reactions 12, 24, 40
  drug interactions 12
  preoperative assessment, 8–13
    passim
  and tremors 8
  volatile 20–1
anaesthetic department,
    communication with 7
anal dilatation, Lord's 287
anal examination 170–1
anal fissure 170, 171, 296
anal fistula 300–1
anal polyps 289
anal skin tags 170
anal warts 170, 290
analgesia 25
  administration 49–51
  epidural 20, 49–50
  obstetric 26
  relative 31
  TENS machine 51
anaphylactoid drug reactions 12,
    24, 40
anastomosis
  arterial 404–7
  breakdown 47, 52
angelchik prosthesis 206–7
angina 9
ankle block 51
ankle fractures
  AO classification 705
  open reduction and internal
    fixation 704–7
  Pilon classification 705
anorectal polyps 291
antacids 14, 18–19
anterior tibial artery, access 412
antibiotics
  prophylaxis 9, 80–1, 83
  in renal failure 11
anticoagulants 9, 560
anticonvulsants 52
antidepressants 48, 52
antiembolism stockings 83, 560
antiemetics 46, 74
antihistamines 18
antihypertensives 19, 52
antisialogues 18, 25
aortic (aorto-bifemoral)
    bifurcation graft 446–7

aortography 537
apnoea alarm 38
appendicectomy 250–3
  laparoscopic 334–7
  surgical set 100–1
apudomas 12
Arbeitsgemeinschaft für
    Osteosynthese fragen
    (AO) 552–7
arrhythmias 9
arterial anastomosis 404–7
arterial sampling/cannulation
    63–5
arteriovenous fistula 440–1
ASA (American Society of
    Anesthesiologists)
  classification 16
ascites 11
aspirin 25, 48
asthma 10, 25, 45
atopy, 18, 12, *see also* allergic
    reactions
atracurium 27
atropine 18, 27, 44
atropine plus neostigmine 46
autograft 568
awareness 27, 41
axillary node dissection 398–9
axillo-bifemoral graft 434–6
axonotmesis 566

Barton's fracture 602–3
basal atelectasis 44, 52
baskets, stone 127
Belsey Mark IV operation 220–1
Bennett's fracture 627–8
benzodiazepines 18, 30, 48
Bier's block 611
bile duct exploration 230–1
biliary bypass procedures 236–9
bleeding disorders 9
blood gases 45
  arterial sampling 63
  cannulation 64–5
blood pressure monitoring, 37,
    see also hypertension
blue bloaters 10
bone grafts 568
bone healing 552–3
bougies 35
boutonnière deformity 634–5
bowel injuries 533
bowel lavage, on-table 275, 283
boxer's fracture 626
Boyle's anaesthetic machine 22

brachial embolectomy 438–9
brachial plexus block 20, 50, 611
brain laryngeal mask 33
branchial cyst/sinus/fistula 190–1
breast
  abscess 376
  augmentation 400
  fine-needle aspiration 384–5
  impalpable lesions 390
  nipple fashioning 400–1
  open biopsy 388–9
  reconstruction 400–1
  simple mastectomy 394–7
  Trucut biopsy 386
  wide-excision lumpectomy 392
  see also mastectomy
Bristow procedure 584–5
bronchitis, chronic 45
bronchodilators 10, 19, 45
bupivacaine
  for circumcision 476
  local blocks 50
  squirting 50
buprenorphine 25
buscopan 168

caecal injury 533
caecostomy
  for caecal injuries 533
  on-table lavage 275–7
caesarean section 20
calcium-channel blockers 48
cannulation
  arterial 63–5
  central venous 59–62
  peripheral venous 58–9
capnography 38
cardiac injury, blunt 537
cardiac tamponade 537
cardiovascular health 8, 9
cardiovascular surgical set
    102–3
carotid bifurcation, access 408–9
carotid body tumour 426–7
carpal dislocation 618
cast
  bracing 558–9
  hanging 590
catgut 144
caudal block 50
celestin intubation 218–19
central venous cannulation 59–62
central venous monitoring 38
cerebral haemorrhage,
    postoperative 47

chest
  flail 537
  infections 83
  X-rays 12, 45, 86
  see also respiratory
children
  adhesive skin strips 157
  fractures
    distal humerus 646–51
    epiphyseal, classification
      642
    greenstick 642
    radial 652, 656–8
    ulnar 654, 656
  induction 32
  intra-osseous infusion 66–71
chlorhexidine 160, 161, 563
chloroform 25
cholecyst-enterostomy 237
cholecystectomy 226–9
  laparoscopic 328–33
  surgical set 104–5
cholecystostomy 234–5
choledochoduodenostomy 236
choledochojejunostomy 236
chronic obstructive pulmonary
    disease (COPD) 10
cimetidine 18
circumcision 476–7
clonidine 48
Cockett's procedure (varicose
    veins) 473
codeine phosphate 75
colectomy
  sigmoid 266–7
  total 268–9
  transverse 262–3
Colles' fracture 558
colonoscopy 135, 173
colostomy 270–7, 533
  double-barrelled 273
  end 271–2
  loop 271
  opening 275
  palliative decompressive 282
  Paul Mikulicz 273
  transverse 273–4
common femoral
    artery/bifurcation 409
compartment syndrome 548, 549,
    599, 700
confusion 44, 52
consent 89–90
constipation, postoperative 75
continuous positive airways
    pressure (CPAP) 44, 56

coronary artery disease 9
cotton 144
cricothyrotomy 36
  emergency sets 64
  needle 36, 65
croup 32
cryotherapy 51
cyanosis 45
cyclopropane 18
cystectomy 516–18
cystic artery variations 227
cystoplasty 514
cystoscopy 131, 498–500

dantrolene 40
day surgery 42–3
  admission criteria 12–13
  alfentanil 25
  desflurane 26
  preoperative assessment 6
deep vein thrombosis (DVT)
    81–3, 559
dental procedures 31, 81
dentition 8
desflurane 26
dexon 144
dextran 83
diabetic patients 7, 11
dialysis 56
diamorphine 48
diaphragmatic rupture 536
diarrhoea, postoperative 74–5
diazepam 18, 30, 168
diclofenac 25, 49
digoxin 52
diphenoxylate hydrochloride
    75
diuretics 45
dobutamine 54
dopamine 54–5
doppler imaging 83
doxapram 39
drips, tissued 52
droperidol 18
drug
  abuse 12
  allergies 12, 24, 40
  imbalances 52
  interactions 12
  sensitivity 52
duodenum
  endoscopy 169
  perforated ulcer 204–5
  transection 352–3
  trauma 533

elderly patients
  atropine 44
  constipation 75
  fracture of proximal humerus 586, 587
  induction agents 24
elective surgery, definition 16
electrocardiogram (ECG) 37
Ellick evacuator 489
embolectomy
  brachial 438–9
  femoral 452–4
emergency patients 14, 16
EMLA cream 59
endarterectomy 416–17
  carotid 418–20
endoscopy
  gastric 168–9
  instruments/sets 132–5
  upper gastrointestinal 168–9
endotracheal intubation 35
  emergency 27
  facial structure 8
  size, formula 35
enflurane 26
enoximone 55
Entonox (50% nitrous oxide in oxygen) 26, 30–1
epididymal cysts 480–2
epidural analgesia 20, 49–50
epiglottis, large/floppy 44
ether 18, 25
etomidate 24
exercise tolerance 9, 12
extensor tendon injuries 634–5
exteriorization resection method (Paul Mikulicz procedure) 282–3
extracorporeal membrane oxygenation (ECMO) 56
extracorporeal shock-wave lithotripsy (ESWL) 494

face
  masks 33
  physiognomy 8
familial factors 8
fasciculations 27
fasting, preoperative 14
fat embolism 44, 52
femoral embolectomy 452–4
femoral hernia 310–11

femoral nerve block 51
femoral shaft fracture 558
femoro-femoral cross-over graft 456–7
femoropopliteal bypass graft 460–2
femur, intra/supracondylar fracture 684–5
femur, fractured shaft
  intramedullary nailing 680–1
  skeletal traction 682–3
femur, neck fracture
  dynamic hip screw 674–5
  hemiarthroplasty 676–7
  subcapital 672–3
  subtrochanteric 678
fentanyl 25, 30
fibrescope 498
fibular fractures 704
finger
  digit names 610
  fractures 622–7
  injury to tip 638–9
fissure in ano 296
fistula
  in ano 300–1
  establishing arteriovenous 440–1
  mammillary 383
  mucous 273
flexor pulleys 631
flexor tendon injuries 630–3
fluid challenge 54
fluid replacement 75
flumazenil 30
foot
  amputation 471
  pump 560
  see also toe
fractures
  compound
    classification 564
    management 565
  external fixation 556
  Galeazzi 600
    juvenile 654–5
  greenstick 642
  Monteggia 600
    juvenile 654–5
  open reduction and internal fixation 552–7
  reduction 548–9
  see also children's fractures; specific fractures
frusemide 45, 537
fuel cell 38

gall bladder, anatomy 227
gas embolism 40
gastrectomy 222–5
gastric acidity 14, 18–19
gastric emptying 14, 18
gastric endoscopy 168–9
gastric surgical set 106–7
gastric vagotomy, proximal 200–3
gastroenterostomy 197, 354–5
retrocolic isoperistaltic 197
gastrointestinal
endoscopy of upper, 168–9
injuries 533
postoperative problems 74–5
gastropexy
Boerema anterior 220
Collis 220
Hill posterior 220
gastroscopy 30
surgical set 132
gloves
powder 160
punctured 160
glyceryl trinitrate 55, 59
glycopyrrolate plus neostigmine 46
glycopyrrollate 18, 27
Goodsall's rule 300
greenstick fractures 642
Guedel airway 21, 33

H_2–receptor antagonists 14, 18–19
Hadfield–Adair operation 380–2
haematoma, external plexus 289
haemodialysis 56
haemofiltration 56
haemoglobinopathies 546
haemoperfusion 56
haemorrhage
at operative site 47
postoperative 46, 76–7
haemorrhoidectomy 287, 287–8
haemorrhoids 170, 171, 286–9
banding 286
injection therapy 286
thrombosed external 289
hallux, Keller's arthroplasty 666
halothane 24, 32
hand
fractures 622–9
infections 616–17
ligament injuries 626–7
no-man's land 630

position of function 610, 611
treatment principles 610–13
Hartmann's procedure 282
heart
failure 9
murmurs 9
see also cardiac
hemicolectomy
left 264–5
right 258–61
heparin 10, 81, 560
hepatic failure 11
hepatitis 12, 90, 563
hernia
femoral 310–11
hiatus 11, 12, 220–1
incisional 163, 312–13
inguinal 306–9
high dependency unit 42
high-frequency ventilation (HFPPV) 56
high-pressure nozzled injury 617
hip
dislocated 670
replacement 560, 662–3
surgical sets 116–19
homograft (allograft) 568
hospital admission 6–7
human bite injury 617
human immunodeficiency virus (HIV) 12, 90, 563
humeral fractures
distal 592–3
in children 646–51
shaft 590–1
hydrallazine 55
hydrocelectomy 480–2
hydrogen peroxide 563
hyoscine 18, 49
hypertension 9, 46
hypnosis 51
hypospadias 504
hypotension 46
hypothermia 84
hypovolaemia 24
hypoxia 52

ibuprofen 25
ileostomy 244–5
imaging procedures, 12, 86, see also X-rays
incisional hernia 312–13
incisions
abdominal transverse 164

Anderson–Hynes 520
Cernay 516
Czermy 164
fish-mouth 616
Gridiron 166
hand 611, 612
Kocher's 166
Lanz 166
midline 162
paramedian 162–3
Pfannenstiel 164
Rutherford–Morrison 166
skin crease 164
induction
    agents 24–5
    gas 32
    intravenous 32
    procedure 32
    rapid sequence 32–3
infants/neonates
    anaesthesia 32
    gas embolism 40
    list order 7
    see also children
infections
    hand 616–17
    orthopaedic surgery 562–3
    post-splenectomy 249
    postoperative 52
    respiratory 10–11, 44, 52
inguinal block 50
inguinal hernia 306–9
inguinal ligament bypass 458–9
intensive care unit (ICU) 7, 30,
        42, 54–7
intercostal block 50
intermittent mandatory
        ventilation (IMV) 56
intermittent positive pressure
        ventilation (IPPV) 55–6
internal carotid artery,
        aneurysmal 423–5
intestinal distension, severe 26
intra-abdominal bleeding 46
intra-osseous infusion 66, 69–71
intracranial gas 26
intubation
    awake 32
    difficult 10
    endobronchial 35
    endotracheal, see endotracheal
        intubation
    oesophageal 35
    orotracheal/nasotracheal 33
investigations (preoperative)
        12

ischiorectal abscess 298
isoflurane 26

jaundice 11

keel repair 312
Keller's arthroplasty 666
Kessler suture 631
ketamine 18, 20
Kiel graft 568
knee
    arthroscopic examination
        694–5
    instrument set 120
    replacement 664
    see also patella
knot tying
    guidelines 146–7
    instrument tie 156–7
    square knots 148–54
    surgeon's/friction 155–6

laparoscopic
        instruments/equipment
    Austin Moore set 124–5
    bundle 122
    knee set 120
    menisectomy set 122–3
    Muller 124
laparoscopy
    appendicetomy 334–7
    cholecystectomy 328–33
    equipment 136–41
    gas embolism 40
    room set-up 140–1
    stapling devices 344
laparotomy
    for abdominal trauma 532–3
    exploratory 338–9
    surgical set 108–10
large bowel resection, and
        anastomosis 254–7
laryngeal masks 21, 33–4
laryngeal polyps 44
laryngomalacia 44
laryngospasm 44
lasers
    gas-cooled 40
    inoperable rectal cancer 294
lateral cutaneous nerve block of
        thigh 51
left ventricular failure 44
lignocaine 24

lisfranc amputation 471
lithium 12
lithotripsy 30
liver
  failure 11
  trauma 533
lorazepam 18, 30
lord's dilatation 296
lower limb amputations 468–71
lumbar sympathectomy 442–5
lumpectomy, wide excision 392
lunate, dislocated 618
lung cyst 26

McEvedy approach (femoral
    hernia) 310–11
malignant hyperpyrexia 8, 27, 40
malleolar fractures 704
mallet deformity 635
mammillary fistula 383
mammoplasty 400
mastectomy
  Patey 395, 398–9
  radical 399
  simple 394–7
meatal advancement and
    glanuloplasty (MAGPI)
    504–5
Meckel's diverticulum 246–7
median nerve decompression 576
menisectomy surgical set 122–3
mental state 8, 9
meptazinol 25
mesh repair 306
metabolic disease 11–12
metacarpal fractures 625–6
methicillin-resistant
    Staphylococcus aureus
    (MRSA) 81, 88
methohexitone 24
methylprednisone 537
metoclopramide 14, 18, 74
microdochectomy 378
midazolam 30, 168
midazolam plus papaveretum 30
minor operations set 110–11
Mitchell's ostetomy 668–9
mivacurium 27
monoamine oxidase inhibitors 12
morbidity 40–1
morphine sulphate 18, 25, 30, 48,
    49
mortality 40
muscle pains 27, 41
muscle relaxants 26–8

myasthenic syndrome 46
myocardial infarction 47, 52
myocutaneous flap
    reconstruction 400
myxoedema 11–12

nail
  avulsion 304
  wedge excision 304
  Zadik's procedure 304
nail-bed dislocation 638–9
nalbuphine 25
naloxone 39, 44, 48
nausea, postoperative 46, 74
needles 126, 145, 165
neobladder 512
neostigmine 27
neostigmine plus
    glycopyrrolate/atropine 46
nephrectomy 522–4
nephro-ureterectomy 526
nephroscopes 130, 489
nephroscopy, percutaneous
    494–6
nephrotic syndrome 11
nerve injuries, prevention 83
neuroleptic agents 18, 28
neuromuscular monitoring 38
neuropraxia 566
neurotmesis 566
nightstick injury 600
nipple fashioning 400
nissen fundoplication 220–1
nitrous oxide 26
nitrous oxide (50%) in oxygen
    (Entonox) 26, 30–1
nitrous oxide (70%) in oxygen 26
non-steroidal anti-inflammatory
    drugs (NSAIDs) 25, 48
noradrenaline 55
nylon 144

obesity 8
obstetric analgesia 20, 26
oesophageal carcinoma
  celestin intubation 218–19
  oesophagogastrectomy 212–13
oesophageal cardiomyotomy,
    Heller's 192–5
oesophageal endoscopy 168
oesophageal rupture 537
oesophageal varices 350–1
oesophagectomy, Ivor Lewis
    208–11

oesophagogastrectomy
  lower-third carcinoma 212–13
  total 214–17
oesophagojejunostomy 348–9
olecranon fracture 594–5
operating list 6, 7
opiates 18, 25, 30, 46, 48
  administration, 49–51 passim
  nausea/vomiting due to 46
  patches 49
  respiratory depression 44
  in TIVA 20
oral contraception 81
orchidopexy 484–5
orthopaedic surgery 20
  antibiotic prophylaxis 80
  DVT and PE 81
  theatre ventilation 80
  see also specific operations
oscillotonometers 37
ostetomy, Mitchell's 668–9
Oswestry graft 568
overwhelming post-splenectomy
    infection 249
oxygen monitor 38
oxygen therapy 55

paediatric set 112–14
pain
  postoperative 46
  restlessness 44
  see also analgesia; opiates
palmar space infection 617
pancreas
  enucleation of ampullary
      tumours 364
  trauma 534
pancreatectomy
  distal 366
  total 370
pancreatic duct, drainage 366
pancreatic pseudocyst 372
pancreaticoduodenectomy
    (Whipple's operation)
    360–3
pancuronium 27
papaveretum 18, 25, 48
  by PCA 49
  plus midazolam 30
paracetamol 48, 49
paralytic ileus 74
paramedics 26
parathyroidectomy 320–1
parietal cell vagotomy 200–3
Parkinson's disease 8

parotidectomy, superficial 188–9
patella, tension-band wiring
    688–9
patellectomy 690
patient
  consent 89–90
  correct identity 89
  correct operation 89
  host resistance 562
  postoperative care 42
  preoperative assessment 6,
      8–14
  preparation 18–19
  reassurance 18
  shaving 89, 161
  skin preparation 161
patient-controlled analgesic
    systems (PCAs) 49
Paul Mikulicz procedure
    (exteriorization resection
    method) 282–3
PDS 144
peanuts, inhaled 32
pelvic abscess 75
penile block 50
pentazocine 25
peptic ulcers 25, 196
perfusion problems 52
perianal abscess 298
peripheral nerve
  dysfunction after
      fracture/dislocation 614
  repair 614
  trauma 566
peroneal artery, access 412
pethidine 18, 25, 48, 49
phaeochromocytoma 12
phalangeal fractures 622–3
pharaphimosis 478
pharyngeal pouch 186–7
phenol block of sympathetic
    chain 442
phosphodiesterase inhibitors 55
physical fitness (ASA
    classification) 16
physiotherapy 7, 45
pink puffers 10
piroxicam 25
plaster cast 550–1
plates 553
pneumatic compression,
    intermittent 83
pneumococcus vaccination 81
pneumonia, lobar 44, 52
pneumotachograph 38
pneumothorax 26, 40, 44, 51

podophylline 290
polycythaemia 9, 81
popliteal artery, access 411–12
porphyria 8, 24
Portex Mini-Trach 66
positive end-expiratory pressure
    (PEEP) 56
post-phlebitic limb syndrome 81
postoperative
    care 42–3
    complications 44–7, 52
    pain relief 48–51
povidone iodine 160, 161, 563
pregnant women 18, 26
premedication 18
preoperative advice 6
preoperative assessment
    clinics 6
    elective surgery 8–13
    emergency patient 14
pressure sores, prevention 83
pressure transducer 62
prochlorperazine maleate 74
proctoscopy 170–1
proctoscopy/sigmoidoscopy set
    133
profundaplasty 414–15
prolene 144
promethazine (Phenergan) 18
propofol 20, 24, 30, 44
prostatectomy
    retropubic 490–3
    transurethral 486–8
prostatic hypertrophy 11
prosthetic graft infection 80
prosthetic surgery
    theatre clothing 88
    theatre ventilation 88
protamine, heparin reversal 81
pruritus, epidural analgesia 50
pseudocholinesterase 8, 27
pseudocyst, pancreatic 372
pseudomembranous colitis 74
psychotropic drugs, and
    anaesthetic agents 12
pulmonary artery and wedge
    pressure monitoring 38
pulmonary contusion 537
pulmonary embolism 52, 81–3,
    560
pulp abscess 616
pulse oximetry 31, 37, 45
pyeloplasty 520–1
    Anderson–Hynes 521
    Culp 521
    Foley V-Y 521

pyloroplasty (Heineke–Mikulicz)
    197

quadriceps tendon rupture 686–7

racial origin
    preoperative assessment 8
    and tourniquets 546
radial fractures 596–9
    juvenile 652, 656, 658
radio-allergosorbent (RAS) tests
    40
ranitidine 18
recovery room 42
rectum
    abdominoperineal excision
        284–5
    examination 170–1
    inoperatble cancer 294
recurarization 46
regional anaesthesia 20, 49–51
    in COPD 10
    obesity 8
    sedation 30
regurgitation 8, 18, 32, 35
relaxograph 38
renal calculi
    baskets 499
    minimally invasive surgery
        494–7
renal failure
    postoperative 52
    preoperative assessment 11
renal trauma 533
resection, anterior 278–81
resectoscope, irrigating 128–9
respiration, see-saw 44
respiratory depression 44, 48, 50
respiratory function
    assessment 44–5
    preoperative 11–12
    treatment of problems 45
respiratory infections 10–11, 44,
    52
respiratory support 55–6
respirometer 38
restlessness 39, 44
reversal 38–9
rheumatic heart disease,
    antibiotic cover 81
rotator cuff tears 580

salbutamol 19, 45

Salter–Harris classification 642
saphenous vein
    harvesting 464–5
    in situ bypass graft 466–7
    valve excision 466
scaphoid fracture 619
scar, guidelines for a fine 157
scheduled surgery, definition 16
screws 553–4
scrub-up technique 88, 160–1
sedation 30–1
Seldinger guide wire 61–2
septic shock 55
septicaemia 46, 47
settle plates, microbiology 88
sevoflurane 26, 32
shaving 89, 161
shivering, postoperative 46
shock
    haemorrhagic 76
    septic 55
shoulder dislocation 584–5
sickle cell anaemia 8, 546
sigmoid colectomy 266–7
sigmoidoscopy 172–3
    instrument set 133
silk 144
skin
    adhesive strips 157
    clips 157
    preparation 161
small bowel resection, and
        anastomosis 240–3
Smith's fracture 606
sodium citrate 14, 19
sodium nitroprusside 55
sodium tetradecyl sulphate 530
sodium thiopentone 530
sphincteroplasty, transduodenal
        232–3
sphincterotomy, lateral 295
spinal block 20
spinal fracture 556
spleen, trauma 533
splenectomy 81, 248–9
splints, hand 610
stainless steel wire suture 145
staplers
    early 344
    end-to-end 344
    linear 344
    side-to-side 344
stapling techniques
    anterior resection 346–7
    bleeding oesophageal varices
        350–1

bowel resection and functional
        end-to-end
        anastomosis 356–7
    duodenal transection 352–3
    gastroenterostomy 354–5
Steinstrasse 494
steroids 11, 19
stockings, antiembolism 83, 560
stomach
    trauma to 534
    see also gastric
stone baskets 127
stone punch 130
subclavian artery, access 408, 410
submandibular gland 182–4
surgical cases, classification 16
surgical drains 158
surgical instrument sets
    abscess 96–7
    amputation 98–9
    appendicectomy 100–1
    cardiovascular 102–3
    cholecystectomy 104–5
    endoscopic 132–5
    gastric 106–7
    hip 116–19
    laparoscopic 120–4
    laparotomy 108–10
    minor operations 110–11
    paediatric 112–14
    toenail pack 114–15
    urological 126–9
surgical instruments
    count 89
    sterilization 89
surgical materials,
        disposable/reautoclaved
        88
surgilon 144
sutures
    Kessler 631
    Kessler–Mason–Allen 709
    materials 144–5
    needles 145, 165
    removal 157
    seton 300–2
suxamethonium 27, 33
    apnoea 39
    for laryngospasm 44
    and lithium 12
swab count 89
Swan–Ganz catheters 62–3
sweating, postoperative 46
Syme's amputation 470–1
sympathectomy
    cervical 430–2

sympathectomy (*cont.*)
  lumbar 442–4
  transaxillary 428–9
synchronized intermittent
    mandatory ventilation
    (SIMV) 56

temazepam 18
tennis elbow decompression
    572
tenosynovitis, suppurative 616
tenoxicam 25
thalassaemia 8, 246
theatre
  clothing 88–9, 160, 562
  communication 7
  design 88
  ventilation 88, 562
thigh, lateral cutaneous nerve
    block 51
thiopentone 24, 40
thoracic injuries 536–7
thoracotomy 537
thrombophlebitis 59
thyroidectomy 314–19
  lobectomy 315–16
  para- 320–1
  total 316–18
thyrotoxicosis 8, 11
tibial fractures
  cast bracing 558
  condylar, internal fixatin 696
  external fixation 702
  intramedullary nailing 700
  shaft 698
tibioperoneal trunk, access 412
tobacco smokers 81
toenail, ingrowing 304
toenail pack 114–15
total intravenous anaesthesia
    (TIVA) 20
tourniquets 546–7, 562, 611
tracheal polyps 44
tracheal tug 44
tracheostomy 32, 178–80
  removal 180
tracheotomy, mini- 65–6, 68 fig.
tramadol 25
transcutaneous electrical nerve
    stimulation (TENS) 51
trauma
  abdominal 532–4
  thoracic 536–7
  vascular 531–2
tremors 8

Trendelenburg's procedure
    (varicose veins) 472–3
tricyclic antidepressants 12
trigger finger decompression
    574
trimeprazine (Vallergan) 18
truncal vagotomy and drainage
    196–9
tubocurare 10, 27

ulnar collateral ligament rupture
    636, 637
ulnar fracture 598–9
  in child 656
ulnar nerve decompression 578
upper airway obstruction 10, 41,
    44
ureteric stent 496
ureterocutaneous diversion 512
ureterorenoscope 503
ureteroscopes 131
ureteroscopy 502–3
ureterosigmoidostomy 511–12
urethral stricture
  anterior 506
  posterior 507–8
urethroplasty 504–7
urgent-delayed operation,
    definition 16
urinary conduit 508
urinary diversions 508–12
urinary retention 11, 50, 52
urological instruments 126–9
urological surgery 20, 81
urostomy 508–11

vagotomy, highly selective 200–3
vancomycin 75
vapour-monitoring devices 38
varicose veins 472–3, 530
varus deformity 558
vascular injuries 530–1
vecuronium 27
venepuncture, and obesity 8
venography 83
ventilation, artificial 55–6
ventilator
  disconnect alarm 38
  Manley Pulmovent 23
ventricular failure, postoperative
    47
vicryl 144
vocal cords,
    dislocation/granuloma 35

volatile agents 25–6, 28
vomiting, postoperative 46, 74

warfarin, DVT and PE
    prophylaxis 81, 560
warts, anal 170, 290
water manometer 62
Whipple's operation
    (pancreaticoduodenectomy)
    360–3
wound categories 80

X-rays
    chest 12, 45, 86
    department 7
    gastrointestinal emergencies 86
    preoperative 12, 86
xenograft 568

Z-plasty closure 611, 613
Zadik's procedure (complete
    excision of the nailbed)
    304